Press-Fit Fixation of the Knee Ligaments

Gernot Felmet

Press-Fit Fixation of the Knee Ligaments

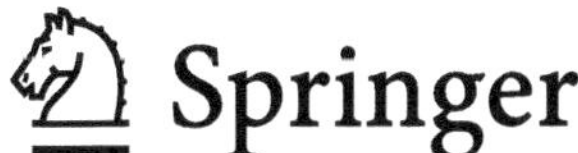

Gernot Felmet
Orthop. Praxis & ARTICO Sportklinik
Villingen-Schwenningen, Germany

ISBN 978-3-031-11908-8 ISBN 978-3-031-11906-4 (eBook)
https://doi.org/10.1007/978-3-031-11906-4

This Springer imprint is published by the registered company Springer Nature Switzerland AG
The registered company address is: Gewerbestrasse 11, 6330 Cham, Switzerland

Foreword 1

Surgical treatment of cruciate ligament injuries began at the beginning of the last century with sutures and autologous replacements, mainly from fascia lata, hamstring tendons, partially damaged menisci, and later with grafts from the patellar tendon and the quadriceps tendon. Implant-free anchorage was described with the patellar tendon after the last world war, in particular by Brückner in Rostock via bolting of the tibial bone graft. Anatomical requirements could not be sufficiently taken into account. A fundamental modification of this principle was first presented at the ESSKA Congress in Stockholm in 1990: the free patellar tendon graft was inverted, the anatomical insertion geometry was accurately reproduced femorally, with the graft block from the tibial tuberosity, and the flat double-bundle structure of the graft corresponded to the natural anterior cruciate ligament. Precise attention to the anatomical cruciate ligament structure and its function also brought about the necessary departure from the physiologically incorrect doctrine of isometry. Very good long-term results of anatomy-oriented surgical techniques also confirm these considerations in new reviews.

The implant-free technique for reconstruction of the knee ligaments with the hamstring tendons presented in this book is the logical development of the basic idea started with the patellar tendon: the body's own tissue heals better if it is not pressed or damaged by implants, the costs of the operation are reduced, and revision operations, which must always be taken into account, are enormously facilitated.

Advocates of these ideas have always struggled in cruciate ligament surgery under the disregard (for competition) from industrial producers of fixation materials, for obvious reasons that, however, simply overlook or set aside the basic idea of biologically optimized surgery.

In this highly interesting and recommendable book for all knee surgeons, in addition to the general principles of knee ligament surgery, the author's special implant-free technique with the semitendinosus tendon is described in detail and is eye opening.

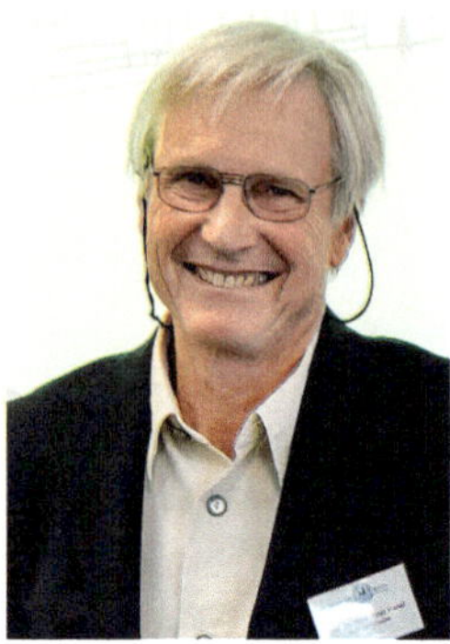

Klinik Sanssouci
Potsdamm, Berlin, Germany

Peter Hertel

Foreword 2

The knee joint is one of the most fascinating and complex human joints. Its complexity arises from the variability of its anatomy. As Werner Müller, the godfather of European knee surgery, once stated, the anatomy of the knee joint is variable and the only constant is its variability. Its complex function is the result of the optimal interplay of bony structures such as femur, tibia, patella, and fibula, as well as soft-tissue structures such as its ligaments, tendons, muscles, and joint capsule.

Generally, each function of the knee is the result of a complex teamplay of numerous anatomical structures together. In our daily activities, the knee carries a large part of our body weight, allowing a wide range of motion for flexion–extension and internal–external rotation. The main principles of knee kinematics are rolling, gliding, and rotation. The knee joint offers a six degrees of freedom range of motion. Rotational movement consists of flexion–extension, internal–external, and varus–valgus. Translational movement is possible in anterior–posterior and medial–lateral directions, as well as via compression and distraction. All these freedoms of motion are combined in a complex function within the envelope of motion.

Restoration of anatomy is the most important key to knee surgery and cannot be overestimated. Only if the surgeon knows what the normal anatomy is can anatomy be restored in the injured knee. Outcomes after knee surgery are only as good as our knowledge of anatomy and our understanding of knee function.

One major factor is the surgical technique and the question whether such a technique closely restores the patient's individual anatomy, while not harming other structures or leaving burned bridges such as the tunnels in anterior cruciate ligament (ACL) surgery. The anatomy of the ACL insertion site varies in size and shape, but we still fail to consider this variability in terms of graft sizes and positioning. Remnants of the native ACL can also vary in size and utility. The surgeon needs to decide whether to resect or at least partially incorporate ACL remnants into the reconstructed ACL.

In this book we have the pleasure of reading from a great knee surgeon with vast experience in reconstructive knee surgery all about biological and anatomical ACL reconstruction techniques with press-fit anchoring and bone filling of the tunnels, which the author has developed and successfully tested over the last few decades. Furthermore, this book describes the much greater scope of the use of bone dowels and also provides various solutions for revision surgery. "Save the ACL with the healing response" reminds you to handle biological resources carefully. At the same time, bioregenerative and reparative measures with PRP-analogous substances are used, which hopefully can provide us with even better tools in the future. In addition to all points, a well-founded examination and quality control after the surgical work are carried out, and the author gives a very comprehensive look at rehabilitation and the return to sport and competition—shaped by his many years of experience.

The book is a historical review and gives a positive outlook on common biological and anatomical ligament reconstructions in the knee joint. The pragmatic guidelines included make it a handbook of diagnostics, surgery, revision, and rehabilitation for every knee surgeon.

I hope you enjoy reading this fantastic book and keep your eyes wide open for future advancements in reconstructive knee surgery. "That is what learning is. You suddenly understand something you have understood all your life, but in a new way."

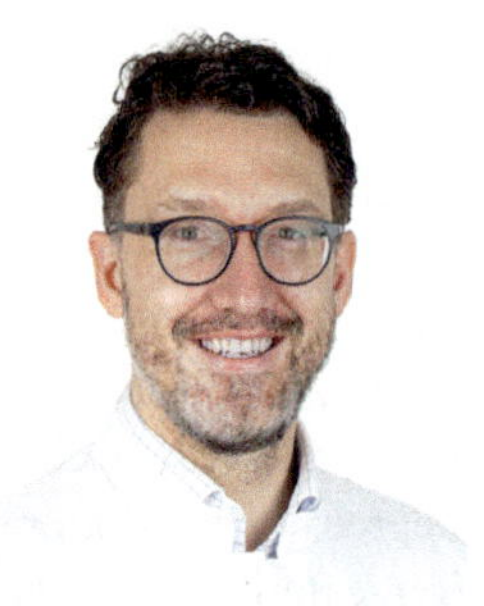

Michael T. Hirschmann

Department of Orthopedic Surgery
and Traumatology
Kantonsspital Baselland
Bruderholz, Switzerland

Department of Clinical Research, Research
Group Michael T. Hirschmann, Regenerative
Medicine and Biomechanics
University of Basel
Basel, Switzerland

Foreword 3

In ancient times, knee ligaments permanently occupied the famous *h'iatroi*, physicians such as Avicenna, Hippocrates, the Persians, and the Egyptians. Herodicus, the *híatros* of the Olympic athletes, in competition with Hippocrates from the neighboring island of Kos, as an ancient sports physician, certainly had good knowledge of these ligaments.

In 1543, Andreas Vesalius in his world-famous book, "*On the fabric of the human body in seven books*" showed the human anatomy with accurate drawings, including the knee anatomy with the cruciate ligaments.

These have fascinated modern-day orthopedic surgeons in sports traumatology so much that they tried to reinvent the anatomical situation shown by Vesalius 500 years earlier, looking for anatomical and technical solutions to reconstruct this short anterior cruciate ligament (ACL), which is so important in sports, to provide biomechanically sufficient, long-lasting, satisfactory results, as close as possible to the original. Here is a partial list of names of great knee surgeons involved in ligamentary stabilization of the knee. Each of them sought a different approach to the main goal: ACL reconstruction. Among them, Cabot, Lindemann, Trickey, Augustine, Wittek, zur Verth, Slocum and Larson, Helfet, Hughston, O'Donoghue, Trillat, McIntosh, Ellison, and many others attempted with ligaments, soft tissues, and peripheral tendons to dynamically stabilize the knee joint. Some tried to find a solution to the problem of anterior instability by using bone corrections such as osteotomies. Most, however, continued to rely on tendon and ligament transfers. Then, ligament augmentation devices such as Kennedy's LAD and other implanted, artificially strong ligaments such as Goretex were used, but even these very strong ligaments, which are much tougher than a normal ACL, tore in the joint at the exit of the tibial canal.

At the time when patellar bone-tendon-bone (BTB) and hamstrings were competing, various industry-developed devices were used for fixation to make the procedures easier, better, and faster.

In addition to good results, tunnel widening and loosening of implants occurred, leaving noticeable holes and making revisions difficult. This was the time when BTB reconstructions became more prominent again, with the advantage of rapid bone-to-bone consolidation at the ligament ends. Brückner's technique was now the leading example of BTB procedures, including those without foreign fixation materials, and Hertel was an early presence with the press-fit reconstruction technique.

Uninfluenced by the techniques established up to that time, this book is based on a surgical approach that is very efficient in terms of design. The author discusses all aspects of injury analysis, modern diagnostics, and therapy as if in a checklist. The special key to his press-fit anchorage is to consistently conserve biological resources. With the system, the ligaments can be reproduced close to the anatomical ribbon-like insertion. The author also precisely describes the use of knee kinematics for logical graft tensioning. In addition, modern treatment strategies such as "save the ACL," the healing response, and PRP-autologous therapy are presented. The author deals just as intensively with individual graft selection, rehabilitation, and return to sport and competition, which is why this book is once again highly recommended.

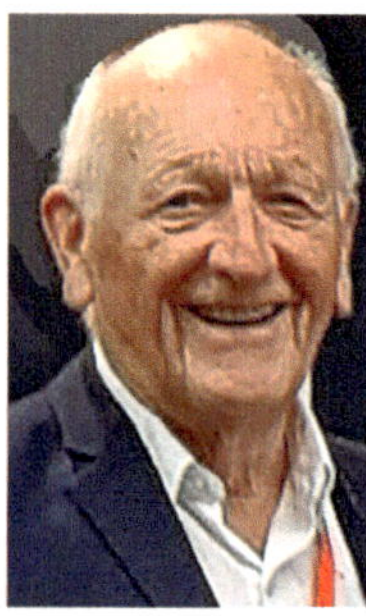

Orthopaedic Surgery Emeritus
at the University of Basel
Basel, Switzerland

Werner Müller

Foreword 4

Implant-free press-fit fixation techniques were used in the early years of cruciate ligament surgery, as there was little material available except for K-wires and screws for achieving a rigid fixation of a graft inside a bone tunnel. In the early 1960s Jones and Brückner were associated with bone–patellar bone–tendon grafts but it was Peter Hertel from Berlin who introduced anatomical bone–tendon–bone implant-free fixation to the world of cruciate ligament specialists during an ESSKA meeting in Stockholm in 1990. Over the following years, more and more implants were developed to achieve rigid graft fixation, some of them disturbing the collagen architecture close to the tunnel entrance. Soon, high revision rates were found for femoral titanium screws securing a hamstring tendon within the femoral tunnel.

Gernot Felmet's focus was on the use of bone blocks for all kinds of grafts close to the tunnel entrance and allowing "ribbon-like" fixation using autologous tissue.

In daily practice, most hospitals in Germany suffer from poor reimbursement of anterior cruciate ligament (ACL) reconstructions, especially in outpatient settings. Only high-volume centers manage to be economically viable, leaving hospitals with high implant costs, poor quality control of tunnel placement, and therefore high revision rates.

Gernot Felmet has done an outstanding job of developing instruments for bone stock preservation and has followed his dream of biologically superior graft fixation for all available ACL grafts. He has managed to preserve his ideas at a time when the orthopedic community was fixed on double tunnels or anterior lateral ligament reconstruction.

This book focuses on the next generation of ACL surgery: safe, anatomical, biological, and efficient, with low costs.

All this will then leave us with good healing results that will allow us to focus on rehabilitation and return to sports, with a decreased likelihood of graft re-rupture and contralateral ACL injury.

I wish Gernot a bright future and all the readers a joyful encounter with Gernot's work of the last 25 years!"

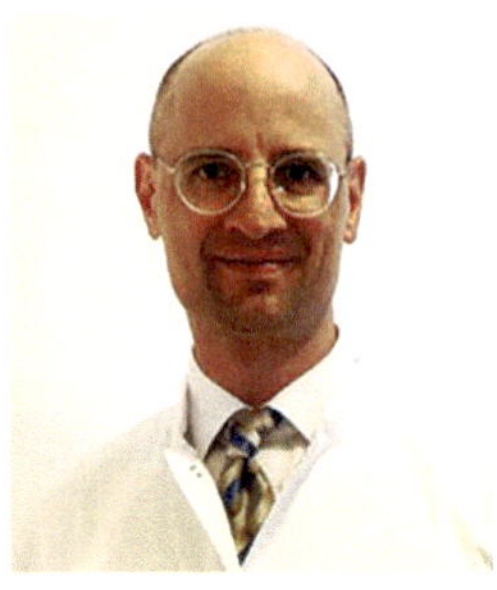

Agaplesion Ev. Klinikum Schaumburg
Obernkirchen, Germany

Michael Jagodzinski

Foreword 5

In addition to demonstrating a unique biological ligament reconstruction technique at the knee, laxity tests and their respective reproducibility are described in a structured manner. It is gratifying that cone beam CT high-resolution imaging quality controls under axial loading were used extensively to verify the results. These demonstrated the exceptional anatomical quality of the anterior cruciate ligament reconstruction technique described here. All the important basics of rehabilitation around the knee are underscored with the author's own valuable manual examination techniques and his extensive experience. This book is therefore recommended to anyone working on the injured or postoperative knee as a sports scientist, physiotherapist, or as an orthopedic surgeon.

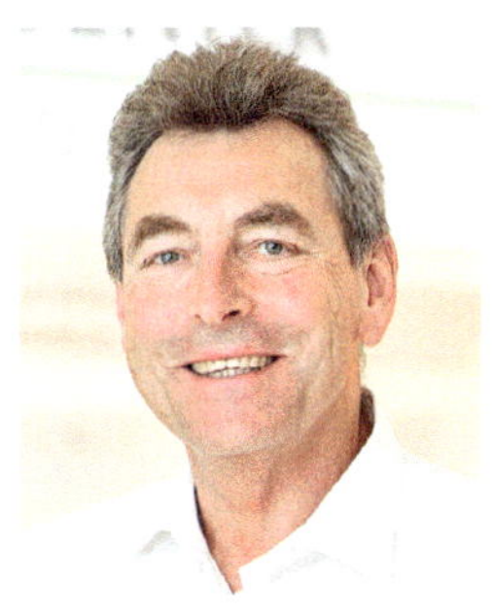

Heinz Lohrer

(Past) Director of the Institute for Sports Medicine
and Olympiastützpunkt (OSP)
Frankfurt am Main, Germany

University of Freiburg
Freiburg im Breisgau, Germany

Preface

This book describes purely biological ligament reconstructions of the knee joint without foreign material involving reconstruction of the anatomy. Since the 1980s, a small group of joint surgeons have been describing excellent results in cruciate ligament reconstruction using biological and purely foreign material-free techniques. The author describes the path and solutions of enthusiastic sports orthopedic surgeons, as well as his own technique, "ribbon-like" self-tensioning, which replaces or complements established procedures. The anatomy, modern understanding of biomechanics, and history of cruciate ligament surgery make the book a concentrated pragmatic manual for diagnostics, indications, and planning of surgical techniques for revision procedures, possible complications, and solutions with "Plan B." In addition to prevention in sports and participation in competitive sports, the modern elements of rehabilitation and return to sports are presented for every knee surgeon.

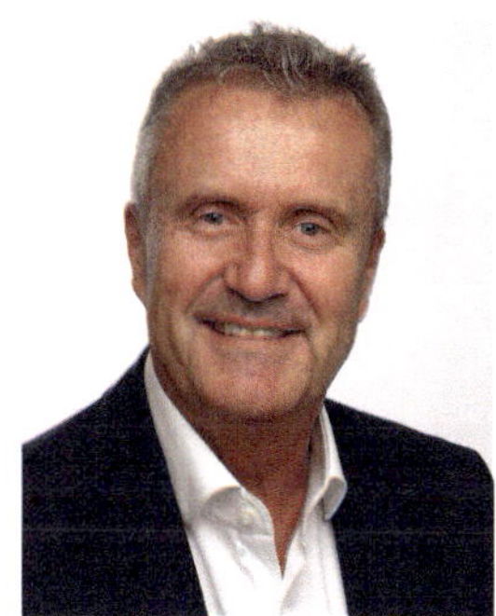

Gernot Felmet
Villingen-Schwenningen
Germany

Acknowledgements

Acknowledgements go to my family, my children and my wife, the team at the Artico Sports Clinic, Senior Physician Alexander Gassert, without whose patient and unwavering support over the past 30 years the developments as well as this book could not have been realized. So it is dedicated to them, as well as to my friends and colleagues who supported me.

Contents

1 Anatomy and Biomechanics

Knowledge about the anatomy is an important prerequisite for understanding the knee with capsular ligament structures, their biomechanical properties and their influence on joint kinematics. Therefore, this first chapter is a guide through the main anatomical structures of the knee ligament apparatus, as well as their biomechanical and articulated kinematic tasks, and explains the latest findings and understanding.

1.1 Anterior Crucial Ligament

The anterior cruciate ligament (ACL) and the posterior cruciate ligament (PCL) stabilize in the central area of the knee the anterior and posterior translation surrounded by the capsule and ligaments, protected and controlled by the thigh and lower leg muscles (Fig. 1.1a) [1]. The ACL rises on the lateral posterior femoral condyle diagonally through the intercondylar fossa and is inserts in the eminentia intercondylaris. Both the ACL and the PCL are enveloped by the synovial membrane (Fig. 1.1b). Anatomically, without preparation and arthroscopically, the ACL is almost not seen flat, but rather oval to round (Fig. 1.2a, b). Under the synovial membrane, it consists of many individual structural bundles; however, in the current literature from biomechanical investigations and reflections, a more ribbon-like or multi-bundle functional classification is established [3–5].

Anatomy is basic to understanding biomechanical function; therefore, it is important to represent the latest aspects from the last 20 years. Since 2000, different ideas developed about the function of the ACL as a double bundle, the multiple bundle, and later the ligamentous anatomy. Many working groups described the femoral insertion as an oval area with a longitudinal diameter of about 18 mm and a transverse diameter of 11 mm. The tibial insertion was described with a triangular ("duck foot") insertion area, with 17-mm expansion in the sagittal plane and 11-mm extension in the transverse plane [3] (Fig. 1.3). In addition, the ligament was divided into functional portions anteromedial (AM) and posterolateral (PL) bundles [6]. In 2012, the anatomy of insertion of the ACL was focused on and discussed again by the findings of Robert Smigielski et al. [7]. This working group described one significantly flatter progression ("ribbon-like") of the ACL with a flat, rectangular femoral and C-shaped tibial approach [7] (Fig. 1.4a–c). Smigielski et al. described a flat, almost rectangular femoral

G. Felmet, *Press-Fit Fixation of the Knee Ligaments*, https://doi.org/10.1007/978-3-031-11906-4_1

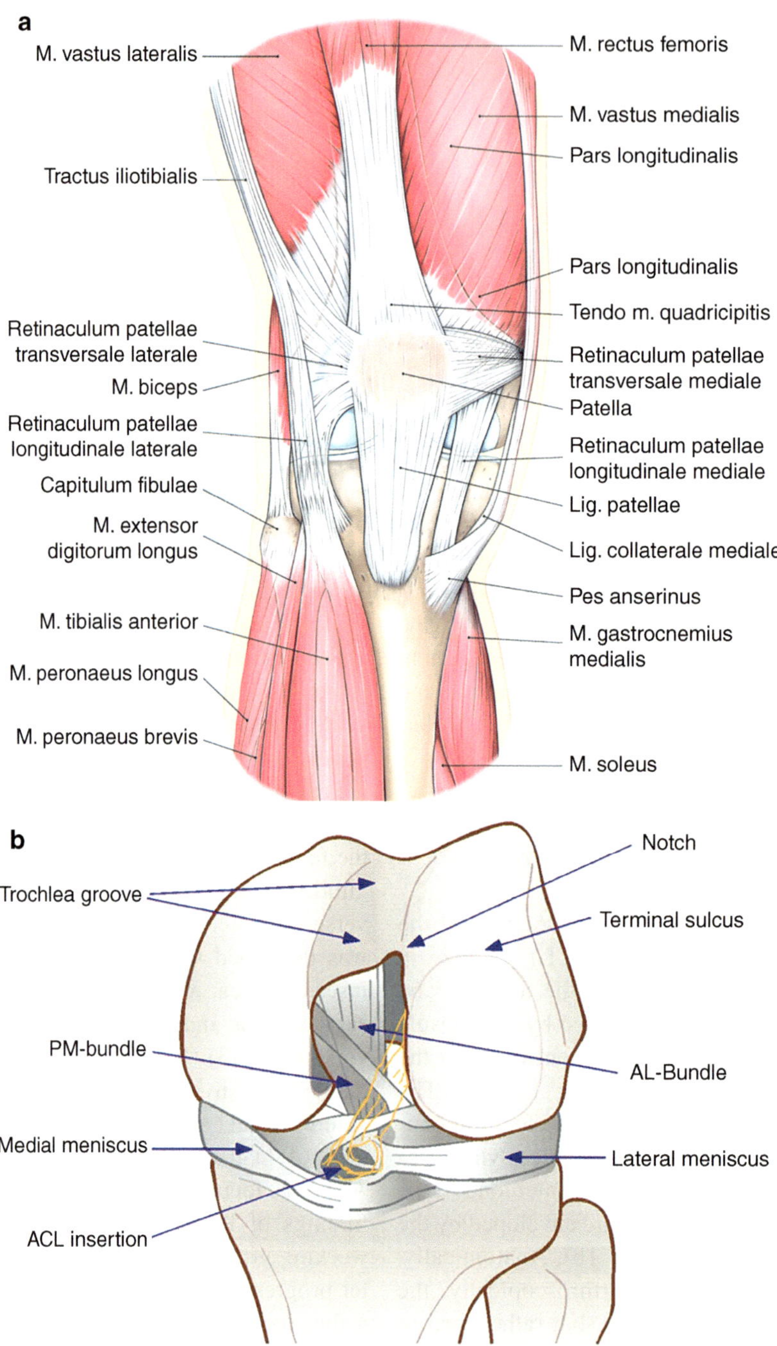

Fig. 1.1 (**a**) Right knee from anterior, from Jagodzinski et al. [1]. (**b**) Anterior cruciate ligament (ACL) with tibial insertion and posterior cruciate ligament (PCL) from anterior with anterolateral (AL) and posteromedial (PM) bundle, Wrisberg ligament and Humphrey ligament in a left knee, adapted from Anderson et al. [2]

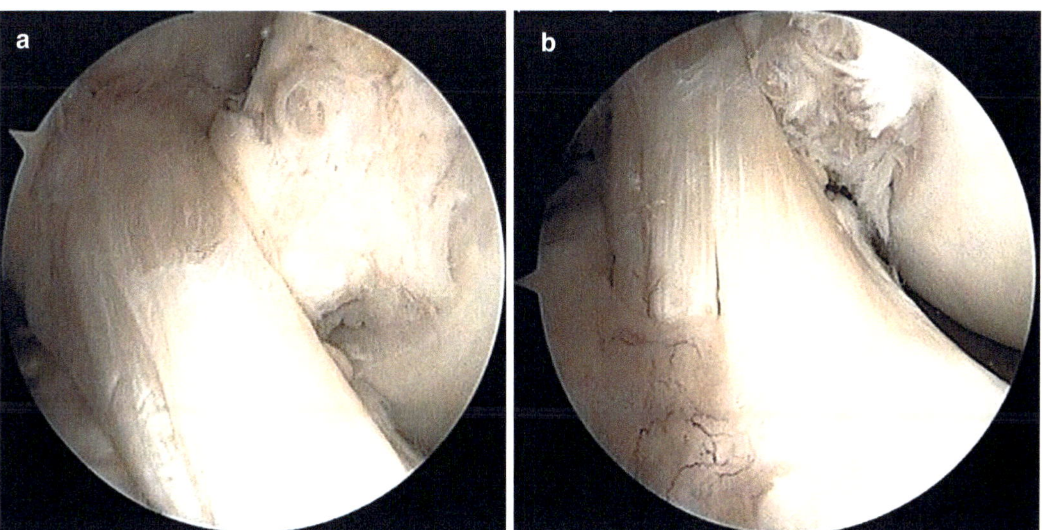

Fig. 1.2 (**a**) Anterior cruciate ligament in frog position from anterior in an oval mode in the femoral insertion in a right knee. (**b**) Flat tibial insertion right knee

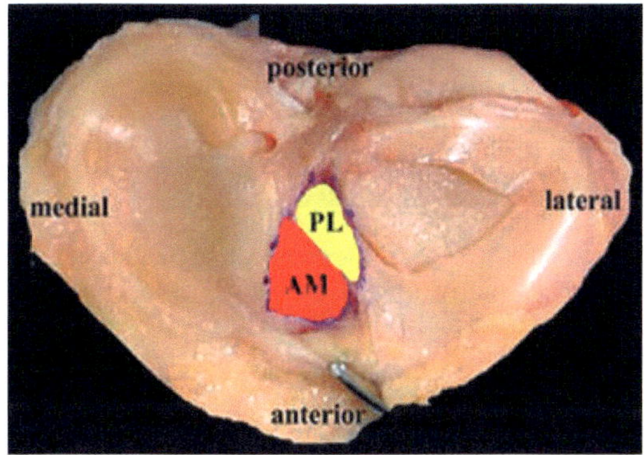

Fig. 1.3 Tibial insertion of the anterior cruciate ligament of anteromedial (AM) and posterolateral (PL) bundle as a duck foot [6]

insertion with an extension of 11–17 × 3 mm [7] (Fig. 1.5a, b). The tibial insertion was described by Siebold et al. as mostly C shaped, with only functionless fatty fibers in the original PL bundle insertion zone [8, 11]. The C form of the tibial insertion is individual and varies between men and women. Individual anatomical variations make it difficult in the case of reconstruction. Tibial landmarks and the "tibial square model" may assist in individualized bone tunnel placement [10, 12] (Fig. 1.6).

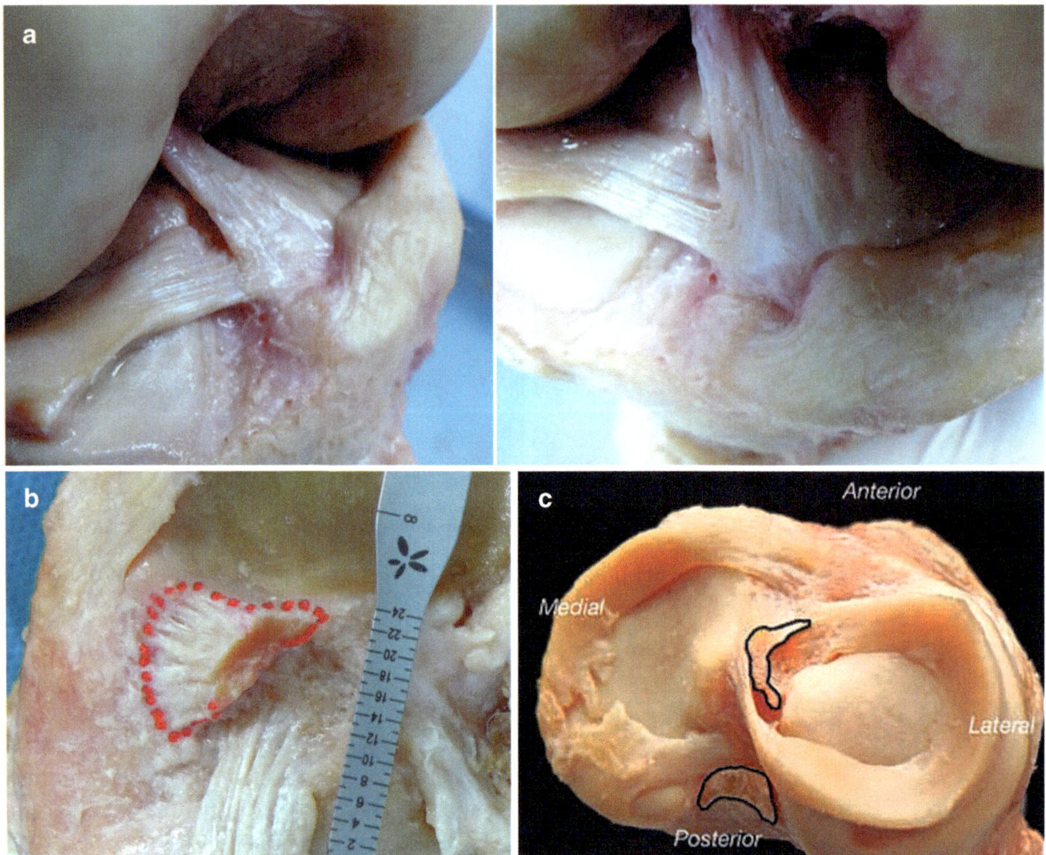

Fig. 1.4 (**a**, **b**) C-shaped tibial insertion, fat and synovial tissue removed by Siebold et al. [8]. The anterior horn of the lateral meniscus drives underneath the anterior cruciate ligament (ACL). The medial meniscus inserts right in front of the ACL [9]. (**c**) Anatomical preparation and dissection of the ACL by Robert Smigielski et al. in a C-shaped tibial insertion [7, 10]

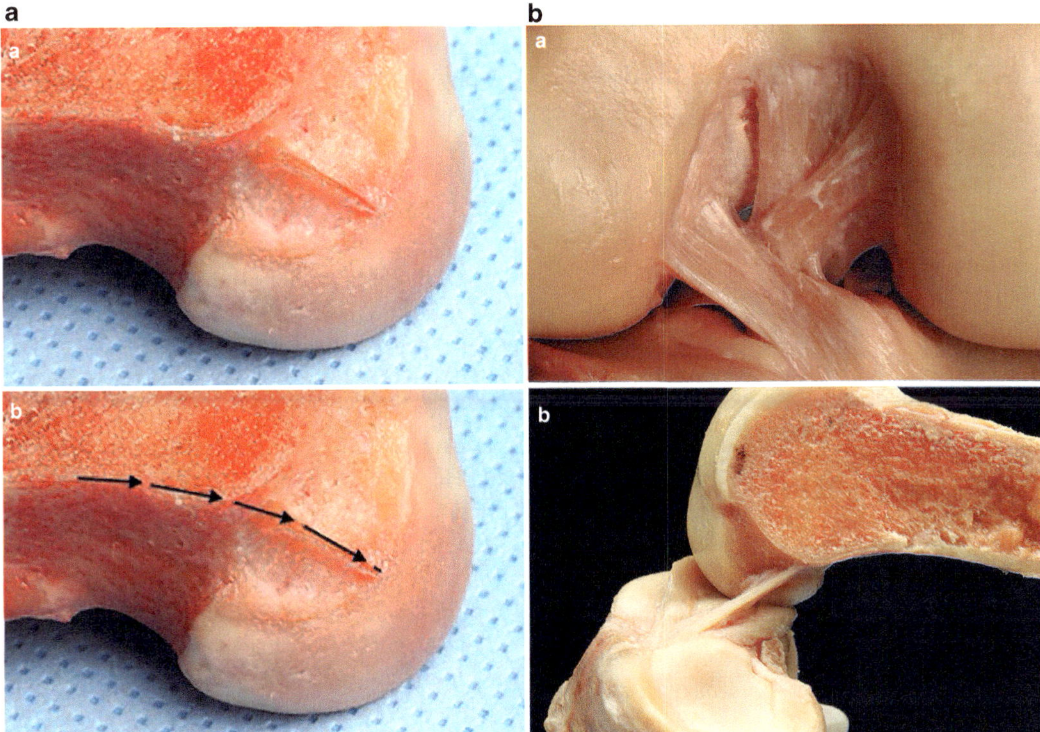

Fig. 1.5 (**a**) The direct insertion of the ribbon-like anterior cruciate ligament fibers is in continuity of the posterior femoral cortex (a) (arrows b) [7]. (**b**) Femoral insertion after resection of the synovial tissue (a, b) by Robert Smigielski [7]. He presents a flat ribbon-like femoral insertion in continuity (arrows) of the femoral cortex as a curved line

Classification of Tibial Insertion

Type I — elliptically

Type II — triangularly

Type III — C - shaped

Fig. 1.6 Classification of the tibial insertion by Guenther et al. [12]

1.2 Biomechanics

The biomechanical properties of the knee joint can be divided into two parts:

a. Structural properties (e.g., the ligament structures or reconstructed ligaments) and
b. Joint kinematics.

The structural characteristics of the original ACL are with a maximum pull-out force of 2160 (±157) N and a stiffness of 242 (±28) N/mm (Table 1.1). The physiological burden of the ACL was indirectly calculated in different studies when running with 169 N and with activation of the knee extensors when climbing stairs given as 445 N. The ACL consists of many individual bundles. Biomechanical investigations and considerations describe functional bundles divided into an AM and PL bundles established [3–5]. The bundle design is due to the tibial insertion of the individual bundles [3, 11]. This functional classification of the ACL into a two-bundle structure is an understanding of the complex function that has been simplified and is currently undergoing high scientific acceptance [3, 11]. In vitro investigations showed that the AM bundle in particular tenses with increasing flexion over 30°, whereas the PL bundle tightens near complete knee extension in less than 30° flexion [5, 11]. The PL bundle also seems to stabilize particularly against rotational forces [4, 22, 23]. Kinematic studies with selective separation of the two ACL

Table 1.1 Biomechanical properties of the anterior cruciate ligament (ACL) and tendons to replace the ACL in different shapes, diameters and fixations [13]

Subject	Maximum load to failure (N)	Stiffness (N/mm)	Ref.
Biomechanical properties of tendons, grafts and fixation techniques			
Intact ACL (with femur and tibia)	2160 (±157)	242 (±28)	[14]
Two gracilis strands	1550 (±369)	370 (±108)	[15]
Two semitendinosus	2641 (±320)	535 (±76)	[15]
Four combined hamstring strands	4090 (±295)	276 (±204)	[15]
7 mm BPTB	2238 (±316)	327 (±58)	[16]
10 mm BPTB	2977 (±516)	424/455 (±57/67)	[16]
15 mm BPTB	4389 (±708)	556 (±67)	[16]
15 mm BPTB	4389 (±708)	556 (±67)	[16]
10 mm QTB	2353 (±495)	621 (±122)	[17]
Interference screw (BPTB)	683–863	76–80	[18]
Interference screw (hamstrings)	534–926	189–316	[19, 20]
Endobutton (hamstrings)	520–1364	35–195	[19, 21]
Interference screw and Endobutton (hamstrings)	1290–1449	307–341	[19]

BPTB bone-patellar-tendon-bone

bundles detected increased rotational instability after separation of the PL bundle [23]. After transection of the AM bundle an increased AP translation resulted in the simulated Lachman test [23].

1.3 Anterior Tibial Translation

Some degree of anterior tibial translation (ATT) is physiologic.

A physiologic ATT in extension of approximately 2 mm at an anterior force of 100 N is reported. The radiographic Lachman test revealed an average ATT of approximately 5.5 mm. During physiologic gait, an ATT of approximately 3 mm was noted [24].

Instability in the sagittal direction can be measured with the KT-1000 or with the Rolimeter/ArticoMeter [25, 26]. This makes it possible to determine the individual ligament laxity.

1.4 Stability in Rotation

The ACL is the primary stabilizer of the ATT of about 86% [27]. The AM bundle with its short fibers seems to have a minor effect on ATT stabilization [28] (Fig. 1.7a, b). Replacing the ACL anatomically, the quadrant method described the femoral attachment described by Bernard and Hertel in the 1990s [29] (Fig. 1.8). The stabilization in rotation of the intact ACL results from horizontal ACL fibers [22, 30]. The inhibition of the internal rotation is not clear. Some authors found no significant internal rotation in the ACL-deficient knee [22, 31]. Other studies found a small but statistically significant increase in both the internal rotation and the pivot–shift phenomenon, although the central structure of the ACL is described as a stabilizer in rotation in complete extension, which fixes the femur in a slightly inwardly rotated position (final rotation mechanism) [32]. This reversed final rotation mechanism of the ACL-deficient knee causes an anterolateral luxation of the tibial plateau with inhibition of the internal tibial rotation by the ACL in complete extension [33]. Combined with this anterolateral luxation an axial shift medially provokes the pivot–shift phenomenon [34, 35] (Fig. 1.9a, b). This kinematic is also influenced by the regional adaptation of knee cartilage morphology and convex-to-convex (lateral) and convex-to-concave (medial) position of the femur to the tibia as an important factor of rotation and alteration in normal gait [36] (Fig. 1.10).

Biomechanical in vitro analysis of rotational stability showed that an isolated dissected ACL did not cause great rotational instability. Rotational instability is determined in the integrity of the lateral collateral ligament (LCL) [22]. Next to the ACL a combined lesion of the lateral capsular structures and ligaments influences the rotational instability [33].

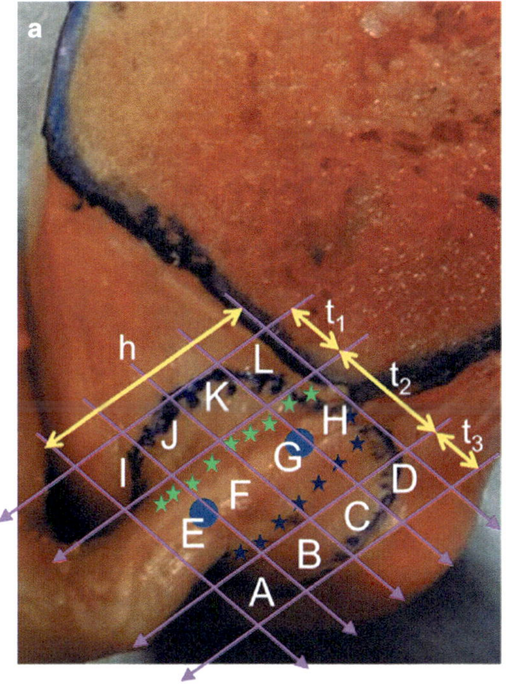

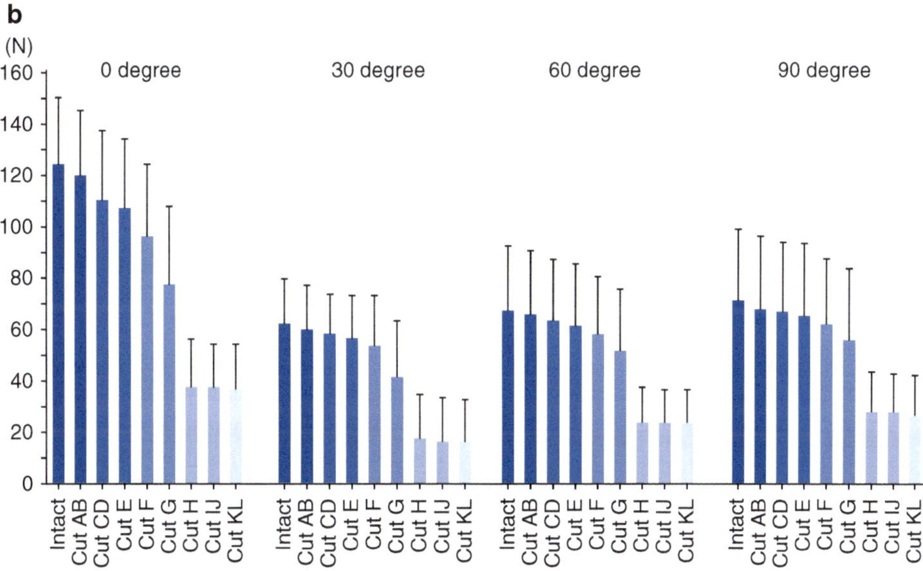

Fig. 1.7 (**a**) ACL attachment and length of fibers as described by Kawaguchi et al. [28]. The blue dots (near E and G) show the center of the anteromedial and posterolateral bundle. The stars show the boundaries between the fibers attaching directly to the bone in (t_2) zone. This is near the line shown by Smigielski [7]. The fan-like extension areas are anterior in (t_1) and posterior in (t_3). (h) describes the length of the femoral attachment. (**b**) Loss of load of the ACL in response to anterior tibial translation after dissection of fiber bundles attaching in different zones. Owing to the path-controlled six-axis robot, this was independent of the cutting order. Fiber bundles *G* and *H* represented the greatest load loss in any degree of flexion [28]

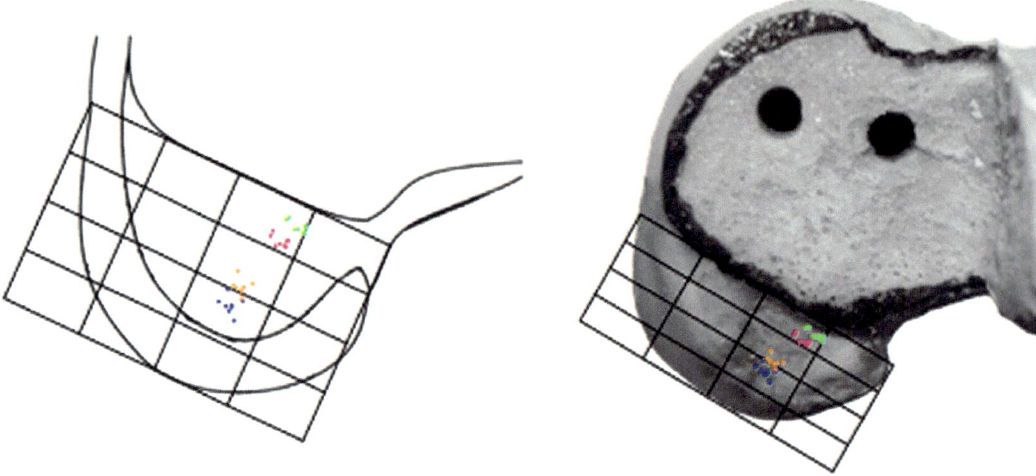

Fig. 1.8 Attachment area (t_2) described by Kawaguchi et al. [28] in the quadrant method described by Bernard et al. in 1997 [29]

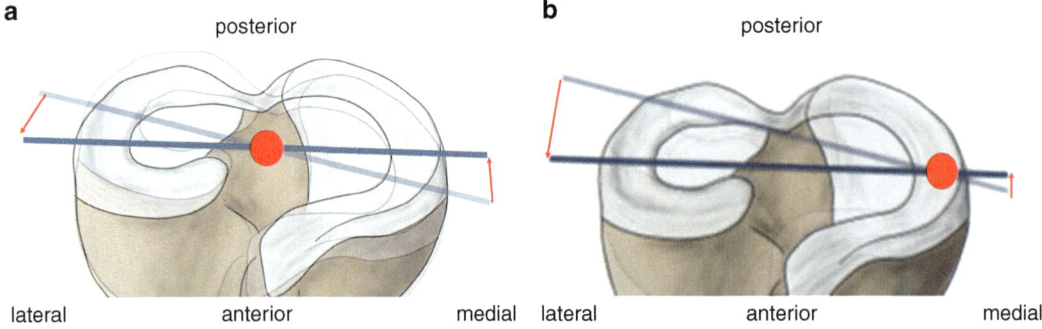

Fig. 1.9 (**a**, **b**) In the anterior cruciate ligament-deficient knee the center and axis of rotation move from central (**a**) to medial (**b**) and causes an anterolateral subluxation of the tibia (**a**, **b**) as a pivot shift [13]

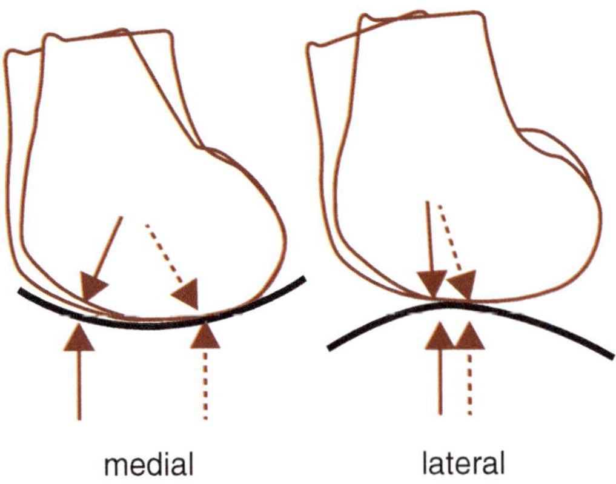

Fig. 1.10 Variation of the area of pressure and contact, convex–concave (medial) to convex–convex (lateral) [36]

After complete transection or tear of the ACL the anterior knee stability is lost with an increased ATT. This instability results in 10–30° knee flexion. During gait and weightbearing the tibia can subluxate ventrally. The physiological ATT of approximately 3 mm increased under ACL insufficiency by 4.7 mm [24].

The instability displaces the center of rotation to the medial joint. The mobility of the lateral tibial plateau by an increased ATT and advanced internal rotation increased [13, 22, 35]. This instability in rotation is examined using the pivot–shift test (Fig. 1.9a, b).

Insufficient extra-articular structures were able to show that as well as the ACL rupture, e.g., a transection of the anterolateral complex (ALL,

Kaplan fibers etc.), there was enlarged rotation instability, although this seems to result in an increased load on the medial structures of the knee joint. Kanamori et al. determined an increase in the tension in the medial collateral ligament (MCL) from 120 to 170% at 30–90° flexion of the knee joint and in the PL structures of 413% at 15° flexion position of the knee joint [37].

Biomechanical tests of pull-out forces and stiffness of the original ACL to different grafts and fixation techniques were started very early by Noyes et al. [38].

The variability depending on age and orientation of the pull-out forces showed different results [14]. Older cadaver knees showed a more than three times reduced maximum pull-out force (658 ± 129 N) and around one third reduced stiffness (180 ± 25 N/mm). Subsequent studies tried to find the perfect graft format. The currently used grafts document the individual biomechanical properties (Table 1.1) [13].

Anterior cruciate ligament deficiency changes the mechanical forces on the articular cartilage with a change of the rotary axis and increasing shift [39]. Specific gait changes are a part of a non-physiological mechanism on the cartilage and progression to osteoarthritis [40–45].

The ACL is an important primary stabilizer of the ATT and reduces the internal rotation in the early beginnings of knee flexion. Two functional bundles work with different elongation.

1.5 Posterior Cruciate Ligament

1.5.1 Anatomy

The PCL is the strongest ligament with a tensile strength of more than 1500 N. It runs from a fan-shaped approach at the lateral ventral border of cartilage of the medial femoral condyle to the sloping plateau between the dorsal central edge of the medial and lateral tibial plateau. The dorsal edge of this sloping plateau is about 1 cm below the level of the tibial articular cartilage and in the frontal plane at the height of the dorsal edge of the tibial plateau. Commonly, the PCL is crossed ventrally by the "Humphrey ligament," incipient from the posterior horn of the lateral meniscus. Dorsally, the PCL is crossed angulated by the anterior meniscofemoral ligament "Wrisberg ligament" [2] (Fig. 1.11). These two rather weak ligaments reinforce the function of the PCL.

The vascular supply of the PCL is mainly from the top margin of the popliteum obliquum ligament obliquely from the proximal side of the popliteal artery to the artery genus media. Owing to good collateralization with the circumflex vessels interruptions of the arteria genus media or their branches are very rarely associated with negative consequences (e.g., after arthroscopic transseptal access or surgery to the PCL). The distance of the arteria poplitea from the rear lower edge of the oblique approach plateau in an extension of approximately 3 mm, in diffrac-

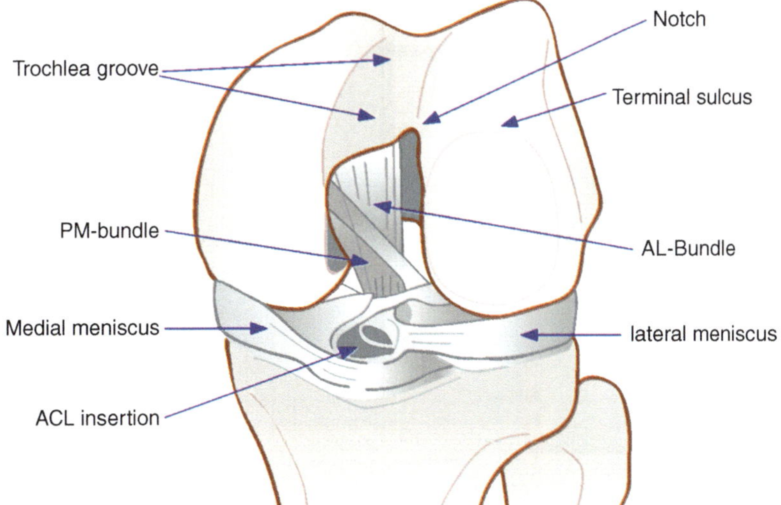

Fig. 1.11 Posterior cruciate ligament from anterior with anterolateral (AL) and posterolateral (PL) bundles, Wrisberg ligament and Humphrey ligament from anterior, adapted from [2]

tion of approximately 4 mm, and increases by capsule distension (over rinsing liquid) and operative capsule release to over 10 mm. The distance is even larger in the central height of the PCL (11.3 mm before and 17.6 mm after release). This explains the relatively low risk to the posterior neurovascular structures and posterior septal area [46].

Two functional bundles are also described in the PCL. The central anterolateral bundle is much stronger. It comes from the frontal upper area of the femoral insertion in the notch and ends posterior to the tibia. The posteromedial bundle is shorter and weaker and comes from the dorsal proportions of the femoral insertion area and ends at the deeper dorsal edge of the tibial insertion [2] (Fig. 1.11).

1.5.2 Biomechanics

In an extended knee position the PCL is not under maximal tension. Only the posteromedial bundle is under moderate tension. Its central and superior stabilization function is in the flexed knee position with both bundles.

The injury-relevant biomechanics of the PCL is determined by tension in flexion and rotation. The bending position with an external impact or without contact in the absence of muscular protection triggered by translation are typical factors of PCL rupture. Transection experiments of the PCL confirm [47, 48]:

a. Slight dorsal displacement of the tibial head in knee extension;
b. Stronger dorsal displacement in knee flexion;
c. Reduction of the shift in flexion by internal or external rotation.

While dissecting the PL structures the PL instability will also increase in extension [47–49] (Fig. 1.12). In internal rotation the posterior instability is not increased. Dissecting the pos-

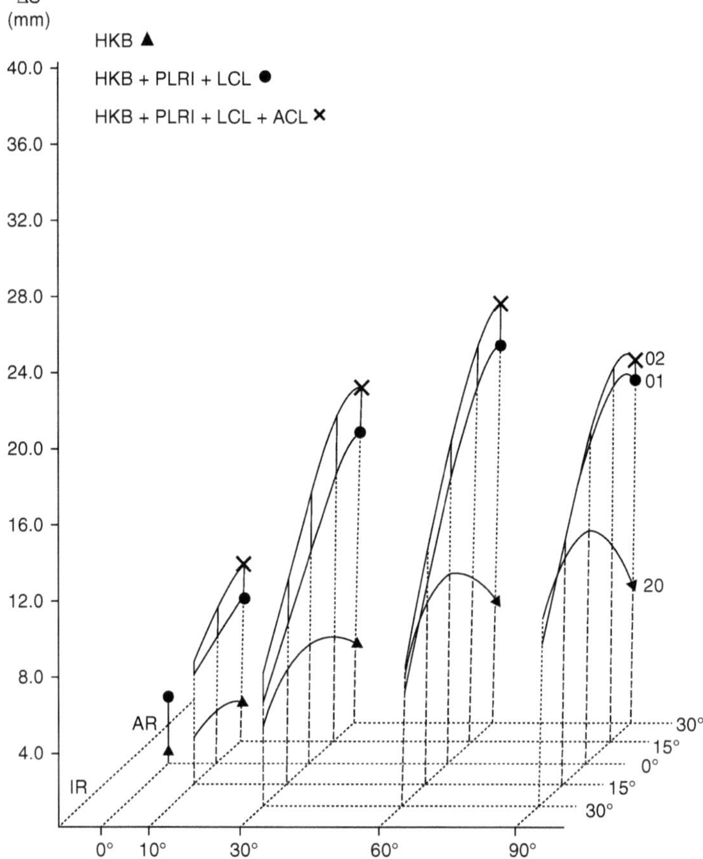

Fig. 1.12 Posterior cruciate ligament (PCL) lesion is combined with posterolateral rotatory instability (PLRI) at the posterolateral corner. *LCL* lateral cruciate ligament, *ACL* anterior cruciate ligament [49, 50]

teromedial structures, posteromedial instability in extension will increase more than PL instability. This complexity of posterior instability changes the center of pivot in 90° flexion. The fulcrum–pivot in 90° diffraction at increasingly complex instability shifts in the PL instability after ventromedial instability, at the posteromedial to centrolateral instability.

1.6 Medial Collateral Structures

1.6.1 Anatomy

The complex of the medial and posteromedial capsular ligament of the knee joint consists of several layers. Structures can be separated into superfascial, fascial and deep layers [51]. A functional description is established from anterior to posterior [1, 52, 53] (Figs. 1.13 and 1.14). Under functional and surgical aspects there are three structures of the posteromedial capsule:

a. Superficial medial collateral ligament (sMCL);
b. Deep medial collateral ligament (dMCL);
c. Posterior oblique ligament (POL).

1.6.1.1 Superficial Medial Collateral Ligament

The sMCL is in the most superficial layer and extends over a length of about 100 mm. This ribbon, which is flat and rhombic-shaped, overlaps the medial joint. The proximal insertion of the sMCL is slightly proximal and dorsal to the medial epicondyle. Two insertions are distally:

1. Proximally: below the tibial plateau with the approach of the semimembranosus muscle;

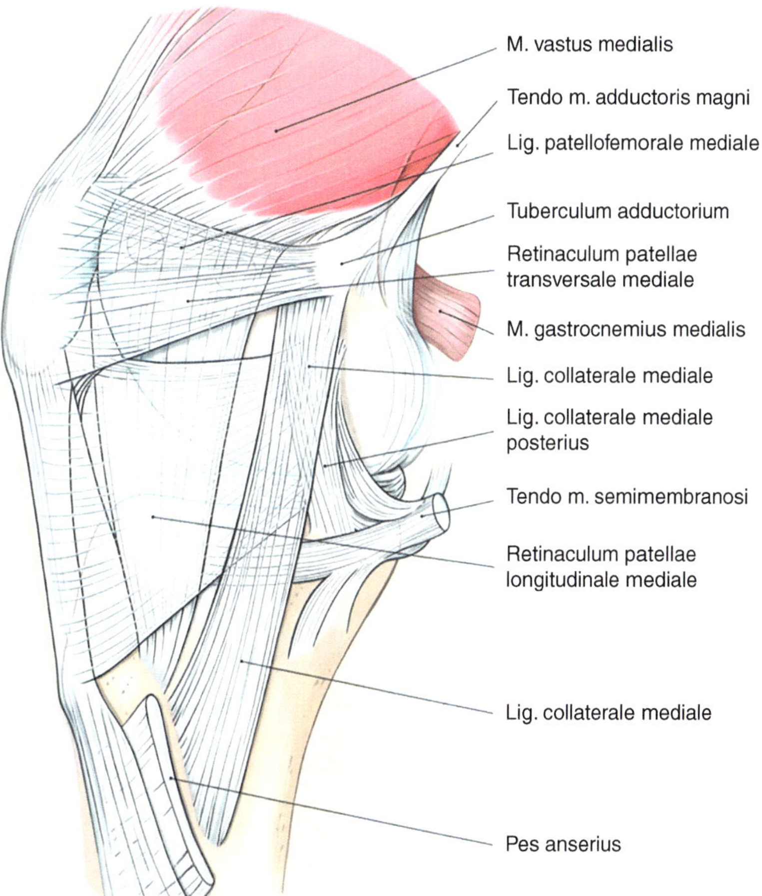

Fig. 1.13 The knee from medial from Jagodzinski et al. with different layers [1]

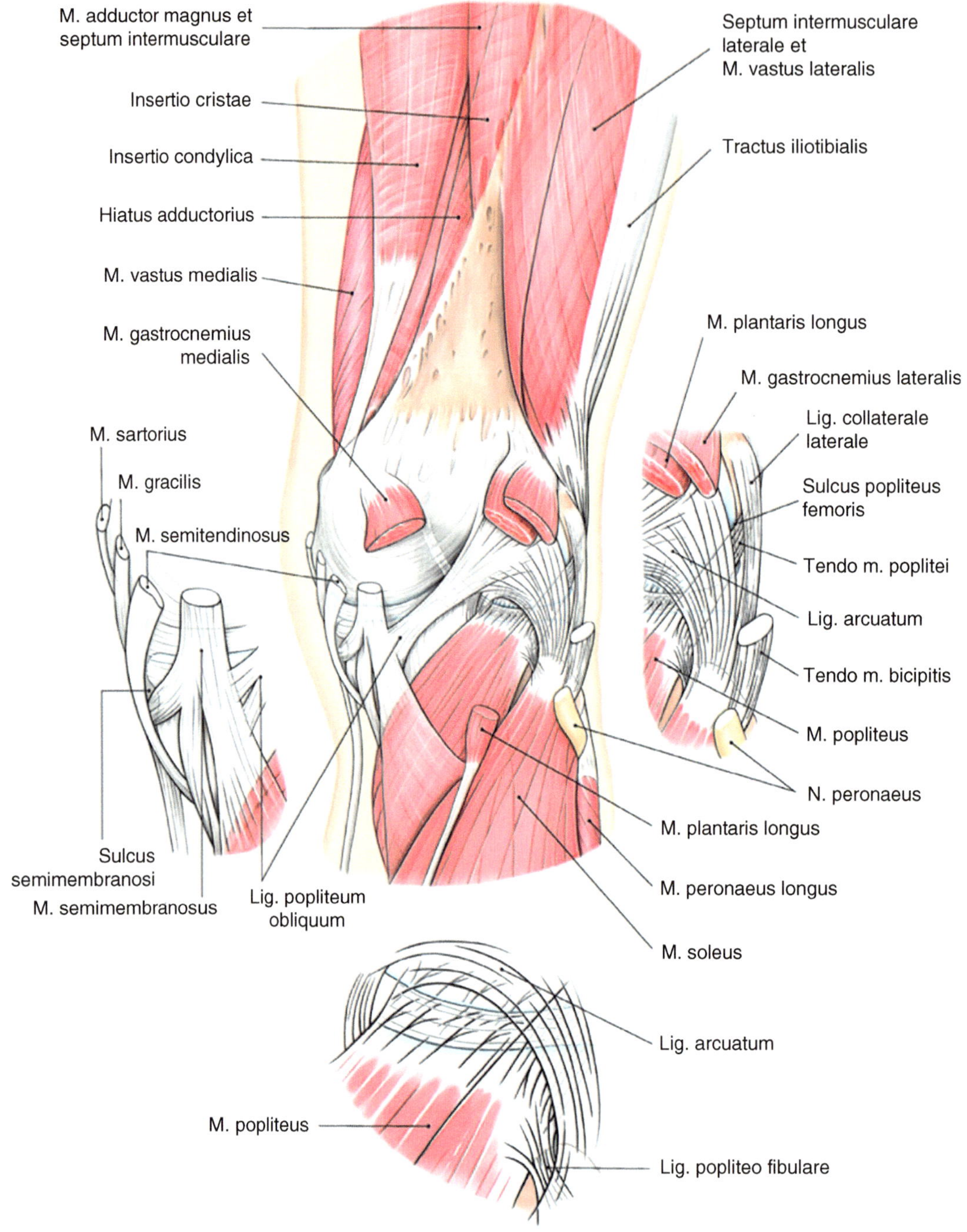

Fig. 1.14 The knee in deep layers from posterior showing the medial and lateral corners, the arcuatum complex [1]

2. Distal: anterior to the posteromedial tibial edge below the pes anserinus.

1.6.1.2 Deep Medial Collateral Ligament

The dMCL extends under the sMCL slightly distal and dorsal to the medial condyle to its tibial insertion, just below the medial tibial plateau. This extends over one significantly shorter distance of about 30 mm with a smaller width (9 mm) than the sMCL. The dMCL has one meniscofemoral (proximal) and a meniscotibial portion (distal). The dMCL connects dorsally to the POL.

1.6.1.3 Posterior Oblique Ligament

The POL inserts distal to the gastrocnemius tubercle with three functional structures:

1. Superficial: parallel and posterior to the sMCL;
2. Central: distal insertion—tibial on the medial meniscus with the posteromedial capsule and the semimembranosus muscle;
3. Capsular: distal insertion with the semimembranosus muscle.

1.6.2 Biomechanics

The anatomical complexity of the medial ligaments symbolizes the complex function in stabilization to different forces on variable positions of the knee joint. With examinations on cadavers the individual ligament structures were examined. Stabilizing effects against valgus stress, ATT, and rotational forces were examined [54, 55].

A separation of the individual structures shows that the proximal portion of the sMCL works especially as a stabilizer against a valgus stress in high flexion and is effective in a close-to-retraction position, whereas the distal portion of the sMCL stabilizes especially in a 60° knee flexion.

Other working groups examined in addition the synergistic influence of combination injuries of the medial ligament complex and the ACL and PCL. A separation of the sMCL with existing ACL insufficiency increased ATT leads in 90° flexion. In a 30° flexion position the sMCL again could not influence the ATT [56]. A synergistic influence of the medial structures on a PCL insufficiency could be shown after combined separation of the POL and PCL with an increase in the posterior tibial translation (PTT) [57]. The transection of the sMCL and dMCL in PCL insufficiency showed no increase in PTT.

The main functions of each medial capsule and ligaments are as follows.

sMCL

- Main stabilizer against valgus stress in full flexion extent (from 30° flexion on)
  a. Proximal part stabilization: near extension and in 90° flexion
  b. Distal part stabilization: 60° flexion position
- Stabilizer against internal and external rotation

dMCL

- Secondary stabilizer against valgus stress in extension and flexion
- Rupture occurs in valgus stress

POL

- Most important stabilizer against internal rotation (especially in extension)
- Stabilizer against valgus stress in knee extension [35, 57] (Table 1.2).

Table 1.2 Function of the medial capsule and different layers of the medial collateral ligament (MCL) [35, 57]

Medial capsule/ MCL	Internal rotation	External rotation	Valgus instability	Anterior tibial translation	Posterior tibial translation
dMCL	/	/	/	(+)	/
sMCL	(+) in flexion	(+ +)	(+ +) in flexion	/	/
POL	(+ +) in extension		(+ +) in extension		(*x*)

dMCL deep medial collateral ligament, *sMCL* superficial medial collateral ligament, *POL* posterior oblique ligament

1.7 Lateral Collateral Structures

1.7.1 Anatomy

The lateral knee is a multilayer complex of capsular, ligamentous, and musculoskeletal structures with importance for stability in knee rotation and translation. The tractus iliotibialis with its superficial structures, runs subcutaneously. Its deep fibers attach at the lateral femoral supracondylar tubercle. They attach as Kaplan fibers at the lateral intramuscular septum. Its deep structures runs to the caput breve of the biceps femoris muscle and also attach at the lateral tibial condyle at Gerdy's tubercle [1, 58] (Figs. 1.14 and 1.15).

The tractus iliotibialis is important for anterolateral stability. Below the tractus iliotibialis are the tendons of the caput longum and caput breve of the biceps femoris muscle. The caput longum inserts directly laterally of the fibula head and is above the fibular insertion of the LCL [58]. An anterior portion is lateral from the LCL and inserts at the lateral tibial plateau. The caput longum and caput breve and the PL fibers of the LCL join as an aponeurotic connection [58]. The caput breve of the biceps femoris muscle has three tendon-like insertions. One capsular part

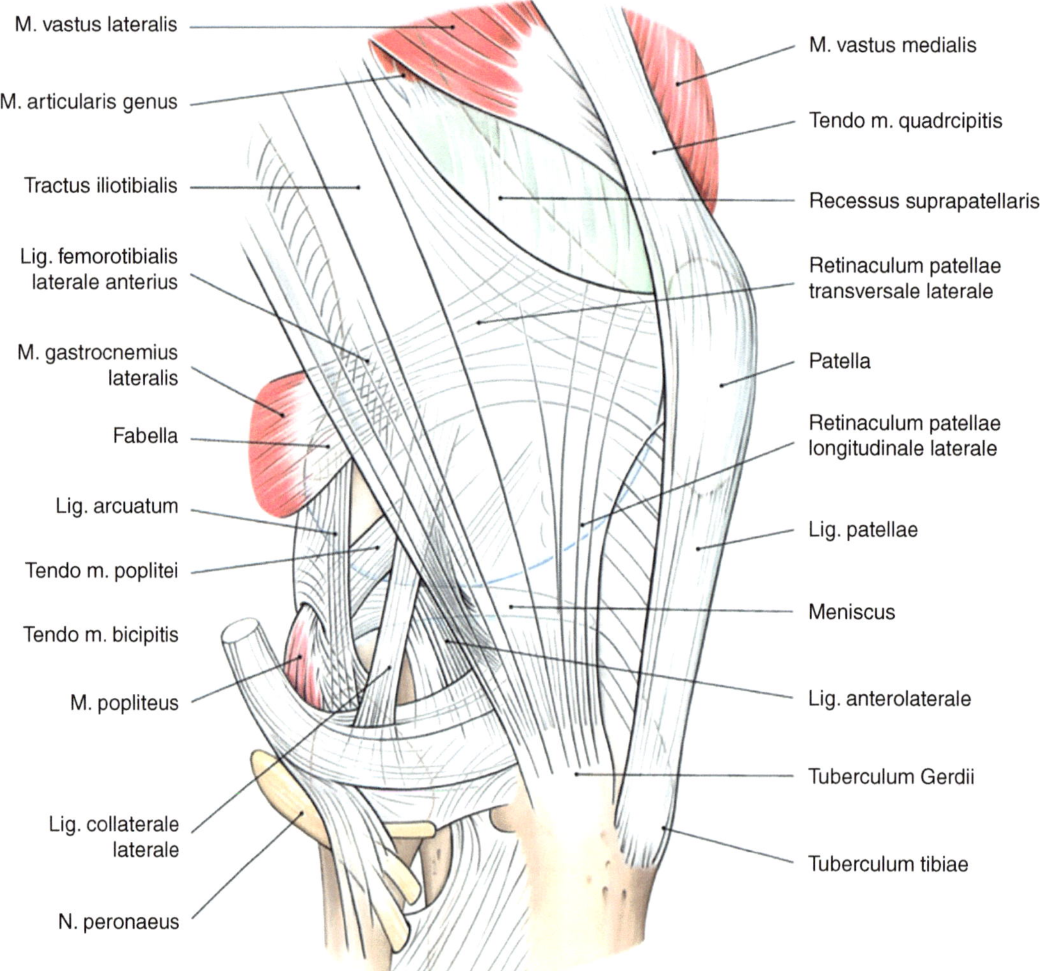

Fig. 1.15 The knee from lateral from Jagodzinski et al. with the arcuatum complex [1]

from the main tendon into the PL capsule inserts laterally to the styloid of the fibula head. The distal part of the capsule forms the fabellofibular ligament [58]. An anterior part inserts with meniscotibial connections to the LCL at the lateral tibial plateau. Posterior to the biceps femoris tendon and 1.5–2 cm distal to the fibular styloid runs the peroneus communis nerve.

The LCL is an extra-articular structure with a length of about 70 mm and inserts at the femoral side dorsal to the lateral epicondyle. At the fibula head it inserts laterally and below the caput longum of the tendon of the biceps femoris muscle.

The tendon of the popliteus muscle is in the sulcus popliteus just distal to the femoral insertion of the LCL. The popliteus tendon starts anterior and distal to the epicondyle lateralis and the femoral insertion of the LCL as an intraarticular structure [59]. It runs distally intra-articularly to the hiatus popliteus and delivers branches to the lateral meniscus. These popliteomeniscal fascicles are dynamic stabilizers of the lateral meniscus. The tendon leaves the interior knee through the lig. coronarium to the popliteal fossa. Different connections follow the musculotendinous part of the popliteus tendon to the fibula through the anterior lig. popliteofibulare. One is directly from of the popliteus tendon to the fibula distal to the fibular styloid through the posterior lig. popliteofibulare [60]. The lig. popliteum arcuatum is a complex of compounds of the fibula head to the fabella, deep capsular structures, and meniscotibial compounds, in their entirety to stabilize the popliteus muscle and its tendon with the capsule, the "arcuate–ligament complex." A further insertion between the anterior proportion of the popliteus muscle and the tibia is lateral to the fovea of the PCL insertion, the "popliteus tendon complex," described together as the "PL corner" [61] (Fig. 1.14).

The broad tendon of the lateral caput of the gastrocnemius muscle is proximal and posterior to the femoral LCL insertion, connecting the meniscofemoral portion of the posterior articular capsule. The tendon of the lateral gastrocnemius muscle with connections to the lig. popliteofibulare is important for PL stability.

1.7.2 Biomechanics

In a variety of studies the function of the PL structures is analyzed [12, 52, 59, 62]. They primary stabilizers against lateral opening and tibial external rotation as well as secondary stabilizers in the functional interaction with the PCL in the PTT (posterior drawer). The PL corner is an important secondary stabilizer of the PTT in a close-to-retraction position with the intact PCL [2]. This effect decreases significantly in knee flexion. In the case of PCL insufficiency the load on the PL structures increases significantly in extension and flexion. In a combined injury of the PCL and the PL structures posterior instability increases, particularly to be observed between 60° and 90° flexion [2].

The popliteus muscle is an important dynamic stabilizer of the posterior knee near complete extension with an intact PCL. In PCL insufficiency an active tensioning of the popliteus tendon could reduce the PTT by 36% [2]. This underlines the importance of the exact imaging and analysis of the injured structures of the PL corner for adequate restoration.

The LCL stabilizes the knee over the entire range of motion. The highest loads could be determined in slight flexion position at 30°. To rupture the LCL in this position about 300 N are necessary [62].

The PL structures stabilize the lateral knee. An insufficiency of the PL structures increases varus instability, which leads to an overload of the PCL. A PL insufficiency that is not addressed can cause a secondary insufficiency of a PCL replacement. Therefore, careful diagnostic and surgical planning of the PL corner is mandatory. The dynamic stabilizers of the lateral knee joint, such as the tractus iliotibialis, the biceps femoris muscle, and the lateral head of the gastrocnemius muscle, are of less importance regarding a stabilizing function under varus stress.

Primary tibial external rotation is stabilized by the PL structures and the LCL [49, 63]. The LCL is the main stabilizer in a near-to-extension position. With increasing flexion the tendon of the popliteus muscle and popliteofibular ligaments perform stabilization in a close interaction with the PCL. An isolated insufficiency of the PL structures significantly increases the tibial external rotation. A combined insufficiency of the PCL and PL structures in 90° knee flexion increase the external rotation instability and posterior shift of the tibia.

The primary stabilizers of the tibial internal rotation are on the medial articular side. The PL ligament complex is not an important stabilizer here.

An increased tibial slope in the presence of a compressive axial load has been shown to generate a greater anterior shear force in the tibiofemoral joint. The higher the tibial inclination, the higher the risk of ACL rupture. The lateral tibial inclination seems of greater importance [64, 65]. A higher lateral inclination increases the tibial pivot and tension in the ACL [66, 67]. In clinical investigation a good predictor for acute ACL injury is a "pivot shift" grade 3 with a higher tibial inclination [68, 69]. In a systematic review of clinical evidence of 29 studies a significant increase in the re-rupture rate in the ACL was observed in a posterior slope of 12° or more [70] (Fig. 1.16).

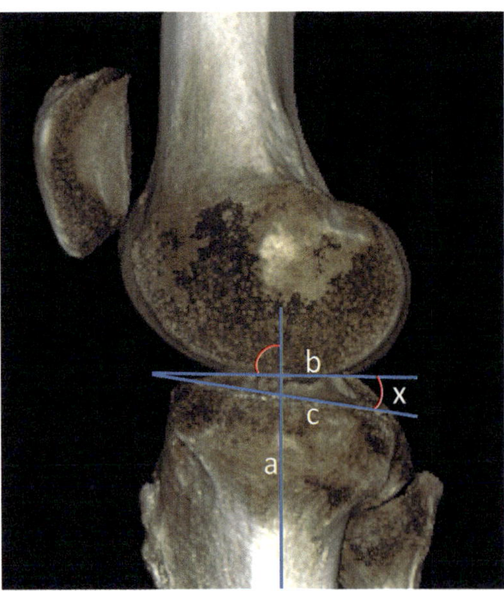

Fig. 1.16 The tibial slope is defined as the angle (*x*) between a line (*b*) perpendicular to the proximal anatomical axis of the tibia (*a*) and a tangent along the tibial plateau (*c*)—here in 3D digital volume tomography [70]

References

1. Jagodzinski M, Friederich NF, Müller W. Das Knie (the knee). 2nd ed. Berlin: Springer; 2016.
2. Anderson CJ, et al. Arthroscopically pertinent anatomy of the anterolateral and posteromedial bundles of the posterior cruciate ligament. J Bone Joint Surg Am. 2012;94(21):1936–45.
3. Petersen W, Zantop T. Anatomy of the anterior cruciate ligament with regard to its two bundles. Clin Orthop Relat Res. 2007;454:35–47.
4. Sakane M, et al. In situ forces in the anterior cruciate ligament and its bundles in response to anterior tibial loads. J Orthop Res. 1997;15(2):285–93.
5. Woo SL, et al. Biomechanics and anterior cruciate ligament reconstruction. J Orthop Surg Res. 2006;1:2.
6. Kopf S, et al. A systematic review of the femoral origin and tibial insertion morphology of the ACL. Knee Surg Sports Traumatol Arthrosc. 2009;17(3):213–9.
7. Śmigielski R, Zdanowicz U, Drwięga M, Ciszek B, Ciszkowska-Łysoń B, Siebold R. Ribbon like appearance of the midsubstance fibres of the anterior cruciate ligament close to its femoral insertion site: a cadaveric study including 111 knees. Knee Surg Sports Traumatol Arthrosc. 2015;23(11):3143–50. https://doi.org/10.1007/s00167-014-3146-7. Epub 2014 Jun 28. PMID: 24972997; PMCID: PMC4611008.
8. Siebold R, et al. Flat midsubstance of the anterior cruciate ligament with tibial "C"-shaped insertion site. Knee Surg Sports Traumatol Arthrosc. 2015;23(11):3136–42.
9. Siebold R, et al. Flat midsubstance of the anterior cruciate ligament with tibial "C"-shaped insertion site. Knee Surg Sports Traumatol Arthrosc. 2014;1:1.
10. AGA-Comitee-Knee-Ligament. ACL rupture – therapy (VKB ruptur - therapie). Zürich: AGA – Society for Arthroscopy and Joint Surgery; 2018. p. 8–142.
11. Siebold R, et al. Tibial insertions of the anteromedial and posterolateral bundles of the anterior cruciate ligament: morphometry, arthroscopic landmarks, and orientation model for bone tunnel placement. Arthroscopy. 2008;24(2):154–61.
12. Guenther D, et al. Variation in the shape of the tibial insertion site of the anterior cruciate ligament: classification is required. Knee Surg Sports Traumatol Arthrosc. 2017;25(8):2428–32.
13. Domnick C, Raschke MJ, Herbort M. Biomechanics of the anterior cruciate ligament: physiology, rupture and reconstruction techniques. World J Orthop. 2016;7(2):82–93.
14. Woo SL, et al. Tensile properties of the human femur-anterior cruciate ligament-tibia complex. The effects of specimen age and orientation. Am J Sports Med. 1991;19(3):217–25.
15. Hamner DL, et al. Hamstring tendon grafts for reconstruction of the anterior cruciate ligament: biomechanical evaluation of the use of multiple strands and tensioning techniques. J Bone Joint Surg Am. 1999;81(4):549–57.

16. Cooper DE, et al. The strength of the central third patellar tendon graft. A biomechanical study. Am J Sports Med. 1993;21(6):818–23.
17. Staubli HU, et al. Quadriceps tendon and patellar ligament: cryosectional anatomy and structural properties in young adults. Knee Surg Sports Traumatol Arthrosc. 1996;4(2):100–10.
18. Kousa P, et al. Initial fixation strength of bioabsorbable and titanium interference screws in anterior cruciate ligament reconstruction. Biomechanical evaluation by single cycle and cyclic loading. Am J Sports Med. 2001;29(4):420–5.
19. Oh YH, et al. Hybrid femoral fixation of soft-tissue grafts in anterior cruciate ligament reconstruction using the EndoButton CL and bioabsorbable interference screws: a biomechanical study. Arthroscopy. 2006;22(11):1218–24.
20. Kousa P, et al. The fixation strength of six hamstring tendon graft fixation devices in anterior cruciate ligament reconstruction. Part I: femoral site. Am J Sports Med. 2003;31(2):174–81.
21. Hoher J, Scheffler S, Weiler A. Graft choice and graft fixation in PCL reconstruction. Knee Surg Sports Traumatol Arthrosc. 2003;11(5):297–306.
22. Diermann N, et al. Rotational instability of the knee: internal tibial rotation under a simulated pivot shift test. Arch Orthop Trauma Surg. 2009;129(3):353–8.
23. Zantop T, et al. The role of the anteromedial and posterolateral bundles of the anterior cruciate ligament in anterior tibial translation and internal rotation. Am J Sports Med. 2007;35(2):223–7.
24. Markolf KL, Mensch JS, Amstutz HC. Stiffness and laxity of the knee–the contributions of the supporting structures. A quantitative in vitro study. J Bone Joint Surg Am. 1976;58(5):583–94.
25. Krautter A, et al. Instrumented arthrometry of the anterior cruciate ligament. A comparison. Biomed Tech. 2012;57:4299.
26. Ganko A, Engebretsen L, Ozer H. The rolimeter: a new arthrometer compared with the KT-1000. Knee Surg Sports Traumatol Arthrosc. 2000;8(1):36–9.
27. Butler DL, Noyes FR, Grood ES. Ligamentous restraints to anterior-posterior drawer in the human knee. A biomechanical study. J Bone Joint Surg Am. 1980;62(2):259–70.
28. Kawaguchi Y, et al. The role of fibers in the femoral attachment of the anterior cruciate ligament in resisting tibial displacement. Arthroscopy. 2015;31(3):435–44.
29. Bernard M, et al. Femoral insertion of the ACL. Radiographic quadrant method. Am J Knee Surg. 1997;10(1):14–21.
30. Zantop T, et al. Anterolateral rotational knee instability: role of posterolateral structures. Winner of the AGA-DonJoy Award 2006. Arch Orthop Trauma Surg. 2007;127(9):743–52.
31. Lane JG, et al. The anterior cruciate ligament in controlling axial rotation. An evaluation of its effect. Am J Sports Med. 1994;22(2):289–93.
32. Hallen LG, Lindahl O. The "screw-home" movement in the knee-joint. Acta Orthop Scand. 1966;37(1):97–106.
33. Kittl C, et al. The role of the anterolateral structures and the ACL in controlling laxity of the intact and ACL-deficient knee. Am J Sports Med. 2016;44(2):345–54.
34. Matsumoto H. Mechanism of the pivot shift. J Bone Joint Surg Br. 1990;72(5):816–21.
35. AGA-Comitee-Knee-Ligament. Diagnostic of the knee ligaments. Zürich: AGA – Society for Arthroscopy and Joint Surgery; 2018. p. 8–74.
36. Koo S, Rylander JH, Andriacchi TP. Knee joint kinematics during walking influences the spatial cartilage thickness distribution in the knee. J Biomech. 2011;44(7):1405–9.
37. Kanamori A, et al. In-situ force in the medial and lateral structures of intact and ACL-deficient knees. J Orthop Sci. 2000;5(6):567–71.
38. Noyes FR, et al. Biomechanical analysis of human ligament grafts used in knee-ligament repairs and reconstructions. J Bone Joint Surg Am. 1984;66(3):344–52.
39. Andriacchi TP, et al. A framework for the in vivo pathomechanics of osteoarthritis at the knee. Ann Biomed Eng. 2004;32(3):447–57.
40. Andriacchi TP, et al. Rotational changes at the knee after ACL injury cause cartilage thinning. Clin Orthop Relat Res. 2006;442:39–44.
41. Andriacchi TP, Dyrby CO. Interactions between kinematics and loading during walking for the normal and ACL deficient knee. J Biomech. 2005;38(2):293–8.
42. Buckland-Wright JC, Lynch JA, Dave B. Early radiographic features in patients with anterior cruciate ligament rupture. Ann Rheum Dis. 2000;59(8):641–6.
43. Daniel DM, et al. Fate of the ACL-injured patient. A prospective outcome study. Am J Sports Med. 1994;22(5):632–44.
44. Lohmander LS, et al. The long-term consequence of anterior cruciate ligament and meniscus injuries: osteoarthritis. Am J Sports Med. 2007;35(10):1756–69.
45. Lohmander LS, et al. Changes in joint cartilage aggrecan after knee injury and in osteoarthritis. Arthritis Rheum. 1999;42(3):534–44.
46. Ahn JH, et al. Increasing the distance between the posterior cruciate ligament and the popliteal neurovascular bundle by a limited posterior capsular release during arthroscopic transtibial posterior cruciate ligament reconstruction: a cadaveric angiographic study. Am J Sports Med. 2007;35(5):787–92.
47. Nannaparaju M, et al. Posterolateral corner injuries: epidemiology, anatomy, biomechanics and diagnosis. Injury. 2018;49(6):1024–31.
48. Bowman KF Jr, Sekiya JK. Anatomy and biomechanics of the posterior cruciate ligament, medial and lateral sides of the knee. Sports Med Arthrosc Rev. 2010;18(4):222–9.
49. Harner CD, et al. Biomechanical analysis of a posterior cruciate ligament reconstruction. Deficiency of the posterolateral structures as a cause of graft failure. Am J Sports Med. 2000;28(1):32–9.

50. Lee HJ, et al. The necessity of clinical application of tibial reduction for detection of underestimated posterolateral rotatory instability in combined posterior cruciate ligament and posterolateral corner deficient knee. Knee Surg Sports Traumatol Arthrosc. 2015;23(10):3062–9.
51. Warren LF, Marshall JL. The supporting structures and layers on the medial side of the knee: an anatomical analysis. J Bone Joint Surg Am. 1979;61(1):56–62.
52. Hughston JC, et al. Classification of knee ligament instabilities. Part II. The lateral compartment. J Bone Joint Surg Am. 1976;58(2):173–9.
53. Hughston JC, Eilers AF. The role of the posterior oblique ligament in repairs of acute medial (collateral) ligament tears of the knee. J Bone Joint Surg Am. 1973;55(5):923–40.
54. Griffith CJ, et al. Medial knee injury: part 1, static function of the individual components of the main medial knee structures. Am J Sports Med. 2009;37(9):1762–70.
55. Wijdicks CA, et al. Medial knee injury: part 2, load sharing between the posterior oblique ligament and superficial medial collateral ligament. Am J Sports Med. 2009;37(9):1771–6.
56. Haimes JL, et al. Role of the medial structures in the intact and anterior cruciate ligament-deficient knee. Limits of motion in the human knee. Am J Sports Med. 1994;22(3):402–9.
57. Weimann A, et al. Reconstruction of the posterior oblique ligament and the posterior cruciate ligament in knees with posteromedial instability. Arthroscopy. 2012;28(9):1283–9.
58. Terry GC, Hughston JC, Norwood LA. The anatomy of the iliopatellar band and iliotibial tract. Am J Sports Med. 1986;14(1):39–45.
59. Watanabe Y, et al. Functional anatomy of the posterolateral structures of the knee. Arthroscopy. 1993;9(1):57–62.
60. LaPrade RF, et al. The posterolateral attachments of the knee: a qualitative and quantitative morphologic analysis of the fibular collateral ligament, popliteus tendon, popliteofibular ligament, and lateral gastrocnemius tendon. Am J Sports Med. 2003;31(6):854–60.
61. Raheem O, et al. Anatomical variations in the anatomy of the posterolateral corner of the knee. Knee Surg Sports Traumatol Arthrosc. 2007;15(7):895–900.
62. LaPrade RF, et al. Mechanical properties of the posterolateral structures of the knee. Am J Sports Med. 2005;33(9):1386–91.
63. Harner CD, et al. The effects of a popliteus muscle load on in situ forces in the posterior cruciate ligament and on knee kinematics. A human cadaveric study. Am J Sports Med. 1998;26(5):669–73.
64. Dejour H, Bonnin M. Tibial translation after anterior cruciate ligament rupture. Two radiological tests compared. J Bone Joint Surg Br. 1994;76(5):745–9.
65. Giffin JR, et al. Effects of increasing tibial slope on the biomechanics of the knee. Am J Sports Med. 2004;32(2):376–82.
66. Feucht MJ, et al. The role of the tibial slope in sustaining and treating anterior cruciate ligament injuries. Knee Surg Sports Traumatol Arthrosc. 2013;21(1):134–45.
67. Simon RA, et al. A case-control study of anterior cruciate ligament volume, tibial plateau slopes and intercondylar notch dimensions in ACL-injured knees. J Biomech. 2010;43(9):1702–7.
68. Song GY, et al. Risk factors associated with grade 3 pivot shift after acute anterior cruciate ligament injuries. Am J Sports Med. 2016;44(2):362–9.
69. Rahnemai-Azar AA, et al. Increased lateral tibial plateau slope predisposes male college football players to anterior cruciate ligament injury. J Bone Joint Surg Am. 2016;98(12):1001–6.
70. Tischer T, et al. The impact of osseous malalignment and realignment procedures in knee ligament surgery: a systematic review of the clinical evidence. Orthop J Sports Med. 2017;5(3):2325.

2 Overuse: Trauma and Mechanism—Knee Morphology Risk Factors

The query regarding the exact accident mechanism helps to analyze the pattern and proportions of the injury. Ligament injuries can be isolated but also more complex. We distinguish between strain, partial rupture, and complete ruptures of the individual structures.

There are intrinsic and extrinsic risk factors for ligament injuries to the knee joint. Intrinsic factors include gender, athlete level, health status (age, weight, pre-injury, fatigue), the anatomy of the knee (measurements of the intercondylar notch, leg axis, ligament stability) and psychological influences (motivation, risk perception, nervousness, gaming experience). Extrinsic risk factors are influences from the environment, but also sports-specific equipment such as footwear and interaction with the game background is, e.g. "football boots and their interaction with the texture of the playing field" is known [1]. The individual injury mechanisms can be roughly divided into contact, indirect contact, and non-contact injuries.

2.1 Anterior Cruciate Ligament

The ACL in general has four common mechanisms of injury:

1. Valgus and internal rotation in the knee when fixed to the ground by changing the direction, taking a long step or a landing after a jump. This mechanism of injury occurs mostly in soccer or handball, often as a non-contact injury, and also occurs preferentially in female athletes when landing a jump (Fig. 2.1a, b).
2. Anterior translation of the tibia to the femur or vice versa in contact sports or traffic accidents or as a noncontact violation during a stopping maneuver of a running athlete with tension of the quadriceps muscle and anterior advancement of the tibia. This is typical in football, but also in skiing [2] and occurs more frequently as an injury mechanism in the context of re-ruptures after ACL replacement.
3. Hyperflexion trauma in the knee frequently combined with a slight external rotation of the tibia, which leads to the example of a backward fall of a skier and by quadriceps tension at the same time as insufficiency of the flexor of the ACL affected by high forces.
4. Hyperextension trauma in violent hyperextension of the knee. The roof of the intercondylar notch is the pivot that the ACL stretches, overstretches, or cuts like a guillotine.
5. A typical mechanism is the forward fall of a skier or an air strike in football, in which the ball is not hit with the foot. In the context of this mechanism partial ruptures of the ACL with the PL bundle often result [1–7].

Knee morphology is a contributor to risk of ACL injury. An increased tibial slope inclina-

G. Felmet, *Press-Fit Fixation of the Knee Ligaments*, https://doi.org/10.1007/978-3-031-11906-4_2

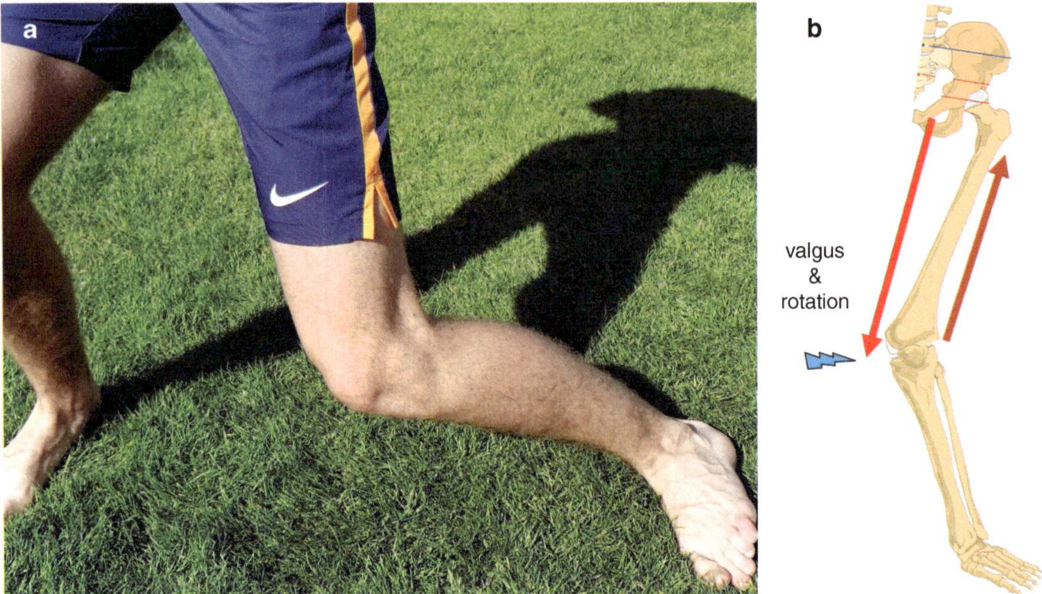

Fig. 2.1 (**a**, **b**) Valgus and internal rotation typical of medial and anterior cruciate ligament lesions

tion is combined with a higher risk of ACL rupture [8]. The lateral tibial inclination seems of greater importance. A pivot shift grade 3 is an excellent predictor of an increased tibial slope [9, 10]. In a systematic review of clinical evidence from 29 studies a significant increase in the re-rupture rate of the ACL was observed in a posterior slope of 12° or more [11] (Fig. 2.2). Other reviews summarized variations in sagittal condylar shape, reduced tibial eminence size, poor tibiofemoral congruity, intercondylar notch stenosis, and reduced ACL size as substantial risk factors for ACL injury. In ACL replacement the morphological risk factors, anatomical landmarks, and femoral and tibial footprints should be considered to improve outcomes in individualized anatomical ACL reconstructions [12, 13].

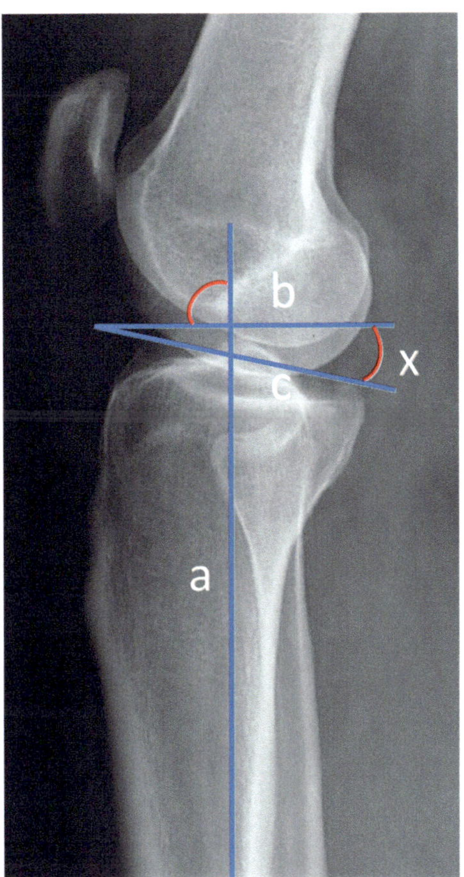

Fig. 2.2 A high tibial slope of 12° or more is a predictor of anterior cruciate ligament (ACL) rupture. It is the angle (*x*) between a line (*b*) perpendicular to the proximal anatomical axis of the tibia (*a*) and a tangent along the tibial plateau (*c*) [11]. Other risk factors are a sagittal condylar shape, reduced tibial eminence size, poor tibiofemoral congruity, intercondylar notch stenosis, and reduced ACL size [12, 13]

2.2 Medial Collateral Ligament

1. Forced valgus stress in the knee joint, often as contact injury.
2. Hyperextension injuries as combination injuries of a valgus/rotational movement with injuries to the ACL and the menisci, also called the "Unhappy Triad" [2].

2.3 Posterior Cruciate Ligament

1. "Dashboard injury" with posterior translation of the tibial plateau in traffic accidents by impact to tibial plateau in the bent knee. In sports the same accident mechanism occurs when falling with direct impact of the tibial head on the ground, typical of football goalkeepers [14] (Figs. 2.3 and 2.4).
2. Hyperextension injuries as combination injuries of a combined varus/rotational movement with injuries of the lateral and posterolateral ligament complex [1, 14, 15].

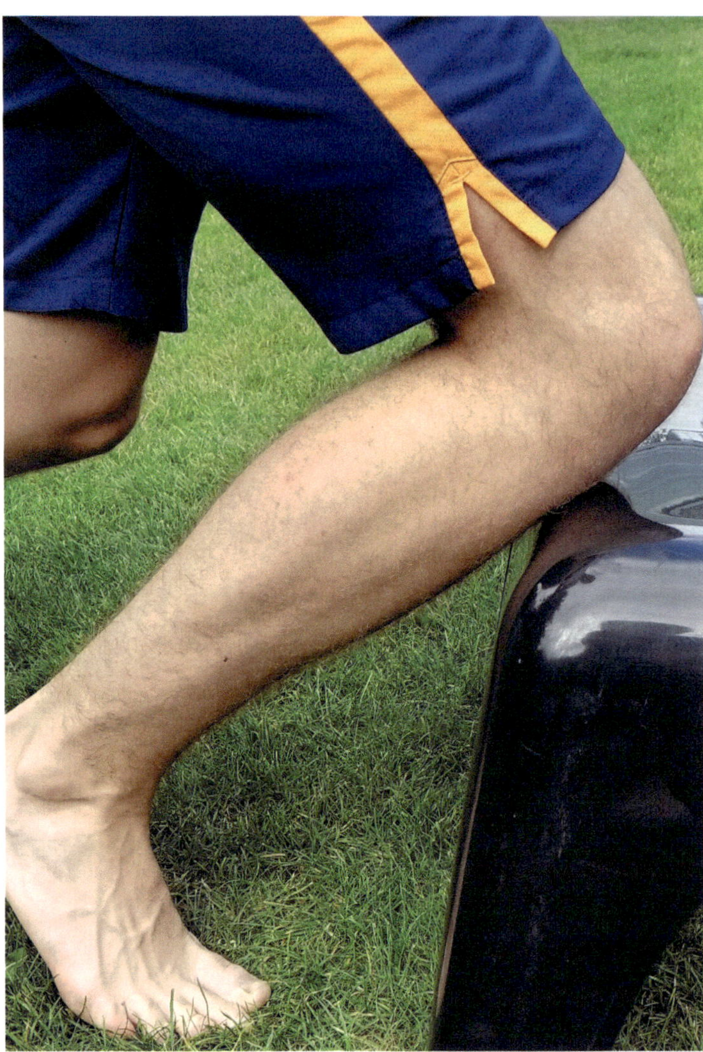

Fig. 2.3 Dashboard injury

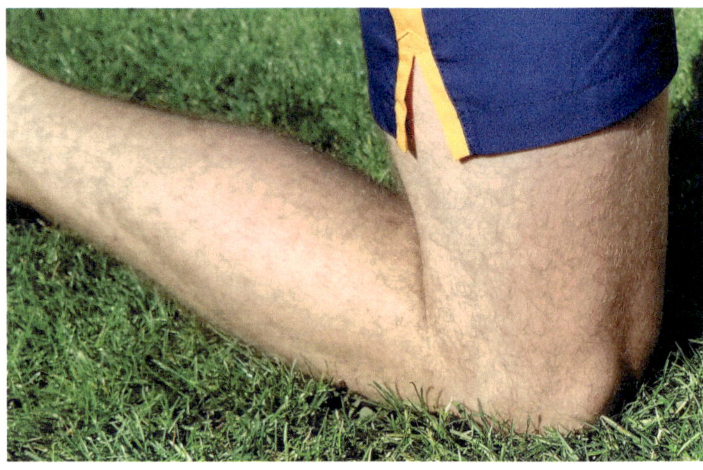

Fig. 2.4 Anterior tibial injury typical of posterior cruciate ligament injury

2.4 Lateral Collateral Ligament

1. Varus trauma in the knee is a frequent contact injury.
2. Hyperextension injuries as combination injuries of a combined varus/rotational movement in combination with injuries of the posterior cruciate ligament and the posterolateral corner [1].

References

1. Nannaparaju M, et al. Posterolateral corner injuries: epidemiology, anatomy, biomechanics and diagnosis. Injury. 2018;49(6):1024–31.
2. Pedersen RR. The medial and posteromedial ligamentous and capsular structures of the knee: review of anatomy and relevant imaging findings. Semin Musculoskelet Radiol. 2016;20(1):12–25.
3. Amis AA, Dawkins GP. Functional anatomy of the anterior cruciate ligament. Fibre bundle actions related to ligament replacements and injuries. J Bone Joint Surg Br. 1991;73(2):260–7.
4. Mehl J, et al. Evidence-based concepts for prevention of knee and ACL injuries. 2017 guidelines of the ligament committee of the German Knee Society (DKG). Arch Orthop Trauma Surg. 2018;138(1):51–61.
5. Petersen W, Zantop T. Partial rupture of the anterior cruciate ligament. Arthroscopy. 2006; 22(11):1143–5.
6. Ettlinger CF, Johnson RJ, Shealy JE. A method to help reduce the risk of serious knee sprains incurred in alpine skiing. Am J Sports Med. 1995;23(5):531–7.
7. Alentorn-Geli E, et al. Prevention of non-contact anterior cruciate ligament injuries in soccer players. Part 1: mechanisms of injury and underlying risk factors. Knee Surg Sports Traumatol Arthrosc. 2009;17(7):705–29.
8. Feucht MJ, et al. The role of the tibial slope in sustaining and treating anterior cruciate ligament injuries. Knee Surg Sports Traumatol Arthrosc. 2013;21(1):134–45.
9. Rahnemai-Azar AA, et al. Increased lateral tibial plateau slope predisposes male college football players to anterior cruciate ligament injury. J Bone Joint Surg Am. 2016;98(12):1001–6.
10. Song GY, et al. Risk factors associated with grade 3 pivot shift after acute anterior cruciate ligament injuries. Am J Sports Med. 2016;44(2):362–9.
11. Tischer T, et al. The impact of osseous malalignment and realignment procedures in knee ligament surgery: a systematic review of the clinical evidence. Orthop J Sports Med. 2017;5(3):2325967117697287.
12. Schillhammer CK, et al. Arthroscopy up to date: anterior cruciate ligament anatomy. Arthroscopy. 2016;32(1):209–12.
13. Bayer S, et al. Knee morphological risk factors for anterior cruciate ligament injury: a systematic review. J Bone Joint Surg Am. 2020;102(8):703–18.
14. Schuttler KF, et al. Posterior cruciate ligament injuries. Unfallchirurg. 2017;120(1):55–68.
15. Veltri DM, Warren RF. Anatomy, biomechanics, and physical findings in posterolateral knee instability. Clin Sports Med. 1994;13(3):599–614.

3 Diagnostics and Treatment

Individual history and clinical investigation are basic and important to working up a diagnosis. Knowledge of the medical history, the clinical examination and specific tests usually yield 90% of the diagnosis. Technical investigations are necessary to validate diagnosis and confirm the subsequent treatment.

This checklist may systematically guide diagnostics and planning of further treatment.

The most frequently used clinical symptoms and knee tests for a basic fast check-up are:

1. Ask about the history.
2. Swelling and heat and skin lesions should be checked.
3. Check range of motion and test for blockade.
4. Collateral ligaments are checked in valgus or varus stress from extension to 30–40° flexion (Fig. 3.1).
5. Spontaneous posterior drawer in 70° knee flexion (Fig. 3.2a) and use the instrumented measurement while measuring only the difference side to side. With an active posterior push on the tibia, measure the complete posterior instability side to side (Fig. 3.2b).
6. Anterior drawer in 90°, better "Lachman" Test in 20° bended knee

   Quality:

   1+ > 0–5 mm of anterior displacement—sometimes with an end point

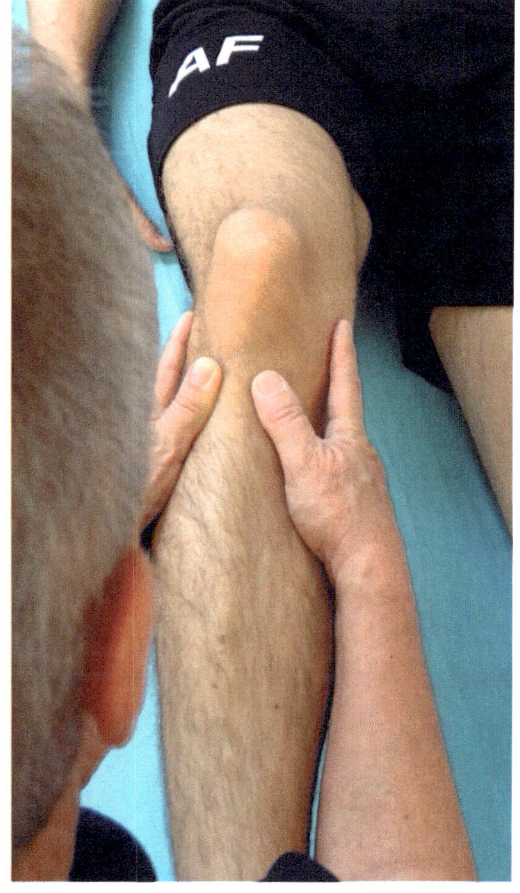

Fig. 3.1 Check the medial and lateral collateral ligaments in stress in 0° to 40° knee flexion

G. Felmet, *Press-Fit Fixation of the Knee Ligaments*, https://doi.org/10.1007/978-3-031-11906-4_3

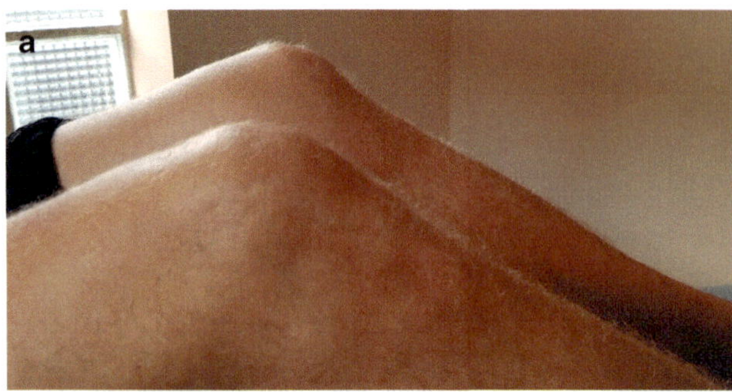

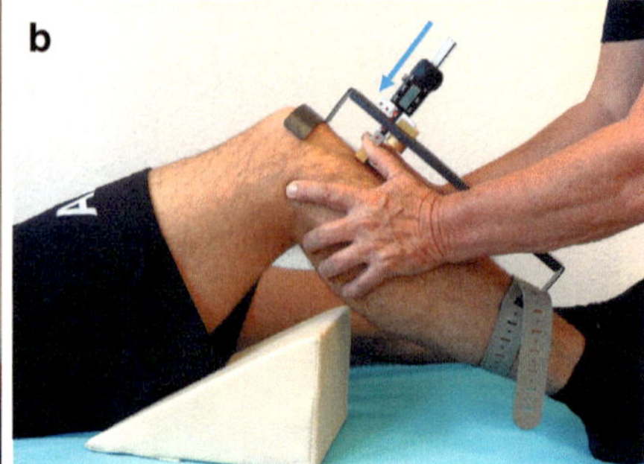

Fig. 3.2 (**a**, **b**) Spontaneous posterior instability in 70° knee flexion compared side to side (**a**). With an active push on the tibia head (blue arrow) measure the complex instability with the Articometer (Digital Rolimeter) (**b**)

2+ > 5–10 mm of anterior displacement—with no end point

3+ > 10 mm of anterior displacement—with no end point [1, 2]. (Figs. 3.3a, b and 3.4a–c). for PL bundle

7. Both transversal stability tests should be performed instrumented with for example KT 1000, Laximeter, Rolimeter, or Articometer (developed by the author) [3, 5] for greater reproducibility, reliability, and ease in documentation.
8. The pivot shift [6]. Depending on the experience of the examiner, but helpful for the extent of instability (Fig. 3.5)—following this subluxation [7, 8] also use the jerk test, Lemaire test, Slocum test, Losee test.
9. Anterolateral and anteromedial instability: outward/inward rotation, 90° knee flexion, fixed foot.
10. The status of muscles (well trained, little or not).
11. Coordination and spontaneous reflective reaction of the vastus medialis of the quadriceps muscle [9, 10] (Fig. 3.6a, b).
12. Spontaneous reflective reaction of the ischiocrural muscles [12, 13] (Fig. 3.7a–d).
13. Meniscus symptoms in typical stress tests (e.g., Steinman I+II, McMurray [14]) (Fig. 3.8a, b)
14. Circulation and neurology are to be checked.
    - History of pre-existing conditions and injuries, malalignments, pre-surgeries; follow-up of the present symptoms (e.g., mechanism or trauma); treatment to date.

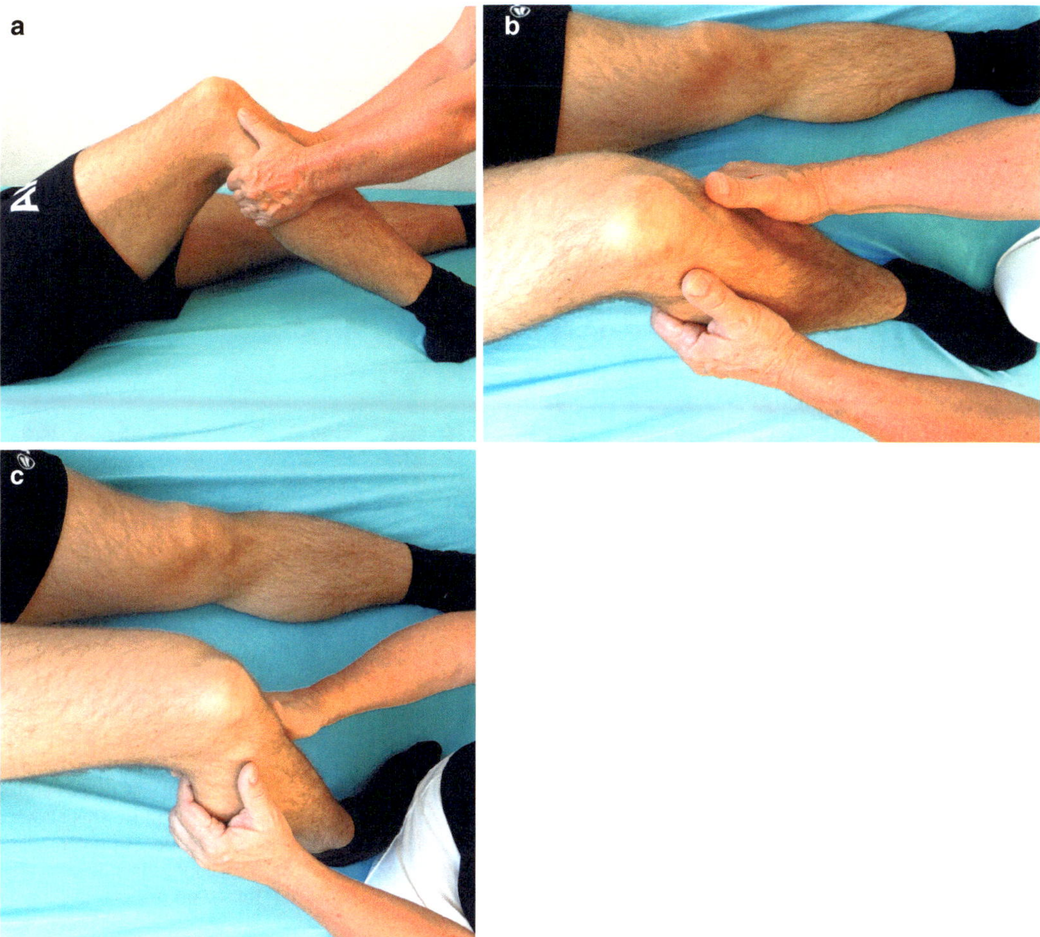

Fig. 3.3 (**a**–**c**) Anterior drawer in 90° knee flexion, pull tibia head to the front (**a**). For anteromedial instability rotate foot outward (**b**) and for anterolateral instability rotate foot inward (**c**)

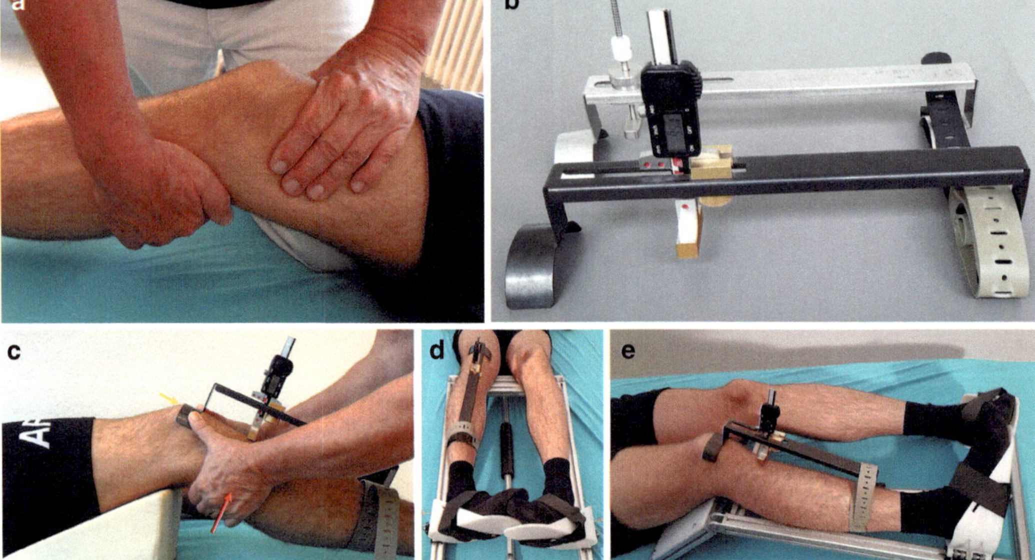

Fig. 3.4 (**a**) Lachman test in 20° knee flexion without instruments [2]. Place the patient's thigh on your thigh and pull the tibial plateau forward. With anterior cruciate ligament deficiency, there is no hard stop combined with greater joint play. (**b**) Instrumented transversal measurement of the knee with the Rolimeter [3] (background) and the digital Articometer [4, 5] (front). (**c**) Lachman test in 20° knee flexion with ArticoMeter and a pillow/soft wedge under the thigh. Set the meter to zero and fix the frame over the patella with both thumbs (yellow arrow). Distally fix it with the elastic band. Push or pull with fingers of both hands the posterior tibia head to the front (red arrow) [5]. Find the maximum distance and difference side to side. A 3-mm difference or more is pathological. (**d, e**) The Artico-Rotameter rotate both feet inward with a defined dynamic stress, knee flexed in 20° Lachman position. The Articometer measures the anterior stability to address the anterior cruciate ligament (ACL) posterolateral bundle and the anterolateral instability. This allows a reliable standard in Lachman position. An anterolateral stability/instability can be checked side to side, e.g., after ACL reconstruction and follow-up for an anatomical function

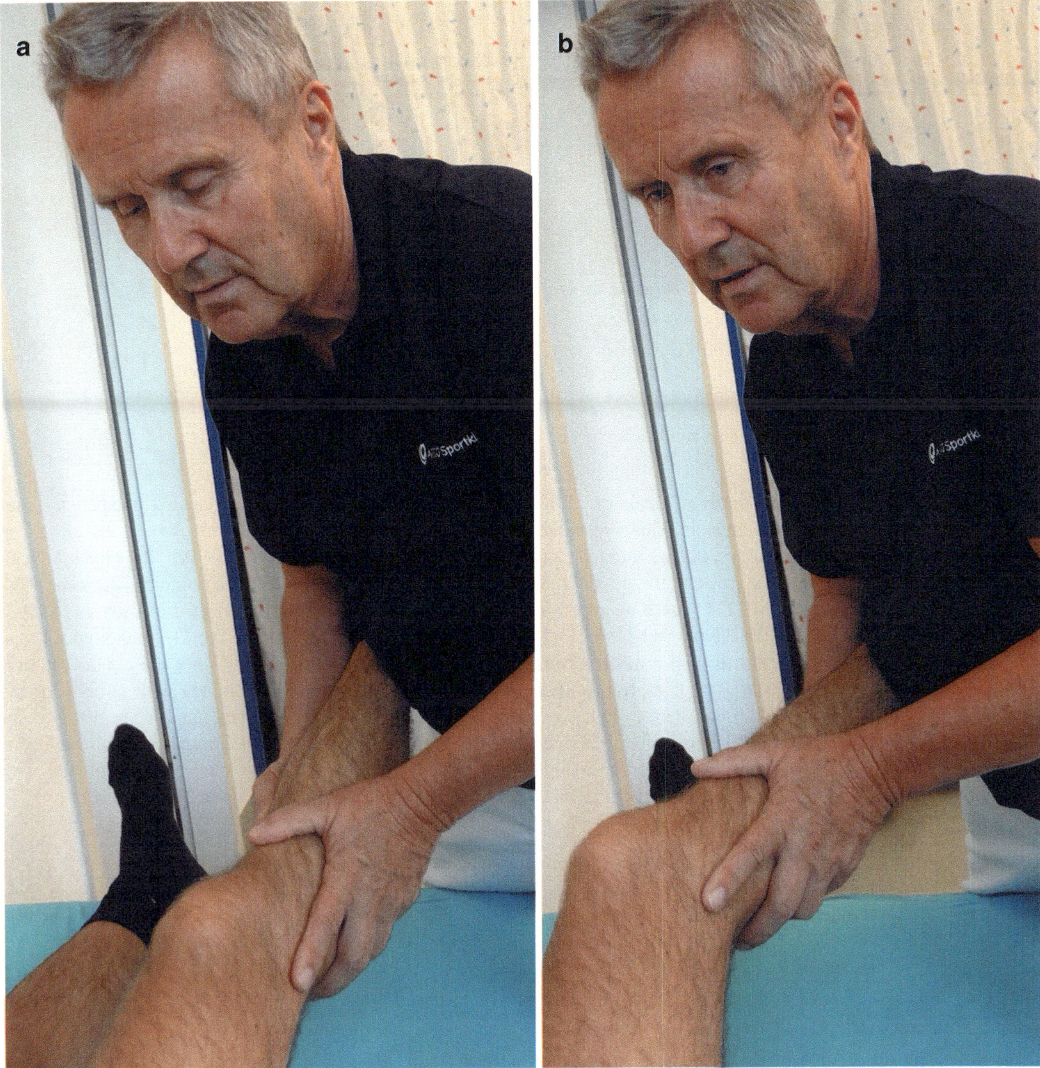

Fig. 3.5 (**a**, **b**) Pivot shift: relaxed knee in extension (**a**). With slight stress into a valgus and flex it (**b**). In deficient anterior cruciate ligament the convex tibia will roll and rotate under the convex femoral condyle

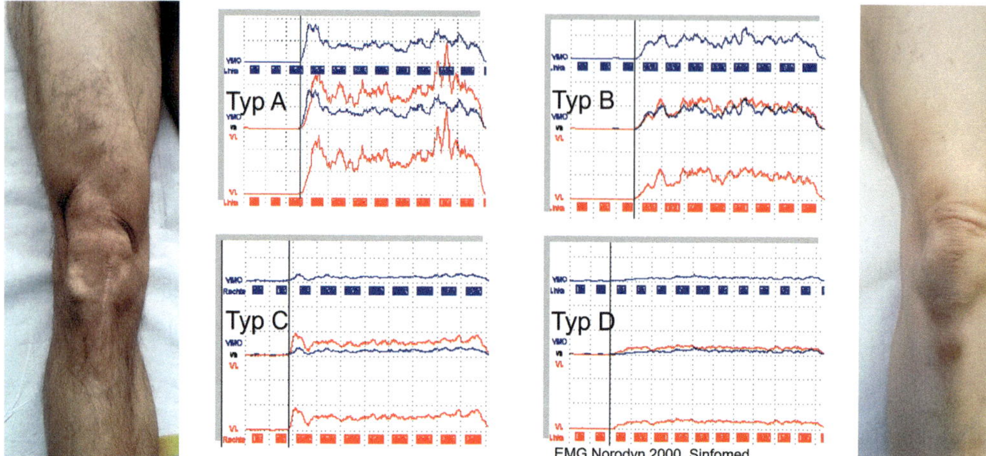

Fig. 3.6 Spontaneous reflective "tense-up" reaction of the vastus medialis of the quadriceps muscle. The electromyography (EMG) describes the reaction of the vastus medialis (blue line) on the time axis parallel to the oblique quadriceps muscle (red line) (**b**) [11]. Tense-up reaction describes four types, two pathological and two physiological patterns. Typ A is to be found in well-trained performance, typ B in regular function. Typ C is found after trauma, surgery, and insufficient training status, often combined with anterior knee pain. Typ D is to be found in neurophysiological deficiency and atrophy of the quadriceps muscle. The typs can be visualized on EMG (**b**), but it is much easier looking at the quadriceps spontaneous tense-up (**a**): Typ A—physiological: vastus medialis tenses up first; oblique quadriceps second. Typ B—physiological: vastus medialis tenses up with the oblique quadriceps muscle. Typ C—pathological: vastus medialis tenses up after the oblique quadriceps muscle. Typ D—pathological: vastus medialis does not tense up—only the oblique quadriceps muscle does; mostly combined with atrophy of the muscles. Left side, a well-trained quadriceps mostly combined with Typ A or B. Right side, atrophy of the vastus medialis in an untrained individual often combined with Typ C, sometimes with no reaction: Typ D

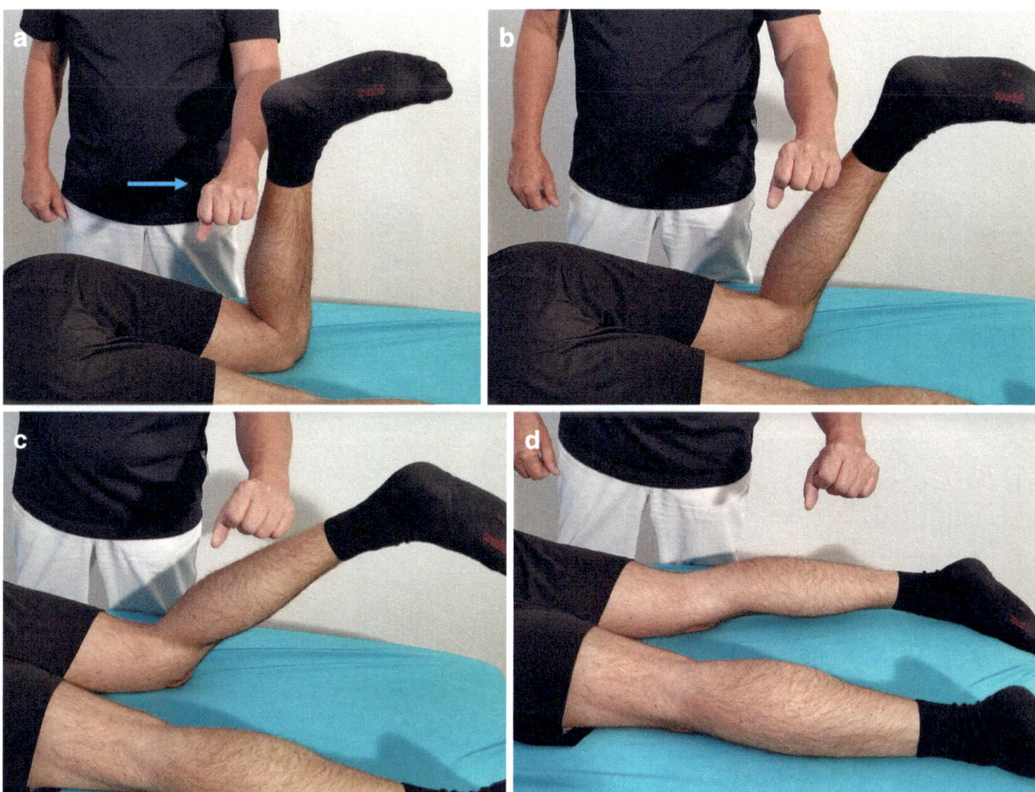

Fig. 3.7 (**a**–**d**) Spontaneous reflective "tense-up" reaction of the ischiocrural muscles lying on the front (**a**). The knee is flexed 90° and the muscles are relaxed (in some patients a handicap). Push the lower leg with a quick and strong hit on the Achilles tendon (blue arrow) to the ground (**a**). Tense-up—reaction describes four types, two pathological and two physiological patterns. Type A is to be found in well-trained performance, Type B in regular function. Types A and B are also positive criteria for returning to play and competition (**a**, **b**). Type C is found after trauma, surgery, and insufficient training status, often combined with anterior cruciate ligament rupture or re-rupture (**c**). Type D is to be found in neurophysiological deficiency and atrophy of the ischiocrural muscle (**d**). The types can be visualized on EMG but it is much easier looking at the ischiocrural spontaneous tense-up (**a**): Type A—physiological—ischiocrural muscles tense-up quickly; the lower leg is not stretched and does not touch the ground (**a**). Type B—physiological—ischiocrural muscles tense up not so quickly—the lower leg is stretched a little and does not touch the ground (**b**). Type C—pathological—ischiocrural muscles tense up later; the lower leg is stretched more but does not touch the ground (**c**). Type D—pathological—ischiocrural muscles do not tense up; the lower leg is stretched completely and touches the ground (**d**)

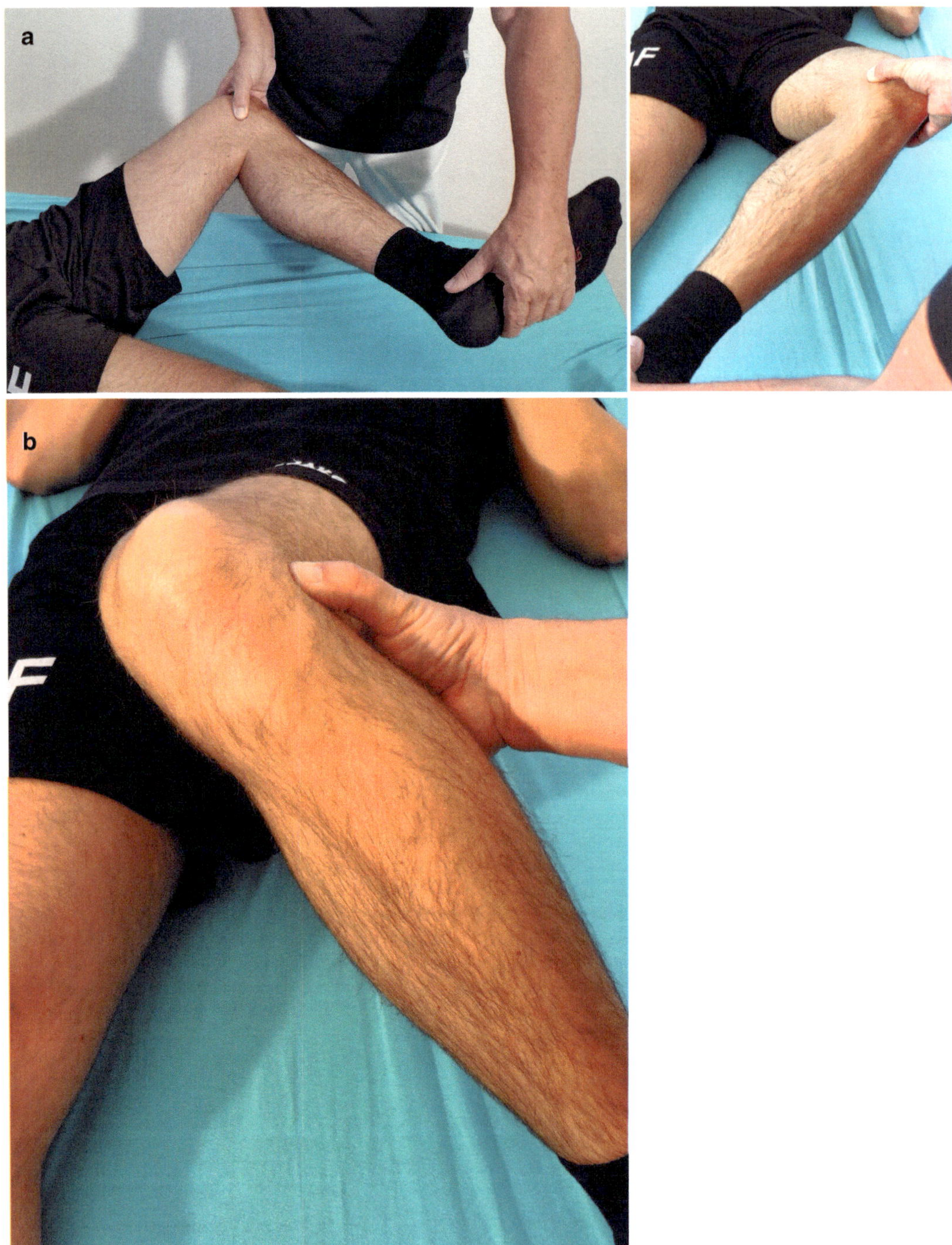

Fig. 3.8 (**a**, **b**) Meniscus symptoms in varus stress, flexion, and rotation of medial meniscus (**a**). In valgus stress, flexion, and rotation of the lateral meniscus (**b**). A combination of Steinmann I+II and McMurray (British surgeon Thomas Porter McMurray (1887–1949) tests [14, 15]

3.1 Anterior Cruciate Ligament

1. Diagnostic:
   (a) Clinical palpation:
   - Examination of the soft tissues (temperature, swelling, skin/superficial/ deep lesion, effusion, and formation)
   - Examination for meniscus signs (medial and lateral meniscus)
   - Active and passive examination with range of motion (extension/flexion/ rotation)
   - Stability tests of the capsule and ligaments (LCL, MCL, patella function)
   - Anterior drawer, Lachman test, pivot shift test, (> ACL)
   - Spontaneous posterior drawer at approximately 70° knee flexion (> PCL)

   (b) Clinical and instrumented stability test
   - Test the stability of ligament structures (PCL, ACL + collateral ligaments, capsule):
   - Examination of anterior tibial translation and ligament attachment in 20–30° flexion (Lachman test)
   - Pivot shift test (subluxation test)
   - Instrumental measurement of anterior tibial translation in side comparison with, for example, the Rolimeter, the Articometer (digital Rolimeter), KT 1000
   - Radiological: stress recording with the Scheuba device (Telos)
   - Varus and valgus stress, anterior/posterior drawer test in 20 and 90° flexion (see below)

   (c) Radiological
   - X-ray examination of the knee joint in two planes with regard to possibly bony distal and proximal tears of the anterior cruciate ligament and other structures
   - Representation of the tunnel position and width including foreign material from the pre-surgery (Fig. 3.9)
   - Radiological: stress recording with the Scheuba device (Telos) anterior/posterior drawer test in 20 and 90° flexion (Fig. 3.10a, b) and varus and valgus stress (Fig. 3.10c, d)

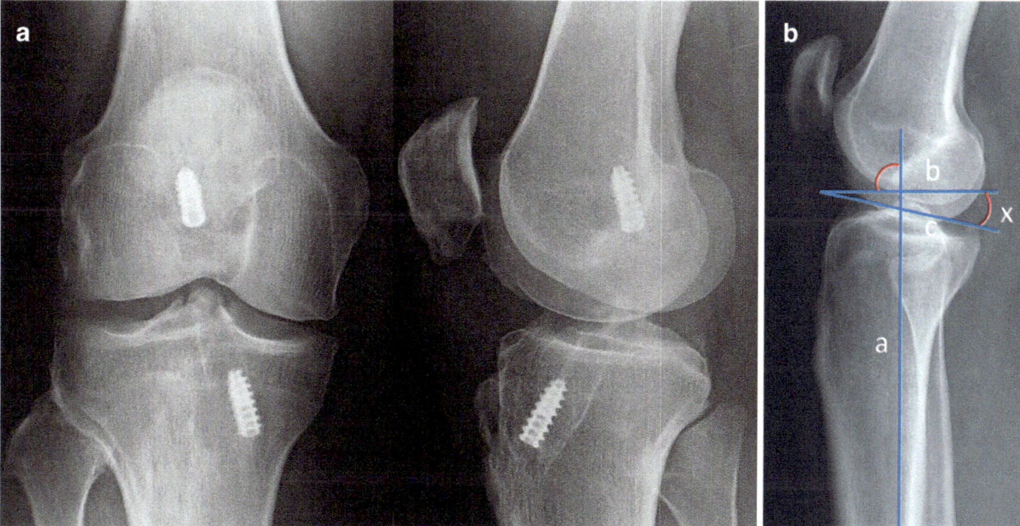

Fig. 3.9 (**a**) Plain X-ray with metal interference screws in high noon position at the femoral side and deep inside the tibial head (in the tibia difficult to remove). Tunnel a little widened. Patella centrally positioned as well as in the trochlear groove. (**b**) The tibial posterior slope of more than 12° has to be considered with a high incidence of anterior cruciate ligament rupture and re-rupture. Plain X-ray in standing [16–19]

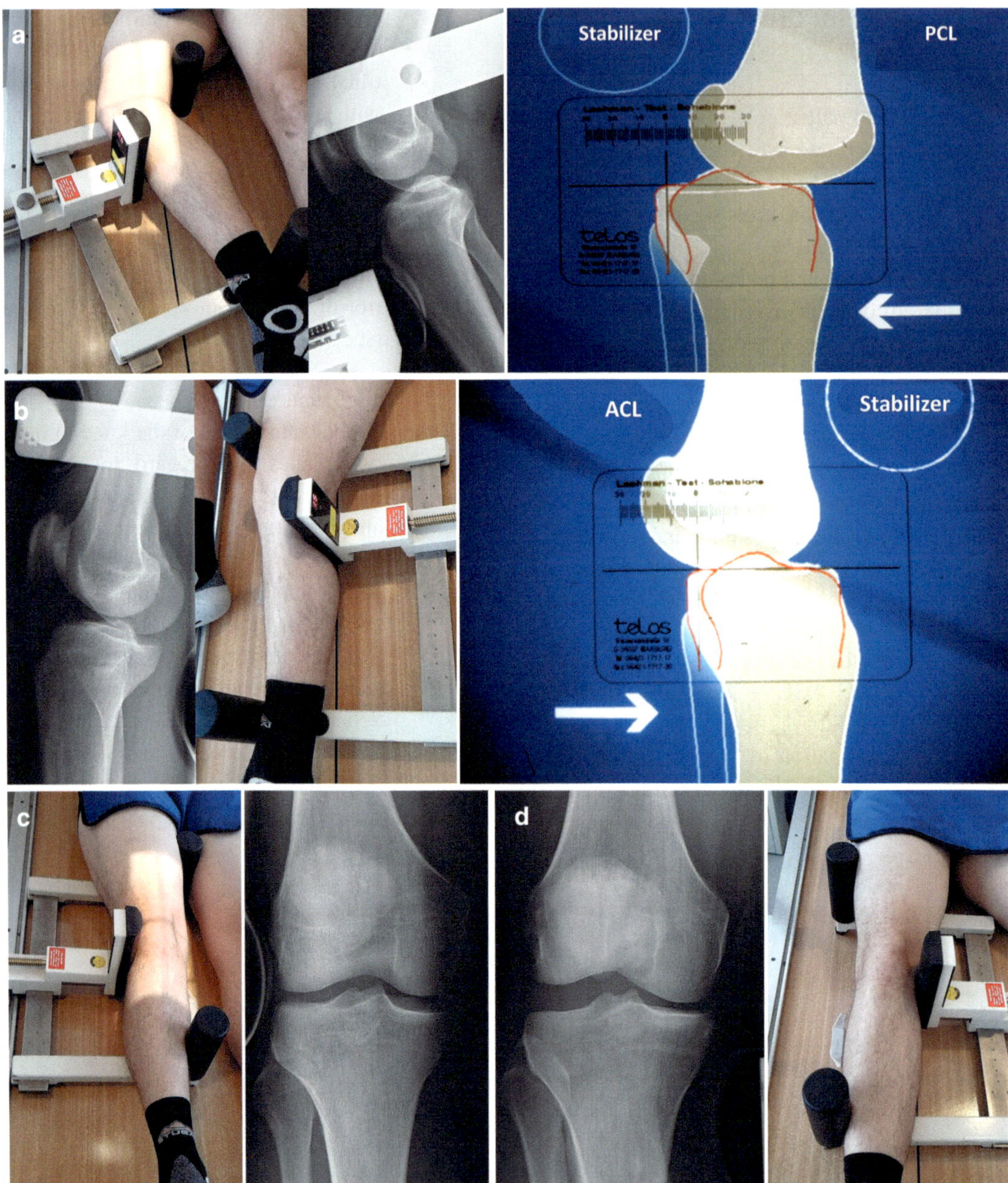

Fig. 3.10 (**a**) Posterior cruciate ligament (PCL)—check: posterior drawer in approximately 70° knee flexion with a Scheuba device with 15 kp stress [20], here with no instability. Use for very early investigations after trauma or for long-term controls. Caveat: not to be used in the early period of conservative treatment. (**a1**) Telos template to measure the posterior transversal drawer. (**b**) Anterior cruciate ligament (ACL)—check: anterior or posterior drawer in approximately 20° knee flexion (Lachman position) with Scheuba device with 15 kp stress [21, 22], here with anterior instability. Use very early after trauma or for long-term controls. Caveat: not to be used in the early period of conservative treatment. (**b1**) Telos template to measure the anterior transversal drawer. (**c**) MCL—check: valgus stress with Scheuba device with 15 kp stress [21, 22], here with no significant instability. Use very early after trauma or for long-term controls. Caveat: not to be used in the early period of conservative treatment. (**d**) Lateral collateral ligament – check: valgus stress with Scheuba device with 15 kp stress, here with significant instability [21, 22]. Use very early after trauma or for long-term controls. Caveat: not to be used in the early period of conservative treatment

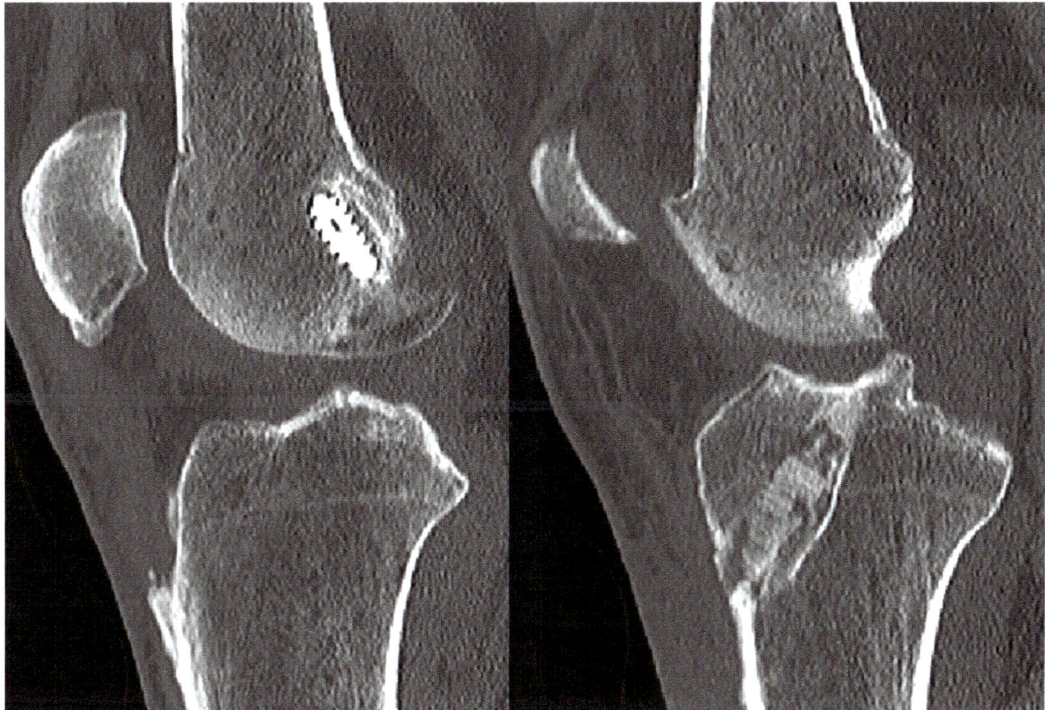

Fig. 3.11 Computed tomography with implants in both tunnels

- MRI (magnetic resonance imaging) scans for imaging bone and soft tissue, e.g., ligaments, capsule, menisci, cartilage, effusion, bone bruise, etc.
- CT (computed tomography), 3D reconstruction possible for detection of fractures, tunnels, foreign material (Figs. 3.11, 3.12, 3.13)
- DVT (digital computed tomography) is a multislice computed tomography (MSCT) device and two cone beam computed tomography (CBCT) similar to CT with another technique and standard higher resolution (0.2-mm slices), possible under weightbearing and 3D imaging with less radiation [23–26] (Figs. 3.14, 3.15, and 3.16)
- pQCT (peripheral quantitative computed tomography) for detection of local bone loss and osteoporotic disease [27] (Fig. 3.17)

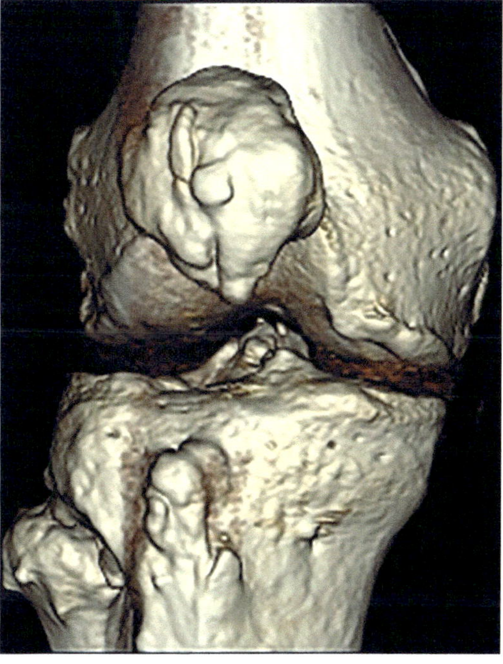

Fig. 3.12 Computed tomography in 3D—reconstruction

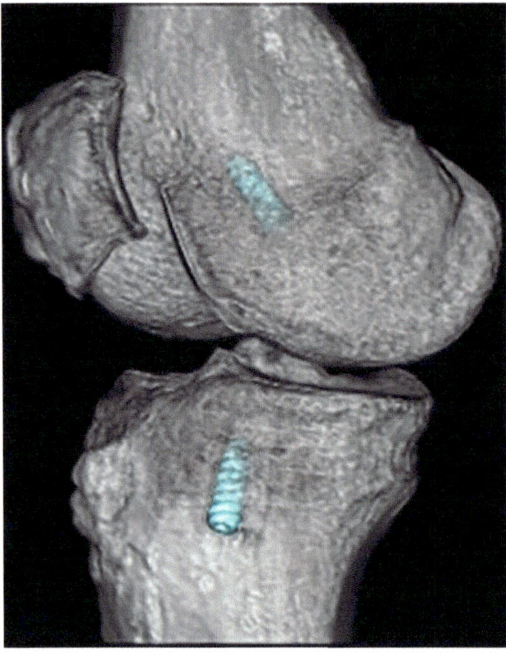

Fig. 3.13 Computed tomography in 3D—reconstruction and filtered layers to show implants

(d) Further diagnostics
- Blood chemistry
- Possibly bone scintigraphy

2. Indication for conservative or surgical therapy

(a) Conservative
- Old age of patient in combination with low physical activity and ambition
- Low instability (Lachman grade A (0–2.9 mm difference side to side)
- Negative pivot shift test

(b) Surgery
- Involvement of meniscus injury, save the meniscus with suture
- Complex instability (e.g., unhappy triad)
- Instability in Lachman grades B and C
- High sporting activity and ambition
- Young age of patients
- Subjective instability (giving-way phenomenon)

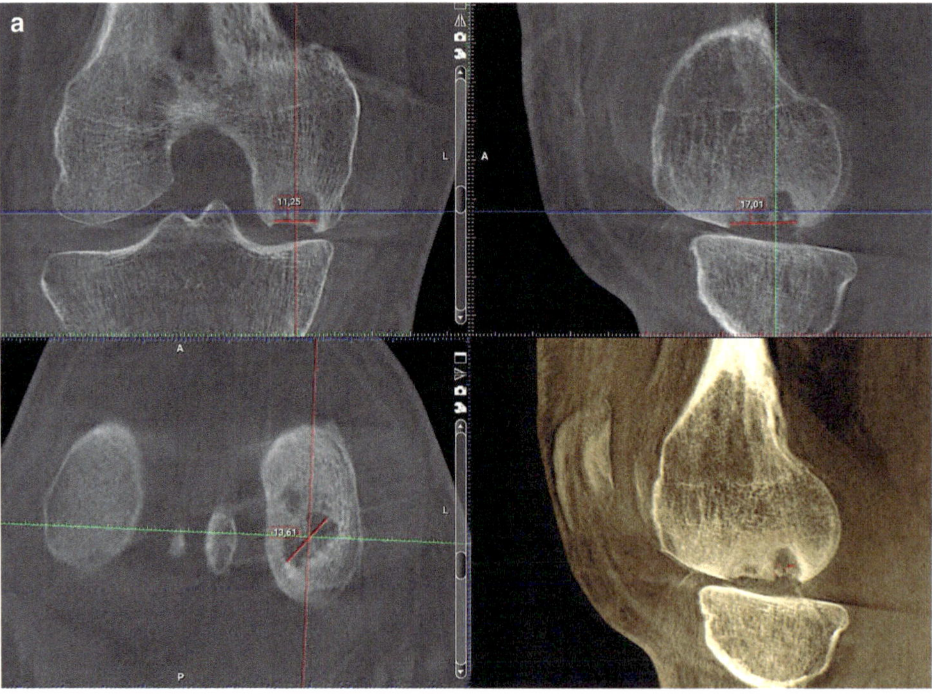

Fig. 3.14 (**a**) Deep osteochondral lesion at the medial femoral condyle with: digital volume tomography (DVT) standing and weightbearing in plain and 3D reconstruction in deeper layers (slices 0.2 mm)—a multislice computed tomography device and two cone beam computed tomography [23–26]. (**b**) DVT allows investigation in standing upright and weightbearing positions pf the knee with a high resolution of 0.2-mm scans for each slice and 3D reconstruction in less than 30 s

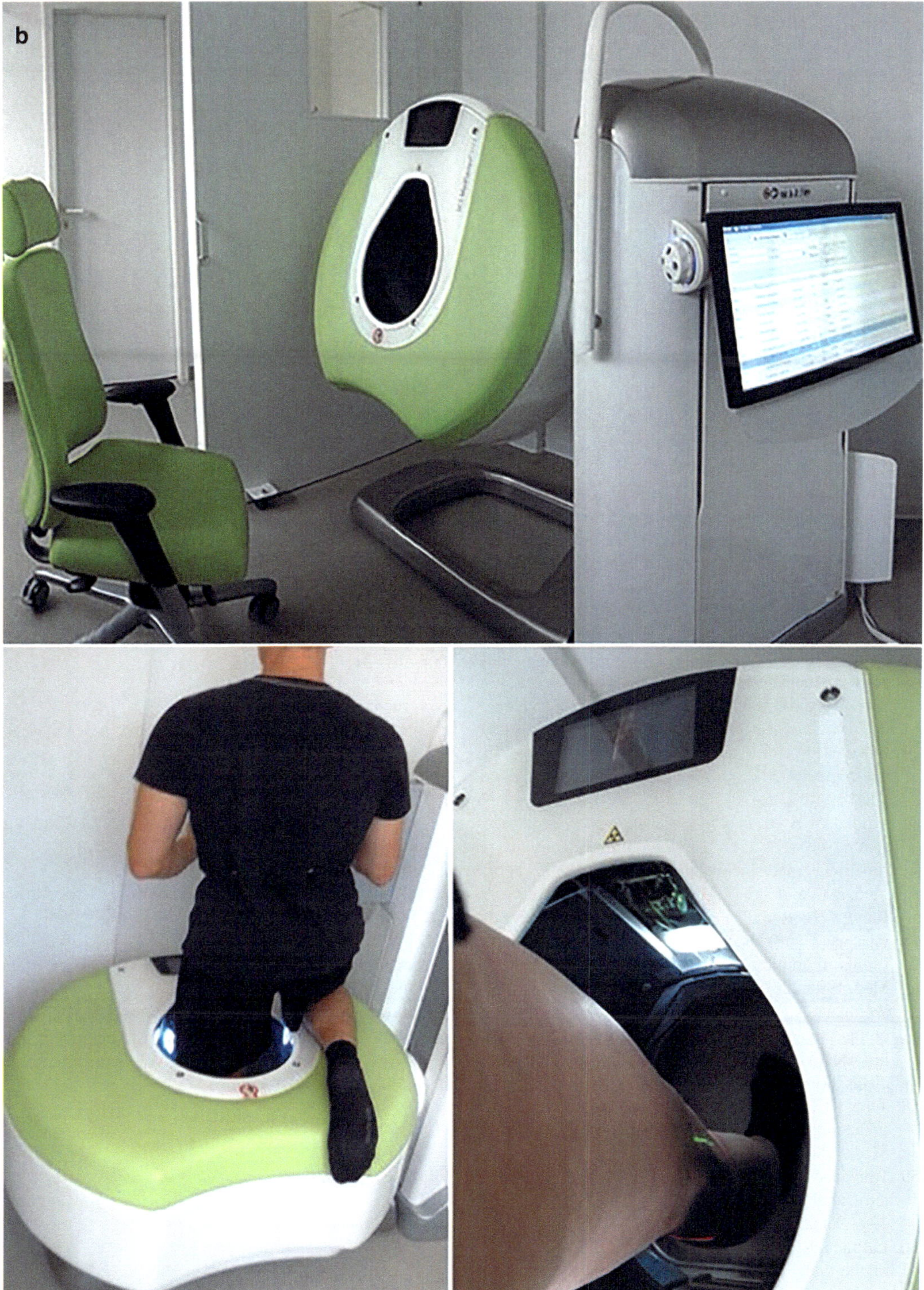

Fig. 3.14 (continued)

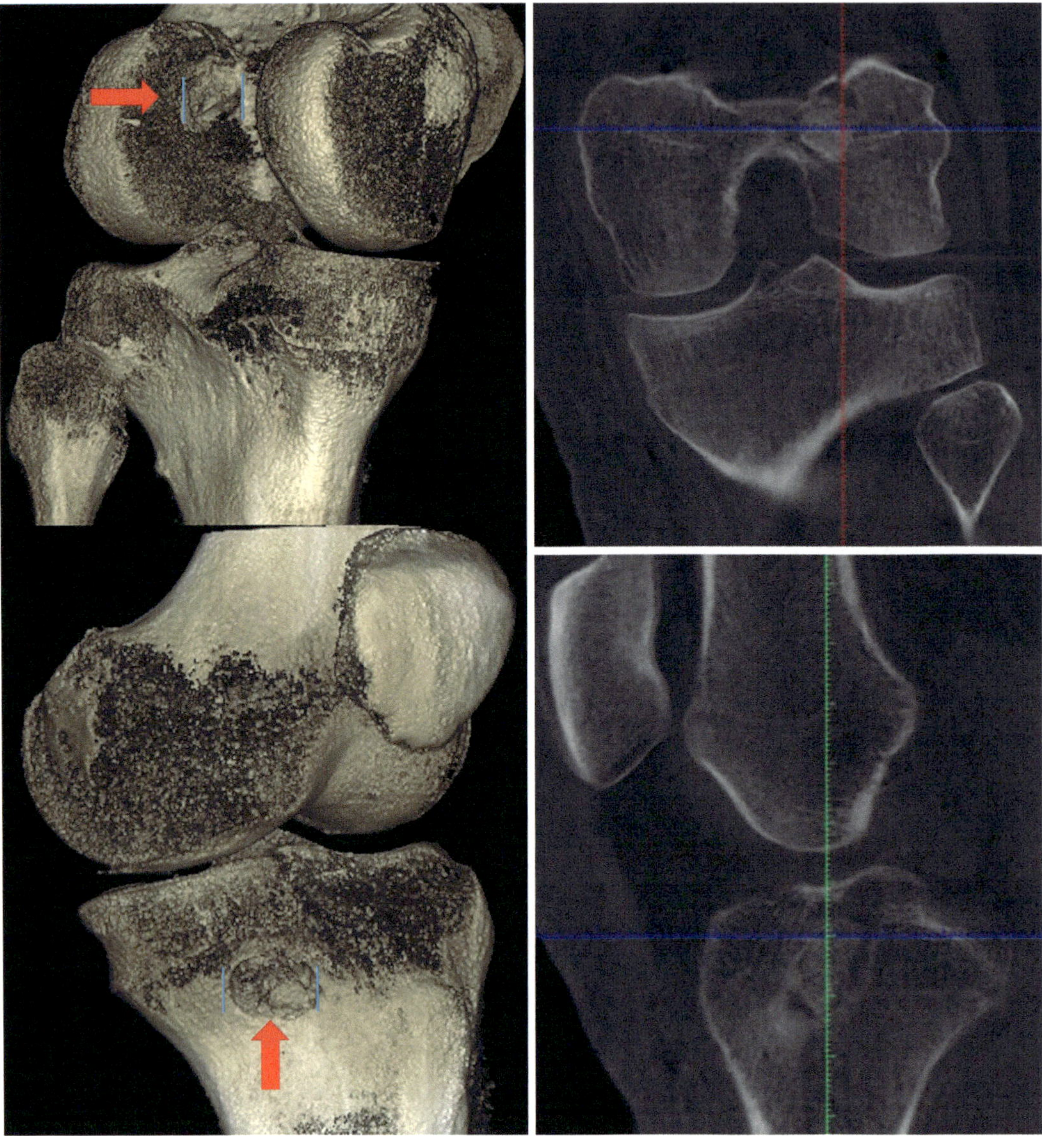

Fig. 3.15 Press-fit anterior cruciate ligament reconstruction with bone dowels. No tunnel enlargement and closed tibial and femoral tunnel. Red arrows show the closed tunnels by bone cylinders: digital volume tomography standing and weightbearing in plain and 3D reconstruction in deeper layers (slices 0.2 mm)

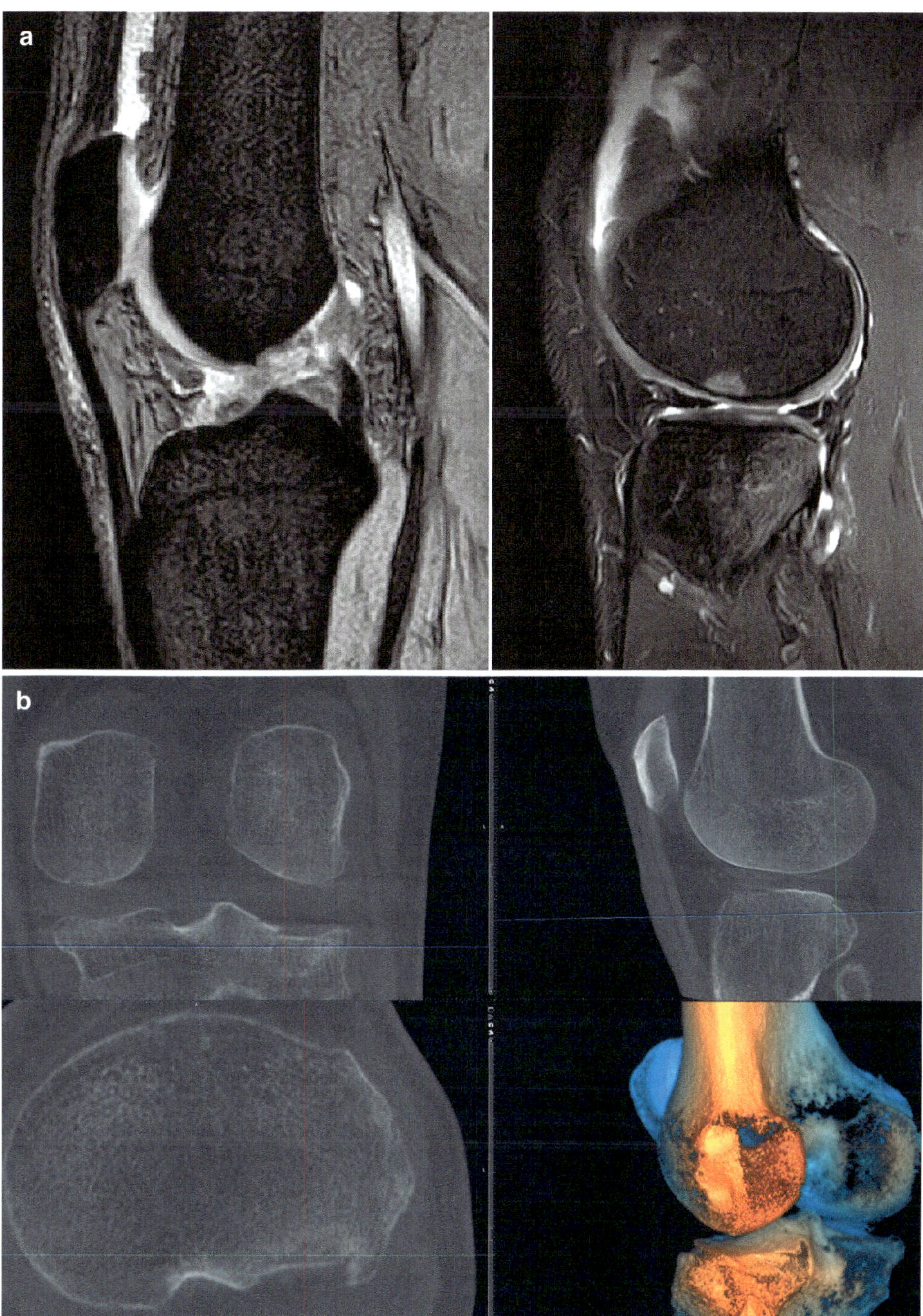

Fig. 3.16 (**a**) Magnetic resonance imaging after a typical anterior cruciate ligament (ACL) trauma: without signal for the ACL, little effusion (**a**). Focal bone bruise at the lateral femoral condyle and focal cartilage lesions (**b**). Typical combined bone bruise at the posterior tibial head for Segond lesion. (**b**) Digital volume tomography (DVT) after Segond lesion and fracture with impression of 2.26 mm at the posterior lateral tibia in combination with ACL rupture: DVT, a multislice computed tomography device, and two cone beam computed tomography [23–26] standing and weightbearing in plain and 3D reconstruction in deeper layers (slices 0.2 mm) [23–26]. (**c**) The tibial posterior slope of more than 12° has to be considered of high incidence of ACL rupture and re-rupture. 3D DVT in standing [16–19]

Fig. 3.16 (continued)

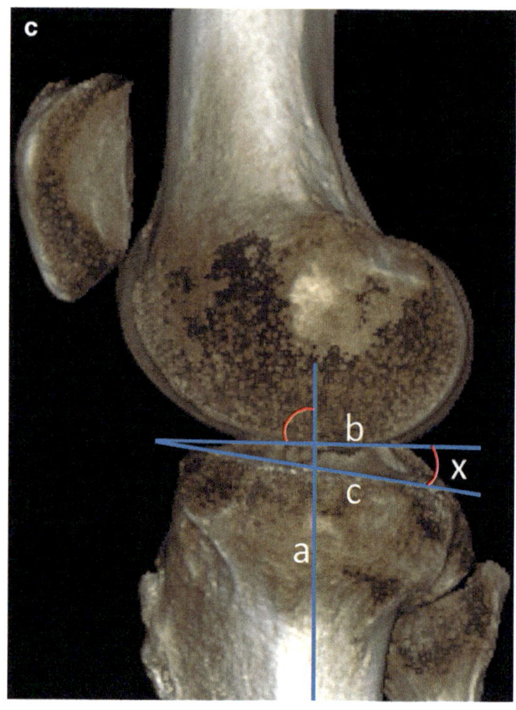

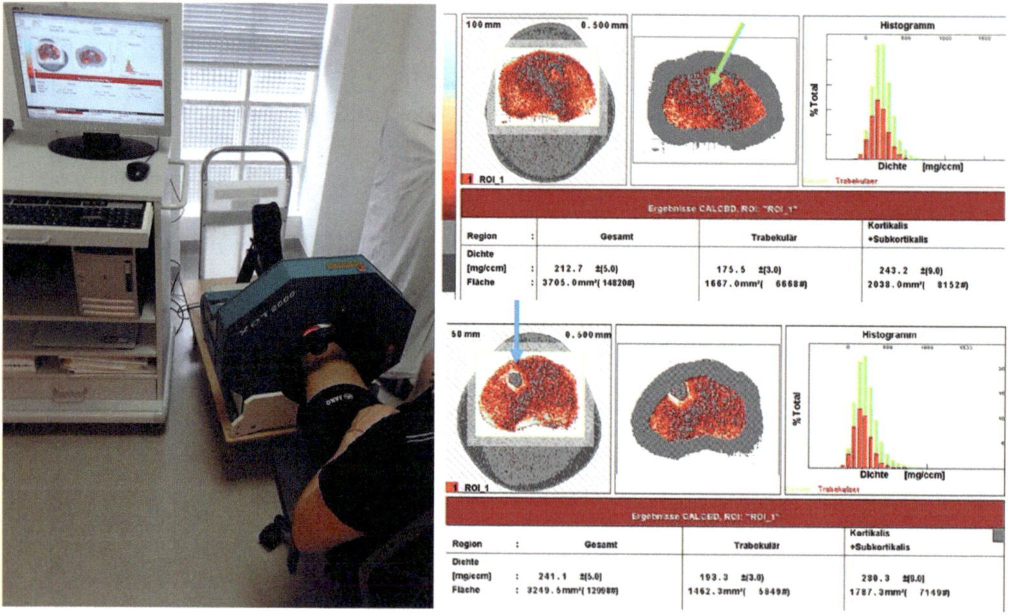

Fig. 3.17 pQCT (peripheral Quantitative Computed Tomography) measurements with low radiation show the loss of mineralization after anterior cruciate ligament rupture in the tibial head (green arrow) and shows the integration and mineralization after all press-fit fixation (orange arrow) [27]

- Indication for ACL reconstruction
  Intraligamentary or distal tears
  Period between trauma and Arthroscopy in isolated rupture within the first 6 weeks in young patients and foreign material-free pre-surgery to enable healing response and meniscus suture
  For complex capsular ligament injury, if necessary >6 weeks
- Indication for ACL preservation and healing response
  Ultra-femoral proximal rupture
  Well-preserved distal cruciate ligament stump
  Period between trauma and arthroscopy <6 weeks

3. Revision surgery
   (a) Rerupture
   Diagnostics
   - Diagnostic of anterior cruciate ligament rupture analogous to the primary rupture
   - Checking the sufficiency of the ACL replacement as described above
   - Taking into account the postoperative period, properties of the graft (e.g., hamstrings, patella or quadriceps tendon)
   - X-ray clarification: location (correct, a little wrong, completely wrong) and width of the tunnels
   - Increased tibial posterior slope [16–19] and anatomical variations
   - If necessary CT/DVT is a MSCT device and CBCT similar to CT with another technique and standard higher resolution (0.2-mm slices), possible under weightbearing and 3D imaging with less radiation [23–26]

   (b) Indication
   - Revision in the correct position of the tunnels with instability and/or comorbidity of the knee
   - Revision of a replacement without foreign material and no tunnel enlargement
     - Single-step surgery might be possible, e.g., with oversized bone dowels and press-fit fixation on both sides
   - Revision of a replacement with foreign material and no tunnel enlargement
   - If necessary remove the foreign material, e.g., metal screws
     - Single-step surgery might still be possible, e.g., oversized bone dowel and press-fit fixation on both sides
   - Alternatively the use of a completely different tunnel, as described under "Revision" and cross the new tunnel in the anatomical position inside the knee
   - In case of an incorrect position or extremely enlarged previous tunnels a two-stage revision is recommended. Restore the bone stock with autologous (or homologous) spongiosa chips for a second-stage surgery about 3–5 months later.

3.2 Posterior Cruciate Ligament

1. Diagnostics
   (a) Clinical investigation
   - Examination of the soft tissue as above
   - Examination of meniscal pathology (medial and lateral meniscus)
   - Active and passive examination of extension/flexion
   - Capsule and complete ligament stability
   - Spontaneous posterior drawer in about 70° knee flexion

   (b) Stability measurement
   - Instrumental measurement of posterior tibial translation (PTT) side to side (Rolimeter/Digital Articometer)
   - Reversed pivot shift test (subluxation test)

   (c) Radiological
   - X-ray examination of the knee joint in two planes for fractures or malalignment

- Collateral ligaments in varus/valgus stress
- Posterior drawer stress with the Scheuba device (Telos).
- MRI scan for imaging bone and soft tissue, e.g., ligaments, capsule, menisci, cartilage, effusion, bone bruise, etc.
- CT (3D) fractures, tunnels, foreign material
- DVT is an MSCT device and CBCT similar to CT with another technique and standard higher resolution (0.2-mm slices), possible under weightbearing and 3D imaging with less radiation [23–26].
- pQCT for detection of local bone loss and osteoporotic disease [27]

(d) Further diagnostics
- Blood chemistry
- Possibly bone scintigraphy

2. Indication for conservative or surgical therapy

(a) Conservatively
- Fresh lesions with slight instability (grades A = <5 mm and B = <9 mm difference side to side posterior tibial translation
- Fixed posterior drawer
- Active PCL brace (PCL JACK, Albrecht) for 12 weeks

(b) Surgery to be discussed
- Medium- and high-grade instability (grades B and C >10 mm difference side to side posterior tibial translation and
- Combined instability
- Subjective instability
- Higher level of activity
  - If indicated for surgical treatment of the PCL (>analogous ACL procedure)
    Intraligamentary or distal tears
    Period between trauma and surgery >6 weeks
  - Healing response (not analog ACL)
    Also intermediate rupture
    Existing cruciate ligament stump
    Period between trauma and arthroscopy <6 weeks

3. PCL revision

(a) PCL insufficiency or rerupture
- Check-up of PCL insufficiency analogous to primary rupture
  - Checking the instability as described above for PCL. Keep in mind early laxity postoperatively, properties of the graft (hamstrings vs. quadriceps tendon)
  - X-ray location and width of the tunnels
- Indication (analogous to ACL revision)
  - Indication for revision is dependent on the tunnels
  - Revision after initial treatment without foreign material, no tunnel enlargement, correct tunnels, and good bone stock, a single-stage surgery analogous to the primary technique, possibly oversized bone dowels for press-fit fixation on both sides
  - Remove foreign material if possible
  - In case of enlarged and wrongly positioned tunnels a two-stage revision is recommended. Restore the bone stock with autologous (or homologous) spongiosa chips for a second-stage surgery.

3.3 Collateral Ligaments (Medial and Lateral)

1. Medial collateral ligament (MCL)

(a) Diagnostics
- Clinical palpation
  - Examination of the soft tissues as above
  - Examination for meniscal symptoms (medial and lateral meniscus)

- Active and passive examination of range of movement (extension/flexion)
- Clinical stability test
  - Check the stability of the MCL by valgus stress in extension, 0°, 20–30° knee flexion or more
  - Test the stability of all ligament structures of the knee joint (ACL, PCL, LCL)
- Radiographically
  - X-ray examination of the knee in two planes for fractures or malalignment
  - Collateral ligaments in varus/valgus stress side to side
  - MRI scan

(b) Indication for conservative or surgical therapy
- Conservative
  - Stretching, partial rupture, and complete proximal rupture with protection against valgus stress (brace)
  - No bony tears
- Surgery
  - Bony lesions distal and proximal
  - Multiligamentary combination injuries
  - Functionally relevant chronic instabilities
  - Distal (tibia side) rupture

2. Lateral collateral ligament

(a) Diagnostics
- Clinical palpation
  - Examination of the soft tissues as above
  - Examination for meniscal symptoms (medial and lateral meniscus)
  - Active and passive range of motion extension/flexion of the knee
- Clinical stability test
  - Testing the stability of the LCL in varus stress in 0° extension and 20–30° flexion or more
  - Test the stability of the other ligament structures of the knee joint (ACL, PCL, MCL)
- Radiographically
  - X-ray examination of the knee joint in two planes for fractures or malalignment
  - Collateral ligaments in varus/valgus stress side to side
  - MRI scan

(b) Indication for conservative or surgical therapy
- Incomplete lesion and no instability than conservatively
- Complete rupture usually by surgery and reconstruction

Imaging procedures:

Plain X-ray (Fig. 3.9a, b)

- Standard in most trauma
- If possible under body weightbearing
  - Check for fractures
  - Malalignment
  - Degenerative signs: reduced joint gap, osteophytes
  - Translucency (reduced calcification)
  - Loose body
  - Foreign material (Fig. 3.9a)
  - Implants/loosening
  - Ligament reconstructions
  - Tunnel position
  - Tunnel enlargement
  - Posterior slope measurement (Fig. 3.9b)
  - Ligament stability/instability stress function (Scheuba device, Telos) [21, 22]

CT (Figs. 3.11, 3.12, and 3.13)

- Check for fractures
- Malalignment
- Degenerative signs: reduced joint gap, osteophytes
- Translucency (reduced calcification)
- Loose bodies
- Foreign material
- Implants/loosening
- Ligament reconstructions
- Tunnel position
- Tunnel enlargement

DVT is a MSCT device and CBCT similar to CT with another technique and standard higher resolution (0.2-mm slices), possible under weightbearing and 3D imaging with less radiation [23–26] (Figs. 3.14, 3.15, and 3.16).

- Higher resolution, 0.2-mm slices
- 70% less radiation
- Possibly upright under body weightbearing
  - Check for fractures (Fig. 3.16a, b)
  - Malalignment
  - Posterior slope (Fig. 3.16c)
  - Degenerative signs: reduced joint gap, osteophytes
  - Translucency (reduced calcification)
  - Loose or free bodies
  - Foreign material (Figs. 3.14 and 3.15a, b)
  - Implants/loosening
  - Ligament reconstructions
  - Tunnel position (Figs. 3.14 and 3.15a, b)
  - Tunnel enlargement

MRI

MRT (Magnetic Resonance Tomography) (Fig. 3.16)

- Different contrasts and echo weighting for fatty (T1) or water (T2) are used to investigate bone, bone bruise, effusion, cysts, soft tissue, cartilage, ligaments, etc.
- Check for fractures
- Malalignment
- Degenerative signs: reduced joint gap, osteophytes, bone bruise
- Loose or free bodies
- Foreign material (magnetic artifacts)
- Ligament reconstructions
- Tunnel position
- Tunnel enlargement

pQCT

- Used to measure the bone mineral density at the periphery at the tibial head femoral condyles, also at the lower tibia and the ultradistal radius
- In the follow-up of trauma it helps to find out local osteoporotic development on inflammatory influence [27] (Fig. 3.17)

Sonography

- Soft tissue
- Effusion
- Ligaments
- Menisci
- (Instability)
- Controlled injections

Indications:

Developing the diagnosis opens the way to treatment. Isolated ACL ruptures are to be divided into

- Proximal or "ultra-femoral" ruptures
- Intermediate ruptures
- Distal and tibial ruptures with eminence fractures

Fractures are classified 1–4 by Meyers and McMeever [28]. Treatment and outcome are still being discussed [29–33]. Conservative treatment is suggested in acute type 1 lesions.

Proximal "ultra-femoral" ruptures are described as being successfully treated with a healing response in the first 6 weeks. It can be successful later depending on the quality of the ACL stump [34–39].

Intermediate ruptures are to be treated by ACL reconstruction with autologous or homologous grafts such as hamstring, quadriceps tendon, or patella tendon bone [40–44]. In combined knee dislocation sutures serve as an intermediate alternative [45, 46]. See algorithm (Fig. 3.18) and the technique in Chap. 5.

Biomechanical axis, knee morphology, and an increased tibial posterior slope should be considered [16, 18, 19, 47–49] (Figs. 3.9b and 3.16c).

Posterior cruciate ligament lesions are mostly successful treated conservatively using braces. The dynamic PCL Jack Brace (Albrecht), which are also used in postoperative and rehabilitative treatment, are established [50].

Instability measurement is mandatory such as plain X-ray with a Scheuba device (Fig. 3.10a–d) or a clinical device such as the Rolimeter or

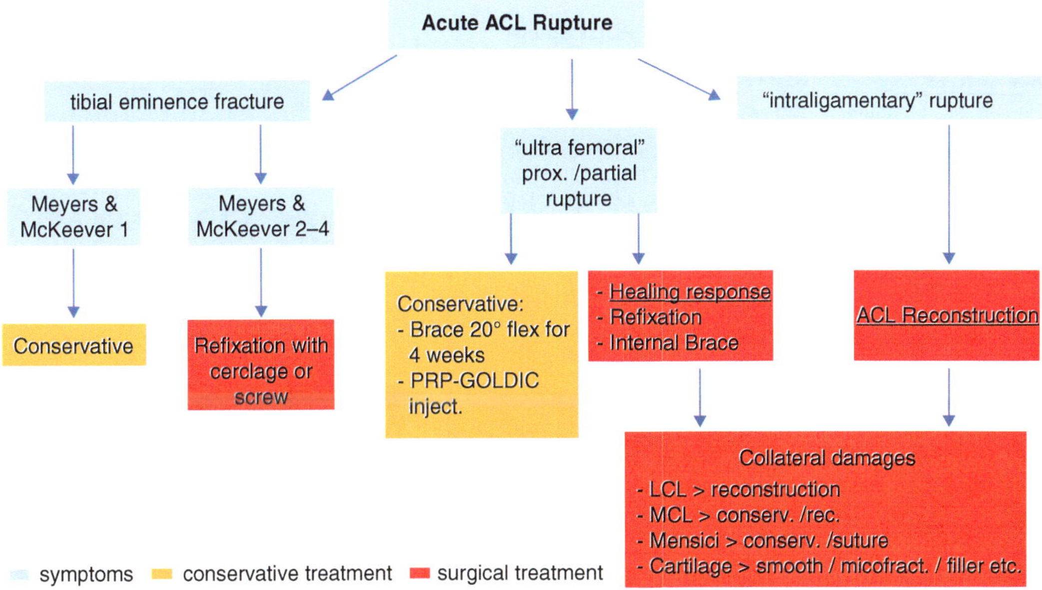

Fig. 3.18 Algorithm of treatment of anterior cruciate ligament (ACL) rupture. *LCL* lateral collateral ligament [39]

Articometer (Fig. 3.4a–d). Transversal laxity compared with the uninjured knee of 10-mm difference is usually treated conservatively like most isolated PCL ruptures. Tibial dislocation fractures are treated by surgical repositioning. Combined isolated ACL and PCL lesions can be treated conservatively—first address the PCL using a dynamic PCL brace for 8–12 weeks. ACL replacement is performed in a second stage. Healing response is a successful alternative in early PCL instability of more than 10 mm. Platelet-rich plasma (PRP) or PRP-analogous gelsolin supports by stimulating growth factors and mobilizing stem cells [51]. Combined lesions are treated using sutures [46] or replacement (Fig. 3.19).

Most isolated medial capsule and medial collateral ligament injuries are treated conservatively. Braces in straight or 20° flexion are used for the first 4–6 weeks. Complex anteromedial instability or chronic instabilities need reconstruction, augmentation, or suture [46] (Fig. 3.20).

Only a small instability of less than 3 mm at the lateral knee joint and lateral collateral ligament (LCL) can be treated conservatively. In these cases PRP or PRP-analogous gelsolin (GOLDIC) support by stimulating growth factors and mobilizing stem cells can be helpful [51–53]. Instabilities of more than 3 mm need surgery as suture, augmentation, or reconstruction [54–57]. Combined instability is seen with ACL rupture [54] (Fig. 3.21).

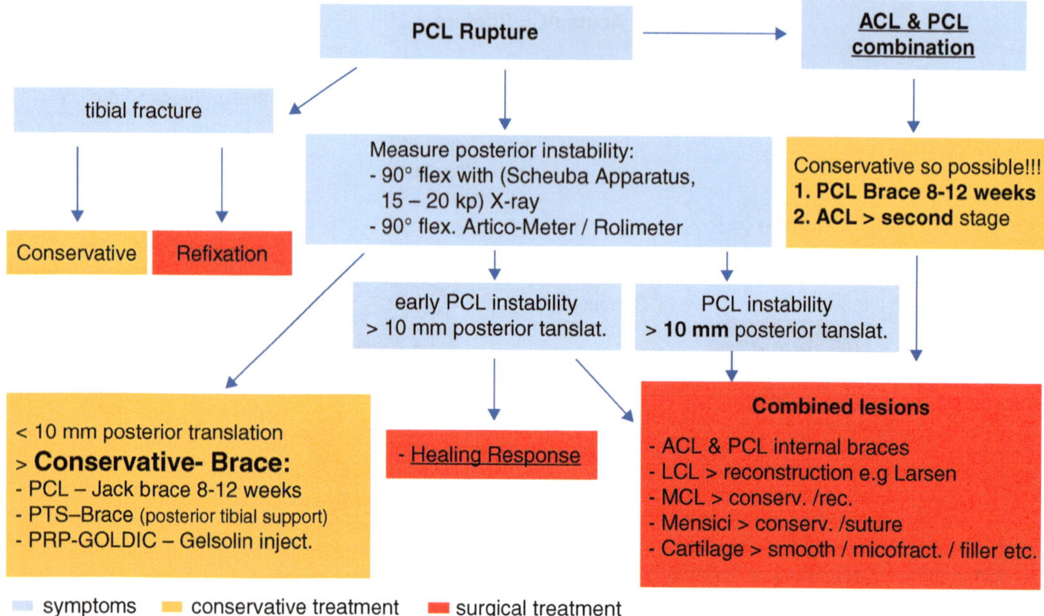

Fig. 3.19 Algorithm of treatment of posterior cruciate ligament (PCL) rupture or combined lesion. *ACL* anterior cruciate ligament, *MCL* medial collateral ligament [39]

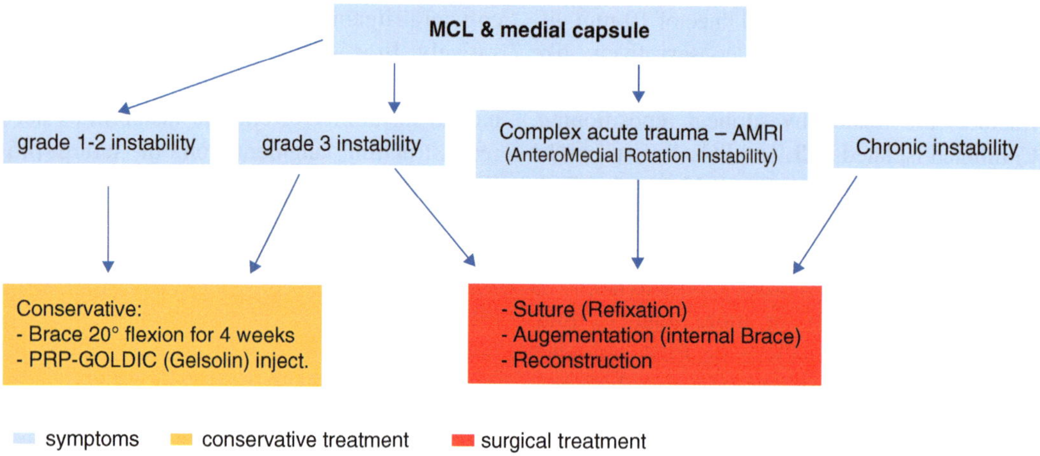

Fig. 3.20 Algorithm of treatment of medial capsule and medial collateral ligament (MCL) [39]

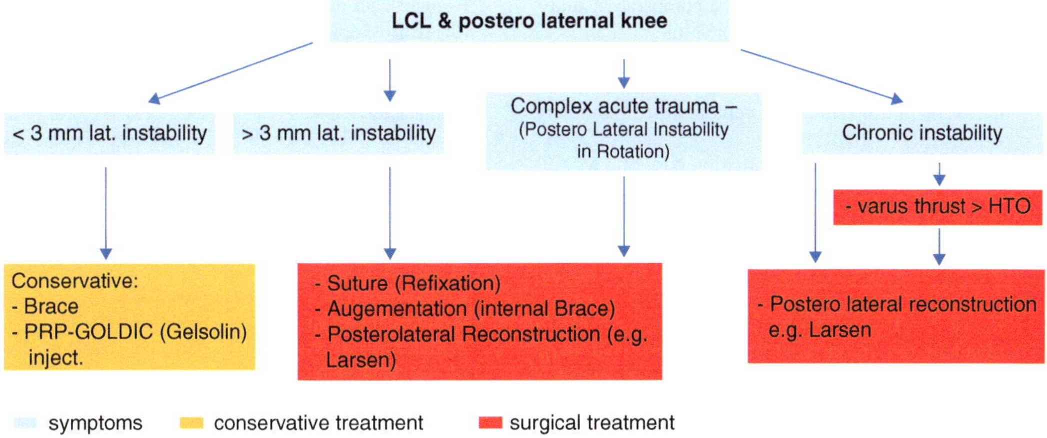

Fig. 3.21 Algorithm of treatment of lateral capsule and lateral collateral ligament (LCL). High tibial osteotomy (HTO) [39]

References

1. Torg JS, Conrad W, Kalen V. Clinical diagnosis of anterior cruciate ligament instability in the athlete. Am J Sports Med. 1976;4(2):84–93.
2. Tanaka K, et al. Human knee joint sound during the Lachman test: comparison between healthy and anterior cruciate ligament-deficient knees. J Orthop Sci. 2017;22(3):488–94.
3. Ericsson D, et al. Test-retest reliability of repeated knee laxity measurements in the acute phase following a knee trauma using a Rolimeter. J Exerc Rehabil. 2017;13(5):550–8.
4. Runer A, et al. The evaluation of Rolimeter, KLT, KiRA and KT-1000 arthrometer in healthy individuals shows acceptable intra-rater but poor inter-rater reliability in the measurement of anterior tibial knee translation. Knee Surg Sports Traumatol Arthrosc. 2021.
5. Krautter A, et al. Instrumented arthrometry of the anterior cruciate ligament. A comparison. Biomed Tech. 2012;57:4299.
6. Galway HR, MacIntosh DL. The lateral pivot shift: a symptom and sign of anterior cruciate ligament insufficiency. Clin Orthop Relat Res. 1980;147:45–50.
7. Müller W. Das Knie – form, funktion und ligamentäre Wiederherstellungschirurgie. Heidelberg: Springer; 1981.
8. Jagodzinski M, Friederich NF, Müller W. Das Knie [the knee]. 2nd ed. Berlin: Springer; 2016.
9. Felmet G. "Aquasprint" in the early functional rehabilitation program after ACL reconstruction. In: Frenzel G, Wuschech H, editors. Arthroskopische Gelenkchirurgie, Gestern-Heute-Morgen Standortbestimmung. Berlin: Kongress Compact Verlag; 2002. p. 188–96.
10. Felmet G. The significance of proprioceptive vibration training in postoperative treatment after ACL reconstruction. Berlin: DGOOC; 2004.
11. Felmet G. Proprioceptive vibrationtraining in ACL rehabilitation [Der Stellenwert des proprioceptiven Vibrationstrainings im Nachbehandlungsprogramm nach Kreuzbandersatz], in DGOOC Berlin, 19–24 October Abtr. E10-1404. 2004.
12. Felmet G. Graft selection in skiing. In: 16th ESSKA Congress, Amsterdam, 14–17 May 2014.
13. Felmet G. NMES in ACL rehabilitation. In: 16th ESSKA Congress Amsterdam, 14–17 May 2014.
14. Gupta Y, Mahara D, Lamichhane A. McMurray's test and joint line tenderness for medial meniscus tear: are they accurate? Ethiop J Health Sci. 2016;26(6):567–72.
15. Meserve BB, Cleland JA, Boucher TR. A meta-analysis examining clinical test utilities for assessing meniscal injury. Clin Rehabil. 2008;22(2):143–61.
16. Feucht MJ, et al. The role of the tibial slope in sustaining and treating anterior cruciate ligament injuries. Knee Surg Sports Traumatol Arthrosc. 2013;21(1):134–45.
17. Napier RJ, et al. Increased radiographic posterior tibial slope is associated with subsequent injury following revision anterior cruciate ligament reconstruction. Orthop J Sports Med. 2019;7(11):2325967119879373.
18. Tischer T, et al. The impact of osseous malalignment and realignment procedures in knee ligament surgery: a systematic review of the clinical evidence. Orthop J Sports Med. 2017;5(3):2325967117697287.
19. Wordeman SC, et al. In vivo evidence for tibial plateau slope as a risk factor for anterior cruciate ligament injury: a systematic review and meta-analysis. Am J Sports Med. 2012;40(7):1673–81.
20. Zink EJ, et al. Gender comparison of knee strength recovery following ACL reconstruction with contralateral patellar tendon graft. Biomed Sci Instrum. 2005;41:323–8.
21. Pape D, et al. Partial release of the superficial medial collateral ligament for open-wedge high tibial osteotomy. A human cadaver study evaluating medial joint opening by stress radiography. Knee Surg Sports Traumatol Arthrosc. 2006;14(2):141–8.
22. Kuster HH, Springorum HW. Contribution to stress X-ray visualization of the fibular ligaments. Arch Orthop Trauma Surg. 1983;101(4):287–90.
23. Koivisto J, et al. Effective radiation dose in the wrist resulting from a radiographic device, two CBCT

devices and one MSCT device: a comparative study. Radiat Prot Dosim. 2018;179(1):58–68.
24. Pallaver A, Honigmann P. The role of cone-beam computed tomography (CBCT) scan for detection and follow-up of traumatic wrist pathologies. J Hand Surg Am. 2019;44(12):1081–7.
25. Koivisto J, et al. Effective radiation dose of a MSCT, two CBCT and one conventional radiography device in the ankle region. J Foot Ankle Res. 2015;8:8.
26. Koivisto J, et al. Assessment of effective radiation dose of an extremity CBCT, MSCT and conventional X ray for knee area using MOSFET dosemeters. Radiat Prot Dosim. 2013;157(4):515–24.
27. Mundermann A, et al. Comparison of volumetric bone mineral density in the operated and contralateral knee after anterior cruciate ligament and reconstruction: a 1-year follow-up study using peripheral quantitative computed tomography. J Orthop Res. 2015;33(12):1804–10.
28. Meyers MH, McKeever FM. Fracture of the intercondylar eminence of the tibia. J Bone Joint Surg Am. 1970;52(8):1677–84.
29. Cannamela PC, et al. Knee extension does not reliably reduce acute type II tibial spine fractures: MRI evaluation of displacement during extension versus resting flexion. Orthop J Sports Med. 2019;7(7):2325967119860066.
30. Chouhan DK, et al. Management of neglected ACL avulsion fractures: a case series and systematic review. Injury. 2017;48(Suppl 2):54–60.
31. Delcogliano A, et al. Tibial intercondylar eminence fractures in adults: arthroscopic treatment. Knee Surg Sports Traumatol Arthrosc. 2003;11(4):255–9.
32. Gans I, Baldwin KD, Ganley TJ. Treatment and management outcomes of tibial eminence fractures in pediatric patients: a systematic review. Am J Sports Med. 2014;42(7):1743–50.
33. Lafrance RM, et al. Pediatric tibial eminence fractures: evaluation and management. J Am Acad Orthop Surg. 2010;18(7):395–405.
34. Felmet G. Healing response – indications and results. In: World Sports Trauma Congress & 7th EFOST Congress, London, 2012.
35. Felmet G. ACL & PCL healing response – indication and results. In: SICOT international orthopedics, Wuerzburg, Germany, 2016.
36. Jorjani J, et al. Medium- to long-term follow-up after anterior cruciate ligament rupture and repair in healing response technique. Z Orthop Unfall. 2013;151(6):570–9.
37. Koch M, et al. Intra-ligamentary autologous conditioned plasma and healing response to treat partial ACL ruptures. Arch Orthop Trauma Surg. 2018;138(5):675–83.
38. Steadman JR, et al. Outcomes following healing response in older, active patients: a primary anterior cruciate ligament repair technique. J Knee Surg. 2012;25(3):255–60.
39. AGA-Committee-Knee-Ligament, ACL Rupture – Therapy (VKB Ruptur - Therapie), AGA-Komitee-Knie-Ligament, Editor. 2018, AGA – Society for Arthroscopy and Joint Surgery – aga-online.de. p. 8–142.
40. Felmet G. [ACL reconstruction with the central third of the patellar ligament and simultanous proximal and distal press fit fixation, ALL PRESS FIT]. In: 14th Kongress der deutschsprachigen Arbeitsgemeinschaft für Arthroskopie AGA, Berlin, 1997.
41. Felmet G. ALL-PRESS-FIT, a new surgical method with femoral and tibial press fit fixation. Arthroskopie. 1999;12:299–304.
42. Felmet G. [ALL PRESS FIT, a near the origin ACL reconstruction with semitendinosus & gracilis tendon, a new surgical technique]. In: 21th Kongress der deutschsprachigen Arbeitsgemeinschaft für Arthroskopie (AGA), Lucerne, Switzerland, 2004.
43. Felmet G. Foreign material-free ACL reconstruction with hollow miller: a biological and anatomic method for every ligament. Tech Orthop. 2013;28(2):166–75.
44. Felmet G, et al. Press-fit ACL reconstruction, in controversies in the technical aspects of ACL reconstruction: an evidence-based medicine approach. Cham: Springer; 2017. p. 247–61.
45. Frosch KH, et al. Primary ligament sutures as a treatment option of knee dislocations: a meta-analysis. Knee Surg Sports Traumatol Arthrosc. 2013;21(7):1502–9.
46. Heitmann M, et al. Management of acute knee dislocations: anatomic repair and ligament bracing as a new treatment option – results of a multicentre study. Knee Surg Sports Traumatol Arthrosc. 2019;27(8):2710–8.
47. Bayer S, et al. Knee morphological risk factors for anterior cruciate ligament injury: a systematic review. J Bone Joint Surg Am. 2020;102(8):703–18.
48. Schillhammer CK, et al. Arthroscopy up to date: anterior cruciate ligament anatomy. Arthroscopy. 2016;32(1):209–12.
49. Wang YL, et al. Association between tibial plateau slopes and anterior cruciate ligament injury: a meta-analysis. Arthroscopy. 2017;33(6):1248–59.e4.
50. Achtnich A, et al. Acute injury of the posterior cruciate ligament with femoral avulsion: arthroscopic ligament repair and bracing. Oper Orthop Traumatol. 2019;31(1):12–9.
51. Schneider U, Wallich R, Felmet G, Murrell WD. Gold-induced autologous cytokine treatment in Achilles tendinopathy. In: Canata G, d'Hooghe P, Hunt K, editors. Muscle and tendon injuries. Berlin: Springer, Heidelberg; 2017. p. 411–9.
52. Schneider U, et al. Intra-articular gold induced cytokine (GOLDIC®) injection therapy in patients with osteoarthritis of knee joint: a clinical study. Int Orthop. 2021;45(2):497–507.
53. Schneider U, et al. Safety and efficacy of systemically administered autologous Gold-Induced Cytokines (GOLDIC®). CellR4. 2021;9:e3132, 2021. p. 1–9.
54. Bonanzinga T, et al. Management of combined anterior cruciate ligament-posterolateral corner tears: a systematic review. Am J Sports Med. 2014;42(6):1496–503.
55. Djian P. Posterolateral knee reconstruction. Orthop Traumatol Surg Res. 2015;101(1):S159–70.
56. Larson R. Isometry of the lateral collateral and popliteofibular ligaments andtechniques for reconstruction using a free tendon graft. Oper Tech Sports Med. 2001;9(2):84–90.
57. Zantop T, Petersen W. Modified Larson technique for posterolateral corner reconstruction of the knee. Oper Orthop Traumatol. 2010;22(4):373–86.

4 History of ACL Reconstruction

The replacement of the anterior cruciate ligament (ACL) is currently one of the most common surgical procedures in orthopedic surgery. Every year about 40,000 ACL replacements are performed in Germany. The incidence of ACL ruptures in the USA is estimated to range from 30 to 78 per 100,000 person-years [1]. This is a short overview of the development of the surgical techniques. The evolution of surgical techniques goes back over more 100 years. Because of copyright it was impossible to underline the important historical steps in pictures. The interested reader may use historical publications and the original literature is cited[1].

The anatomy of the ACL was described and illustrated by the Weber Brothers as early as 1836 in Göttingen, Germany [2]. The work already contained an exact description of the anatomical insertions, the position of the ligaments in the joint, the fiber structure, and the functional bundles. In 1921, Testut and Jakob provided a very detailed anatomical relationship between ACL insertion and the lateral meniscus and tibial plateau [3]. In the international literature the first ACL reconstruction was performed in 1917 by Hey Groves in Bristol, who replaced an ACL with a strip taken from the iliotibial tract (described in [4, 5]). As early as 1895, Robson restored both cruciate ligaments by primary suture in a mine worker in 1903 [6].

In the German-language literature a description of ACL replacement with the iliotibial tract by Giertz from 1913 is reported. In 1914, Grekow described the use of a free fascia lata strip (described in [7, 8]). Zur Verth, a German marine surgeon, used a patellar tendon replacement in 1932 [9].

Maybe because of the confusion of the two world wars and their consequences only a few reports described ACL replacement. Grafts from the patellar tendon [10, 11], the semitendinosus tendon [4, 12], as well as a dynamic gracilis tendon plastic [13] did not enter into the clinical routine of orthopedic–traumatological practice [14].

The semitendinosus tendon and gracilis tendon were already being used by Edwards in 1926 [15], and Lindemann and O'Donoghue resumed the use of these tendons as grafts in 1950 [16]. In 1963, Jones described a new technique using a distally struck graft of the middle third of the posterior tendon [17], followed in 1966 by Brückner with the description of a free patellar tendon transplant from the medial third [18]. This was for many years the "gold standard."

The 1970s produced new trendsetting and developments for the ACL. Torg et al. published the benefits of diagnostics it was first the anterior drawer and later Lachman Test, which has been part of the clinical diagnostics since then [19]. In

[1] However, the chapter has been preserved, at least in outline, for reasons of completeness and the author's deep gratitude to the astute researchers and developers in our field

G. Felmet, *Press-Fit Fixation of the Knee Ligaments*, https://doi.org/10.1007/978-3-031-11906-4_4

1973, Galway and MacIntosh described an exact pivot shift test with clinical correlation with the subjective instability of the patient [20].

Also in 1973, Hughston and Eilers described the posterior oblique ligament at the supply of medial capsule ligament injuries of the knee and published an operative technique for reconstruction of the posteromedial structures, including duplication of the capsule [21]. Various modifications without grafts are described under "Duplication by Hughston" [21–24].

Understanding the pivot shift test with the subjective instability of the patient, many techniques on the lateral side of the knee were developed and published with the goal of eliminating the pivot shift phenomenon [11, 25]. Werner Müller described in his book "The Knee" the use of a quadriceps and patella tendon for anatomical replacement [25] (Figs. 4.1 and 4.2).

A direct address of the ACL itself was not the focus of the surgeons. A systematic 5-year follow-up by Feagin and Curl showed a high rate of ACL insufficiency after suture. They concluded "Do not do primary repairs of the ACL—they fail too often" [26]. Therapy for ACL rupture in the 1970s, whether conservative or by surgery, was very controversially discussed.

The ACL replacement with a patellar tendon graft was described independently by Jones in 1963 [17] and Brückner in 1966 [18]. The graft used originally fixed at the tibial head was too short. Wirth et al. concluded therefore that Brückner´s procedure should be modified as a free graft [27]. Franke then delivered the first

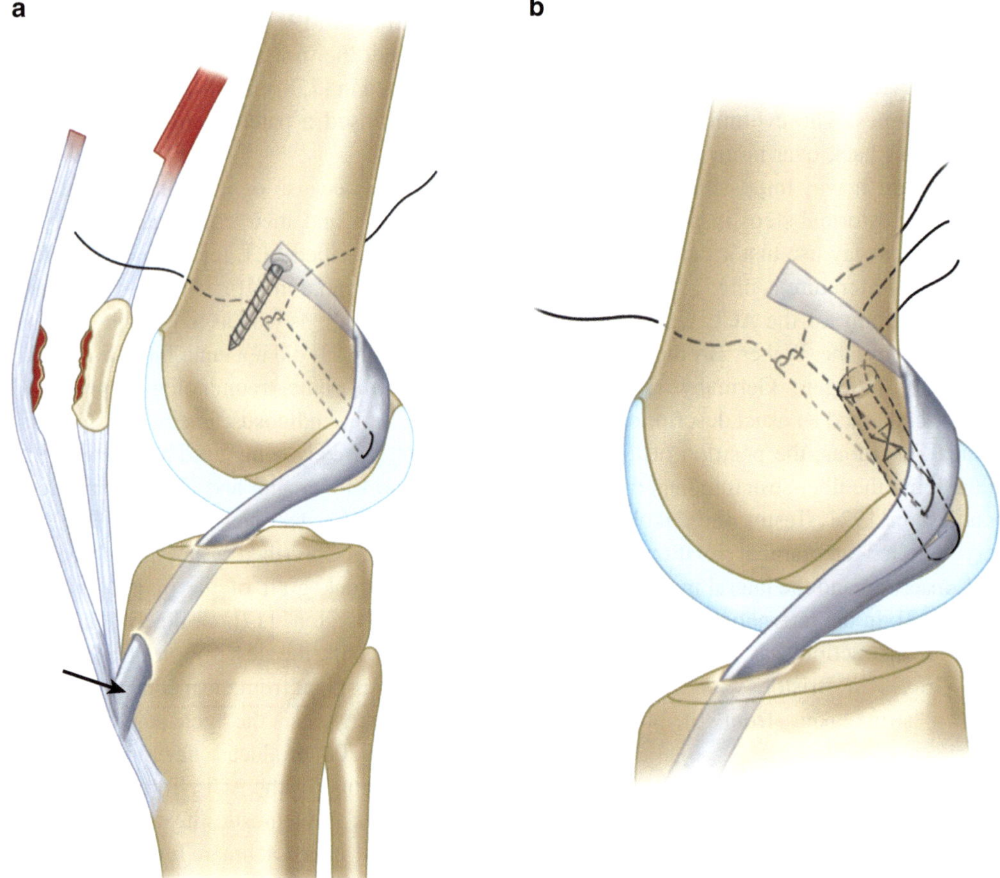

Fig. 4.1 Fixation in a double-bundle reconstruction of the distally fixed patella tendon transtibially guided into a femoral tunnel and over the top (**a**, **b**) [25]

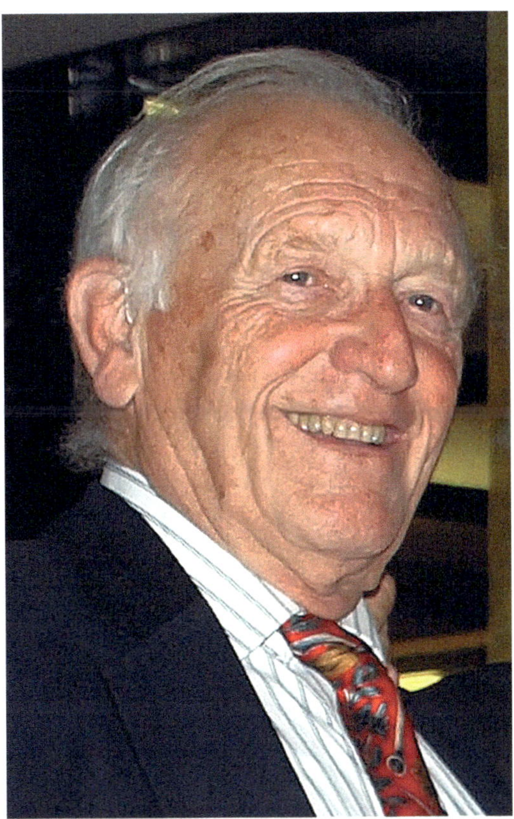

Fig. 4.2 Prof. Werner Müller, head of the section of the Orthopaedic Department at the University of Basel from 1970, Emeritus since 1998

clinical results of a modified Brückner´s technique in 1976 with a free transplant as a patella tendon bone graft with bone plugs from the tibia and patella on each side [28].

In the 1980s this surgical concept was established and designated as the "gold standard" [29]. Bone plugs were fixed partially material free.

In 1987, Lambert and Kurosaka et al. introduced interference screws to block the bone plugs in the tunnels [30, 31]. ACL replacement in the 1980s was performed by mini-arthrotomy. To place the femoral tunnel anatomically, a femoral drill and guiding system was used for a posterior (over-the-top) position.

The fixation was performed either extra-articularly with threads [32] or with bone plugs pressed in the tunnels. In 1982, Clancy was already favoring ACL replacement with simultaneous lateral tenodesis to protect the graft.

In addition to ACL replacement with the patient's own patellar tendon graft, replacement with synthetic materials was propagated.

After introduction of arthroscopy for meniscus surgery in the late 1970s it was a logical and necessary step to perform ACL surgery arthroscopically and to find a prosthetic material. In1982 Dandy et al. described the idea of reducing morbidity with this minimally invasive surgery in combination with a transplant off the shelf [33].

In Europe, especially in German-speaking countries, hopeful reports about ACL replacement with synthetic ligaments had been published [34–36]. In the long term these synthetic grafts showed a high rate of failure and re-ruptures.

The 1990s can be considered the decade of the hamstring graft. Relevant complications after patellar tendon graft such as arthrofibrosis and patella baja and a higher rate of osteoarthritis of the patella and the patella–femoral joint were focused on [37].

The introduction of a titanium plate (Endobutton) paved the way for a simple arthroscopic surgical technique for fixation of a tendon such as the hamstring in a tunnel [38] (Figs. 4.3 and 4.4).

A material-free open press-fit fixation on both sides was reported by Hertel in 1987 [39, 40]. From 1990 up to 2005 different anatomical ribbon-like arthroscopic and minimally invasive ACL reconstructions and press-fit fixation for all grafts were developed by different authors [41–47] (Fig. 4.5). This special history is reported in Chap. 5.

Arthroscopic surgical techniques and ACL replacement have poor morbidity. To simplify surgical procedures, transtibial surgery technology was established. A quick but "wrong way" for a corrrect anatomic ACL replacement to target the femoral anchorage through the tibal tunnel [48].

Insertions far away from the anatomy in a "high-noon" position lead to individual problems [49].

At the end of the 1990s ACL replacement in single-bundle technology guided through an anteromedial femoral tunnel was accepted [50].

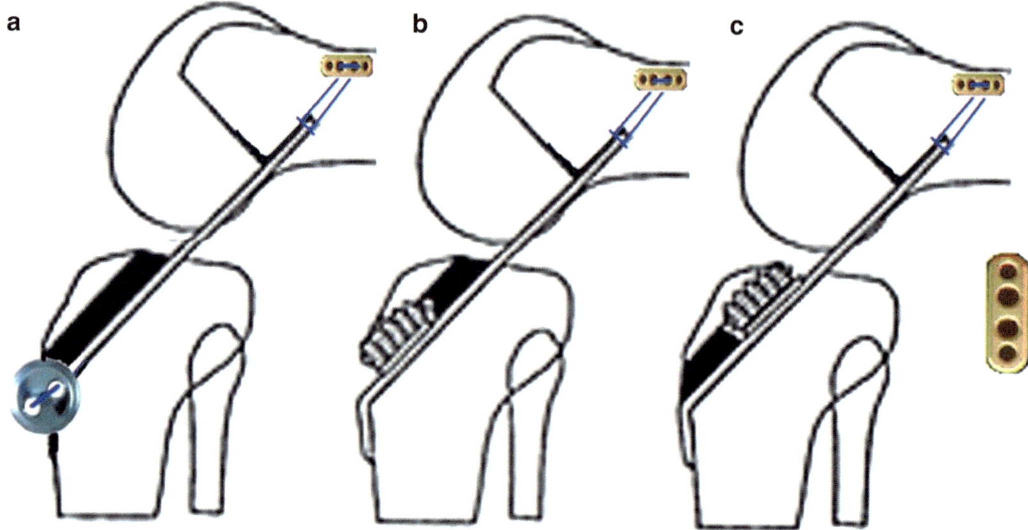

Fig. 4.3 (**a**–**c**) Anterior cruciate ligament reconstruction with Endobutton in the 1990s

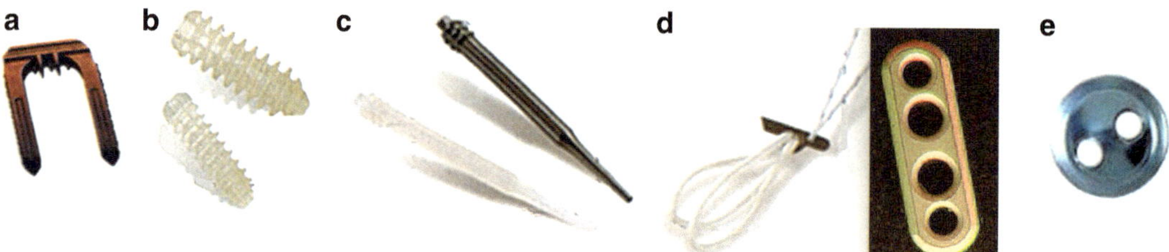

Fig. 4.4 Various fixations have been established such as staples (**a**), interference screws made of metal, non-absorbable, and absorbable materials (**b**), cross pins made of metal, non-absorbable, and absorbable materials (**c**), and in many techniques today interference screws (**b**), Endobutton (**d**), and the suture disk (**e**) are used

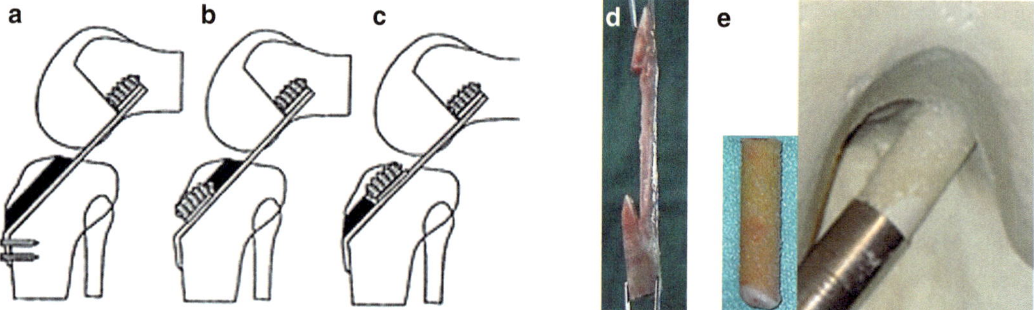

Fig. 4.5 Fixation of the graft was done with staples and interference screws in a distal fixation (**a**) with two interference screws in central position of the tunnels (**b**) and proximal fixation near the joint (**c**). Patella bone-tendon-bone press-fit has been fixed in without foreign material since 1987 [40, 41] (**d**) and with the use of a hollow reamer since 1998 [44] (**e**)

Because of persisting instability in rotation and a positive pivot-shift test in follow-up studies the development of the double-bundle technique followed. The primary goal was better stability in rotation. To mimic the two bundles, each one had to be restored.

Anatomical observations and biomechanical investigations showed a reciprocal tension of the individual fiber bundles. It was shown that particularly the posterolateral bundle transfers higher forces near extension [51]. Different techniques for double0bundle reconstruction were published for the use of the semitendinosus tendon alone or in combination with the gracilis tendon [52, 53].

Femoral fixation was performed with the Endobutton or small interference screws. On the tibial side small interference screws were anchored or outside with a drilled cortical bridge or screw [54].

Many biomechanical studies compared the advantages of the double-bundle technique with those of the single-bundle technique. Clinical comparative studies are often not clear which has better results [55]. Because of greater surgical effort in the double-bundle technique without better results, it did not become a standard technique.

Today, ACL replacement using single-bundle technology guided through an anteromedial portal at maximal knee flexion is well accepted. The experiences and technical developments of double-bundle surgery made individual replacements of isolated anteromedial or posterolateral ACL lesions possible [56, 57].

An individual ACL replacement requires knowledge about the use of established grafts such as quadriceps tendon as a bone–tendon or bone–tendon–bone graft, and quadriceps tendon with and without bone plug and hamstring. Different fixation techniques with interference screws, Endobutton, and drilled bone bridges are established. Also, special press-fit fixation for these grafts has been established for more than 20 years [43].

References

1. Gans I, et al. Epidemiology of recurrent anterior cruciate ligament injuries in national collegiate athletic association sports: the Injury Surveillance Program, 2004–2014. Orthop J Sports Med. 2018;6(6):2325967118777823.
2. Weber W, Weber E. Mechanik der menschlichen Gehwerkzeuge, Göttingen, Germany, 1836.
3. Testut J, Jacob O. Précis d'anatomie topographique avec applications medicochirurgicales. Paris: Octave Doin; 1921.
4. La Galeazzi R. ricostituzione dei ligamenti crociati del ginocchio. Atti Memorie della Soc Lombarda Chir. 1934;13:302–17.
5. Passler HH. History of implant-free anterior cruciate ligament reconstruction. Unfallchirurg. 2010;113(7):524–31.
6. Robson AW. Ruptured crucial ligaments and their repair by operation. Ann Surg. 1903;37(5):716–8.
7. Hesse E. Über den Ersatz der Kreuzbänder des Kniegelenkes durch freie Sehnenstreifen. Verh Dtsch Ges Chir. 1914;43:188.
8. Eberhardt C, et al. History of surgery of the anterior cruciate ligament. Orthopade. 2002;31(8):702–9.
9. Verth Z. Zur Verth in Verh. Dtsch Orthop Ges 1933, German Orthopedic Society 27. Kongress 5–7, September 1932, Mannheim, Germany, pp. 268–72.
10. Campbell TD. Anterior cruciate ligament reconstruction. Using patellar tendon grafts. AORN J. 1990;51(4):944–54.
11. Lemaire M. Ruptures anciennes du ligament croisé antérieur. Fréquence-Clinique-Traitement. J Chir. 1967;93(3):311–20.
12. Macey B. A new operative procedurefor repair of ruptured cruciate ligaments of the knee joint. Surg Gynecol Obstet. 1939;69:108–9.
13. Kaplan E. The iliotibial tract; clinical and morphological significance. J Bone Joint Surg Am. 1958;40(4):817–32.
14. Chambat P, et al. The evolution of ACL reconstruction over the last fifty years. Int Orthop. 2013;37(2):181–6.
15. Edwards A. Rupture and repair of the ACL. Br J Surg. 1926;13:432–8.
16. Lindemann K. Über den plastischen Ersatz der Kreuzbänder durch gestielte Sehnenverpflanzung. Z Orthop. 1950;79:316–34.
17. Jones KG. Reconstruction of the anterior cruciate ligament. A technique using the central one-third of the patellar ligament. J Bone Joint Surg Am. 1963;45:925–32.
18. Brückner H. A new method for plastic surgery of cruciate ligaments. Chirurg. 1966;37(9):413–4.
19. Torg JS, Conrad W, Kalen V. Clinical diagnosis of anterior cruciate ligament instability in the athlete. Am J Sports Med. 1976;4(2):84–93.

20. Galway HR, MacIntosh DL. The lateral pivot shift: a symptom and sign of anterior cruciate ligament insufficiency. Clin Orthop Relat Res. 1980;147:45–50.
21. Hughston JC, Eilers AF. The role of the posterior oblique ligament in repairs of acute medial (collateral) ligament tears of the knee. J Bone Joint Surg Am. 1973;55(5):923–40.
22. Engebretsen L, Lind M. Anteromedial rotatory laxity. Knee Surg Sports Traumatol Arthrosc. 2015;23(10):2797–804.
23. Hughston JC. The importance of the posterior oblique ligament in repairs of acute tears of the medial ligaments in knees with and without an associated rupture of the anterior cruciate ligament. Results of long-term follow-up. J Bone Joint Surg Am. 1994;76(9):1328–44.
24. Jacobson KE, Chi FS. Evaluation and treatment of medial collateral ligament and medial-sided injuries of the knee. Sports Med Arthrosc Rev. 2006;14(2):58–66.
25. Müller W. Das Knie - form, Funktion und ligamentäre Wiederherstellungschirurgie. Berlin: Springer; 1981.
26. Feagin JA, Curl WW. Isolated tear of the anterior cruciate ligament: 5-year follow-up study. Am J Sports Med. 1976;4(3):95–100.
27. Wirth CJ, et al. Plastic reconstruction of old anterior cruciate ligament ruptures by the Brückner procedure. Arch Orthop Unfallchir. 1974;78(4):362–73.
28. Franke K. Clinical experience in 130 cruciate ligament reconstructions. Orthop Clin North Am. 1976;7(1):191–3.
29. Clancy WG, et al. Anterior cruciate ligament reconstruction using one-third of the patellar ligament, augmented by extra-articular tendon transfers. J Bone Joint Surg Am. 1982;64(3):352–9.
30. Kurosaka M, Yoshiya S, Andrish JT. A biomechanical comparison of different surgical techniques of graft fixation in anterior cruciate ligament reconstruction. Am J Sports Med. 1987;15(3):225–9.
31. Lambert KL. Vascularized patellar tendon graft with rigid internal fixation for anterior cruciate ligament insufficiency. Clin Orthop Relat Res. 1983;172:85–9.
32. Shelbourne KD, Nitz P. Accelerated rehabilitation after anterior cruciate ligament reconstruction. Am J Sports Med. 1990;18(3):292–9.
33. Dandy DJ, Flanagan JP, Steenmeyer V. Arthroscopy and the management of the ruptured anterior cruciate ligament. Clin Orthop Relat Res. 1982;167:43–9.
34. Paar O. Management of fresh and older ruptures of the anterior cruciate ligament with the Kennedy modified polypropylene ligament augmented tendonplasty. Preliminary contribution. Chirurg. 1988;59(11):788–92.
35. Park JP, Grana WA, Chitwood JS. A high-strength Dacron augmentation for cruciate ligament reconstruction. A two-year canine study. Clin Orthop Relat Res. 1985;196:175–85.
36. Pässler H, Stadler J, Berger R. First results after 200 old ACL ruptures with a synthetic ligament replacement. Hefte Unfallheilkd. 1987;189:963.
37. Paulos LE, Wnorowski DC, Greenwald AE. Infrapatellar contracture syndrome. Diagnosis, treatment, and long-term followup. Am J Sports Med. 1994;22(4):440–9.
38. Rosenberg T. Technique for endoscopic method of ACL reconstruction. In: Technical bulletin. Mansfield: Acufex Microsurgical; 1993.
39. Hertel P. Technique of an open ACL reconstruction with autologous patella tendon. Arthroskopie. 1997;10:240–5.
40. Hertel P. Anatomic reconstruction of the ACL: a new technique for ACL replacement. In: 4th ESSKA Congress, Stockholm, 1990.
41. Felmet G. [ACL reconstruction with the central third of the patellar ligament and simultanous proximal and distal press fit fixation, ALL PRESS FIT]. In: 14th Kongress der deutschsprachigen Arbeitsgemeinschaft für Arthroskopie AGA, Berlin, 1997.
42. Felmet G. ALL-PRESS-FIT, a new surgical method with femoral and tibial press fit fixation. Arthroskopie. 1999;12:299–304.
43. Felmet G. Foreign material-free ACL reconstruction with hollow miller: a biological and anatomic method for every ligament. Tech Orthop. 2013;28(2):166–75.
44. Felmet G. ACL reconstruction with proximal and distal press fit fixation (ALL PRESS FIT) with SDI (Surgical Diamond Instrument) instruments. Osteosynthese Int. 2000;8(Suppl 1):173–4.
45. Akoto R, Hoeher J. Anterior cruciate ligament (ACL) reconstruction with quadriceps tendon autograft and press-fit fixation using an anteromedial portal technique. BMC Musculoskelet Disord. 2012;13:161.
46. Boszotta H. Arthroscopic anterior cruciate ligament reconstruction using a patellar tendon graft in press-fit technique: surgical technique and follow-up. Arthroscopy. 1997;13(3):332–9.
47. Halder A. Implant free arthroscopical ACL reconstruction in double-press-fit-technique – surgical technique and preliminary results. Arthroskopie. 1997;10(6):298–302.
48. Arnold MP, Kooloos J, van Kampen A. Single-incision technique misses the anatomical femoral anterior cruciate ligament insertion: a cadaver study. Knee Surg Sports Traumatol Arthrosc. 2001;9(4):194–9.
49. Strobel MJ, Castillo RJ, Weiler A. Reflex extension loss after anterior cruciate ligament reconstruction due to femoral "high noon" graft placement. Arthroscopy. 2001;17(4):408–11.
50. Pinczewski L, Roe J, Salmon L. Why autologous hamstring tendon reconstruction should now be considered the gold standard for anterior cruciate ligament reconstruction in athletes. Br J Sports Med. 2009;43(5):325–7.
51. Sakane M, et al. In situ forces in the anterior cruciate ligament and its bundles in response to anterior tibial loads. J Orthop Res. 1997;15(2):285–93.
52. Muneta T, et al. Two-bundle reconstruction of the anterior cruciate ligament using semitendinosus tendon with endobuttons: operative technique and preliminary results. Arthroscopy. 1999;15(6):618–24.

53. Yasuda K, et al. Anatomic single- and double-bundle anterior cruciate ligament reconstruction, part 1: basic science. Am J Sports Med. 2011;39(8):1789–99.
54. Järvelä T. Double-bundle versus single-bundle anterior cruciate ligament reconstruction: a prospective, randomized clinical study. Knee Surg Sports Traumatol Arthrosc. 2007;15(5):500–7.
55. Desai N, et al. Anatomic single- versus double-bundle ACL reconstruction: a meta-analysis. Knee Surg Sports Traumatol Arthrosc. 2014;22(5):1009–23.
56. Ochi M, et al. Anterior cruciate ligament augmentation procedure with a 1-incision technique: anteromedial bundle or posterolateral bundle reconstruction. Arthroscopy. 2006;22(4):463–5.
57. Siebold R, Fu FH. Assessment and augmentation of symptomatic anteromedial or posterolateral bundle tears of the anterior cruciate ligament. Arthroscopy. 2008;24(11):1289–98.

5 History and Techniques of Material-Free and Press-Fit ACL Reconstruction

5.1 Introduction

This chapter presents the history, biomechanical evidence, surgical techniques, and results of press-fit anterior cruciate ligament (ACL) reconstruction, particularly including the evolution of the most developed of all press-fit methods, its creation, and the special steps necessary to use all common grafts on the knee joint. Owing to the dominance of industry-specific, material-based ACL technology, it was and is not easy to spread it, despite very good results. Individual activities and political initiatives, and the necessary luck until the actual establishment of a scientific working group are demonstrated.

Several factors, such as the timing of surgery, graft choice, tunnel positioning, graft tensioning, graft fixation methods, and postoperative rehabilitation protocols, play very important roles in successful ACL reconstruction. Patellar bone-tendon-bone (BTB) and hamstring are the most commonly used grafts with equally successful long-term results [1–4]. The quadriceps tendon (QT) is emerging as an attractive alternative because of its predictable thickness and lowers donor site morbidity [5–12].

Stable graft fixation is paramount for a successful outcome as a graft relies on its initial stability for the first 6–8 weeks. Various absorbable and non-absorbable implants in the form of screws, stables, pins, and buttons have been used. Although these implants provide good initial stability for accelerated rehabilitation, they can be associated with implant migration, osteolysis, and soft tissue irritation. Cost is another important issue and they use signal interference during follow-up imaging. Revision surgery can be particularly challenging. To avoid all these issues with nonbiological implants, Hertel [4] introduced a novel concept of press-fit patellar BTB graft fixation in 1987. The initial description of this technique was for mini-open ACL reconstructions but over last the 2 decades, its use and the influence of other authors have been extended to all arthroscopic graft types and other ligament reconstructions. Biomechanical strength testing results have been promising and various authors have published good long-term clinical results [13–18].

5.2 History and Surgical Techniques of Foreign Material-Free ACL Reconstruction

Bone plugs with a patellar tendon graft were used by Brückner in 1966, Jones in 1963, and Clancy et al. in 1982 [19–23]. Hertel had originally developed a technique for femoral-sided press-fit fixation of a patellar BTB graft in 1989 [24]. This technique uses the bone plugs on either end of the patellar tendon graft for press-fit fixation in slightly undersized bony tunnels. The implantation was to mimic the ribbon-like anatomy. He used the medial third of the patellar tendon. A patellar bone plug was harvested

G. Felmet, *Press-Fit Fixation of the Knee Ligaments*, https://doi.org/10.1007/978-3-031-11906-4_5

in the form of a shallow disk 5 mm in depth and a tibial bone block in an almost square cross section about 0.5 mm wider than the diameter of the femoral tunnel. A mini-arthrotomy was made through the donor site defect. The femoral tunnel was drilled with a 8-mm hollow reamer from inside out and dilated to 9 mm with a tunnel dilator. A tibial bone plug of 9.5 mm is then tapped into the femoral tunnel from inside out, until flush with the joint surface. The tibial tunnel was drilled in a standard fashion with the same hollow reamer. A 5-mm bone block was cut out above the tibial drill hole. The tibial trough was deepened with a chisel. Then, the patellar bone block was driven into the gap of the chisel securing the graft (Fig. 5.1) [24–28].

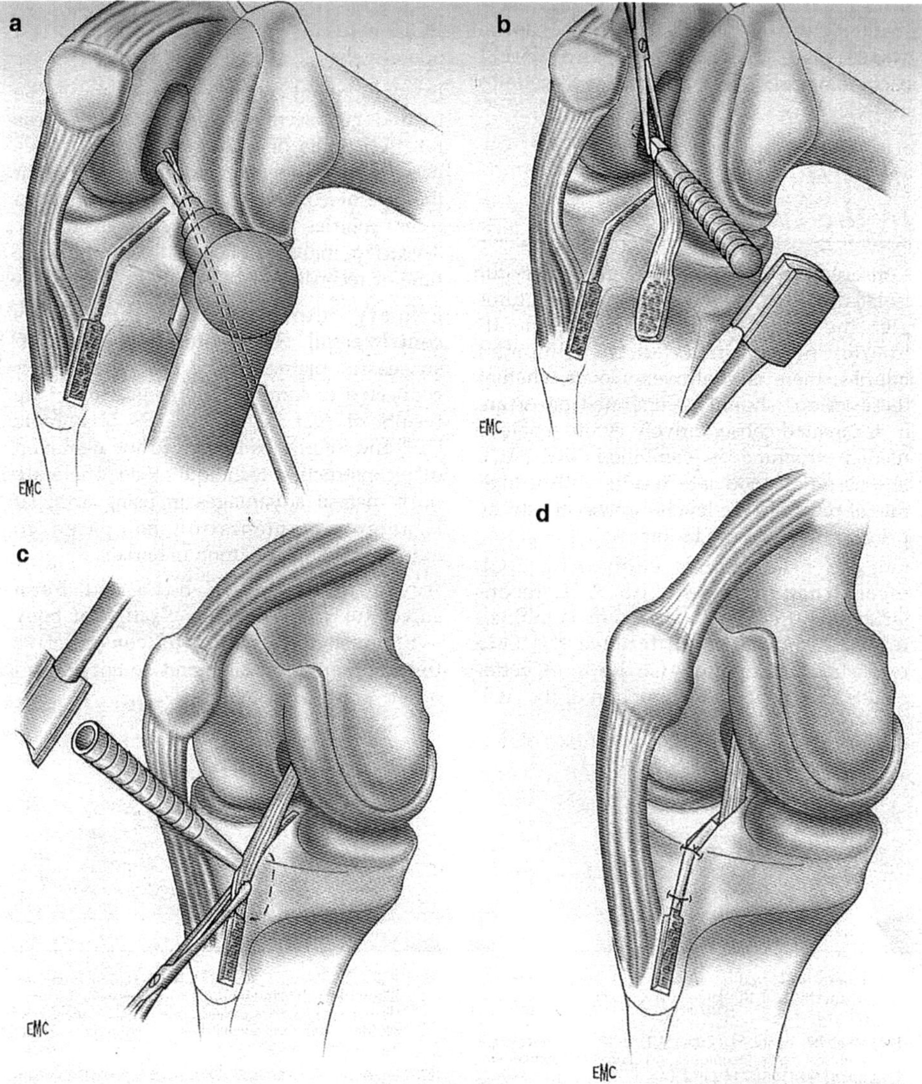

Fig. 5.1 In his first open technique Peter Hertel used the medial third of the patellar ligament. A 5-mm-wide triangular bone segment was taken from the anterior tibial head. A hollow reamer was used to cut the femoral drill hole at 120° knee flexion in front of the palpation hook in the "over-the-top" position (**a**). The tibial bone block of the graft is pushed into the femoral drill hole by a pusher. The patellar corticoligamentous part of the graft is anterior the tibia (**b**). At 20° of flexion the tibial trough is deepened by a chisel and the patellar bone block is driven into the gap created by the chisel, tensioning the transplant distally. The cancellous part of the patellar bone block faces the lateral side, thus providing parallel orientation of the graft fibers (**c**). All gaps are filled with bone blocks and chips. The triangular bone segment is sutured back to its bed (**d**) [27]

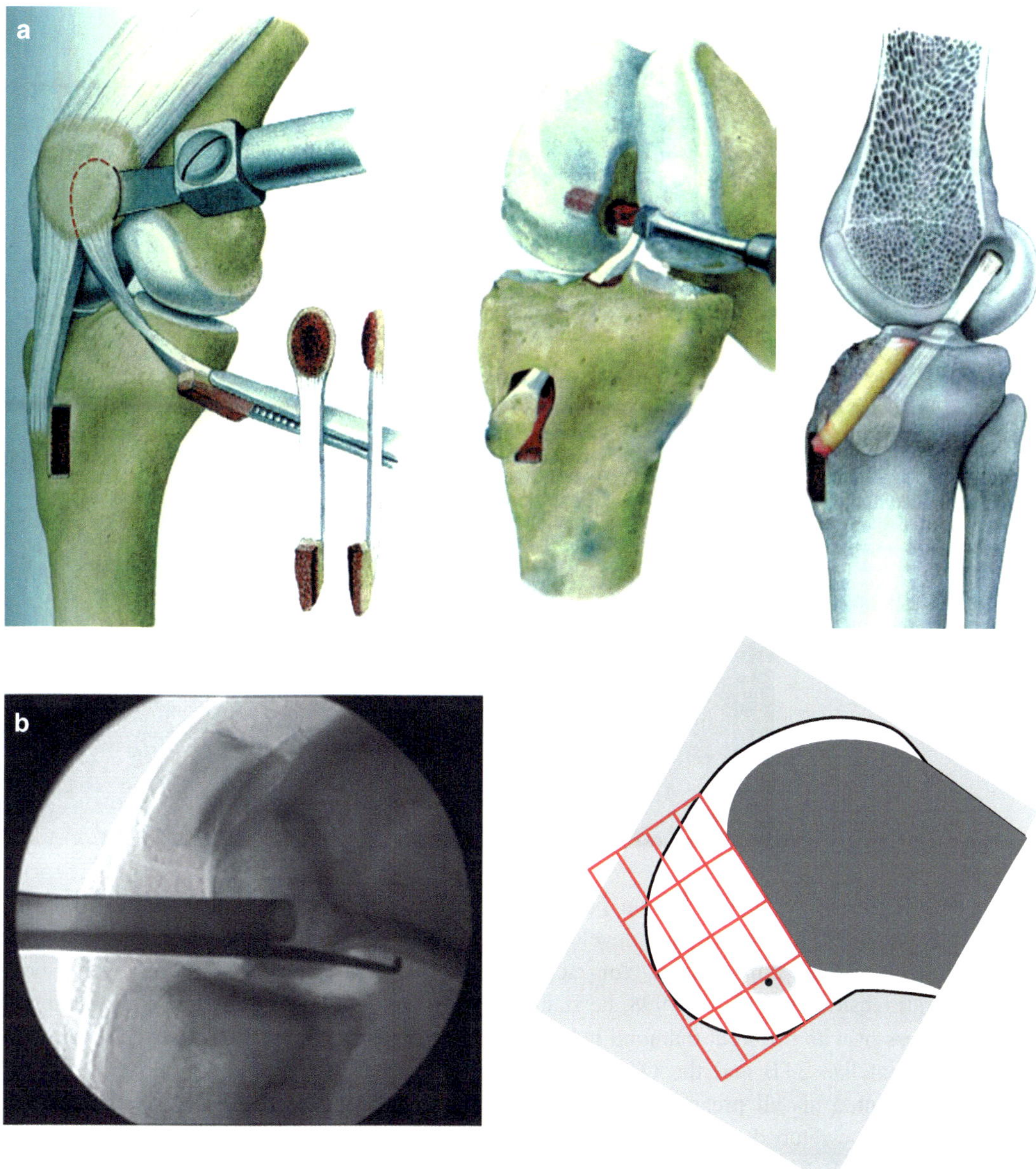

Fig. 5.2 (**a**) Peter Hertel uses the medial third of a patellar bone-tendon-bone graft with a flat structure ribbon like [1, 28]. The graft is tensioned in knee flexion. The patellar bone disk is fixed in this later version without osteotomy through a tunnel and bone cylinder from this tunnel. (**b**) The anatomical insertion is positioned by the "quadrant method" described by Manfred Bernard and Peter Hertel [29]

Later, this technique was modified for arthroscopic use (Figs. 5.2 and 5.3) [23]. For the femoral tunnel Hertel used the quadrant method he described with Bernard et al. [29]. At the same time a material-free patellar BTB fixation was presented by Wuschech [30].

In 1993, Boszotta developed an arthroscopic technique using an oscillating hollow saw for rapid and standardized harvesting of cylindrical bone plugs, ensuring safe and adequate femoral press-fit fixation [31–33] (Fig 5.4). An analogous technique was used for quadriceps and later published in a variation by Barie et al. [7, 34] and Akoto et al. [8]. Gobbi et al. created a single femoral conical press-fit fixation as an outside-in implantation in 1994 [35].

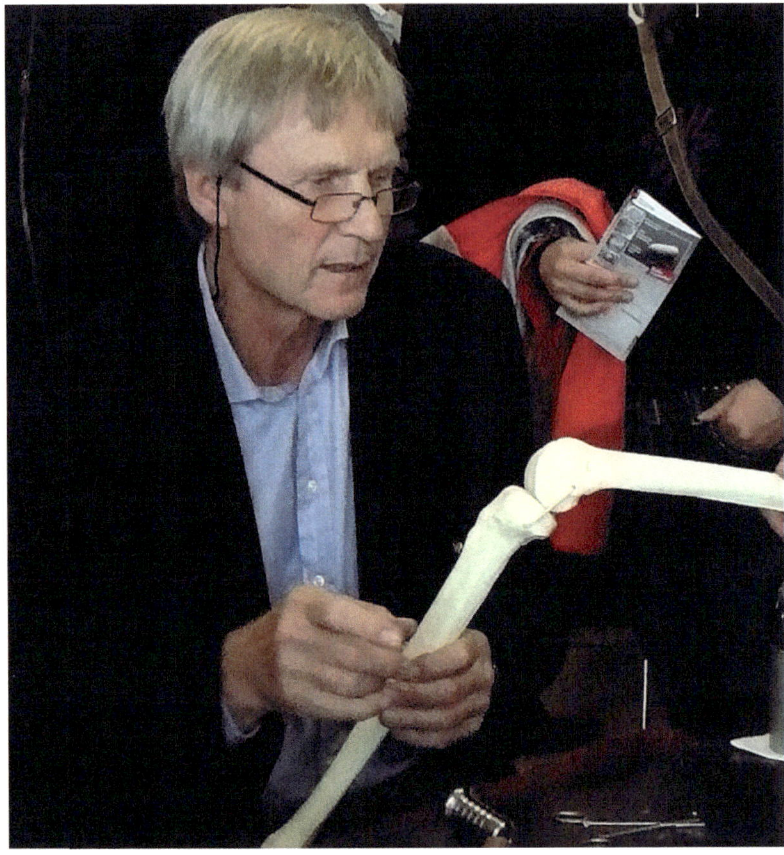

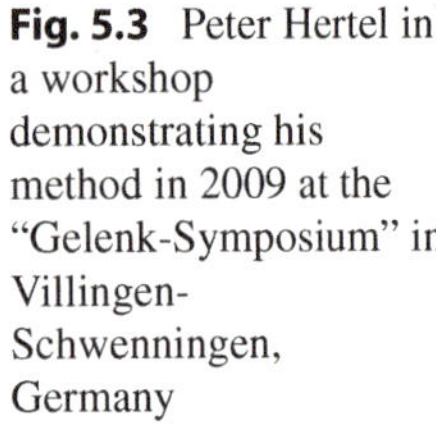

Fig. 5.3 Peter Hertel in a workshop demonstrating his method in 2009 at the "Gelenk-Symposium" in Villingen-Schwenningen, Germany

In 1995, Felmet developed his own patellar BTB "all press-fit" technique and developed bottom-to-top (BTT) implantation for self-adapted graft tension [36, 37]. In 1998, he standardized press-fit with different diamond hollow reamers for patellar BTB and the QT [38]. In 2004, he presented his all press-fit method for hamstrings and new tubed guiding devices for hollow reamers [2, 3, 38, 39] (see also Sect. 5.3).

In 1998, Pässler and Mastrokalos described the first material-free ACL reconstruction with hamstring autograft [40]. The semitendinosus and gracilis tendons were both tied together with a simple knot. A bottleneck-like tunnel is created on the femoral side, in which the knot of the tendon loop is firmly secured just proximal to the cortex of the notch wall at the anatomical insertion, hence avoiding any bungee effect that has been described with suspensory fixations. The tibial side was fixed with sutures over a bone bridge (Fig. 5.5). A variation with a supplemented bone cylinder instead a knot has been reported by Liu et al. [41].

Hybrid fixations are also described, where the femur is press-fit and the tibial side is fixed with implants [35, 42–44]. Prado et al. in 2004 created a femoral implant-free hamstring double-bundle reconstruction over a bone bridge inside out and outside in, which was fixed with an interference (IF) screw on the tibial side [45].

Studies and results from each author of foreign material-free and press-fit fixation of patellar BTB, hamstring, and quadriceps tendon are listed in Table 5.1.

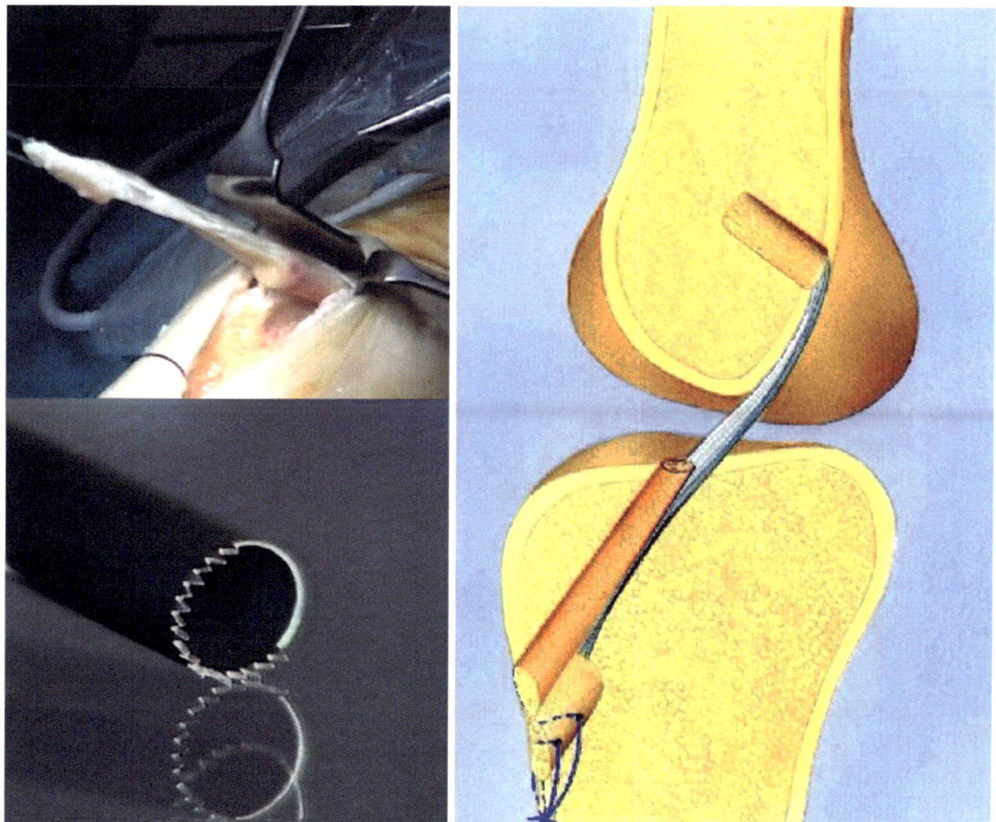

Fig. 5.4 Harald Boszotta from Austria used an oscillating hollow reamer (by Richard Wolf, Knittlingen, Germany) to harvest a patellar bone-tendon-bone graft and preparing the tunnels for press-fit fixation [31]

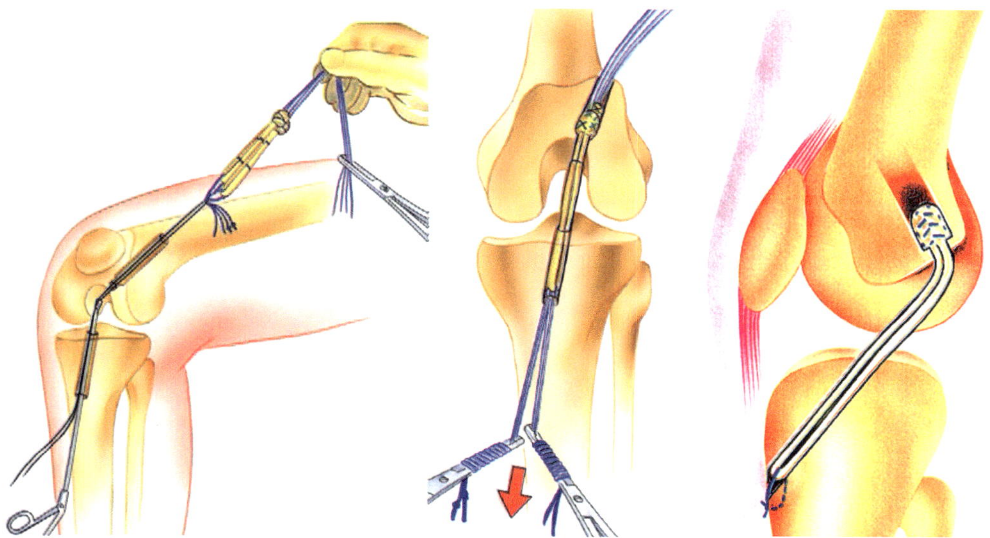

Fig. 5.5 Pässler and Mastrokalos material-free anterior cruciate ligament reconstruction with hamstring autograft [45]. Semitendinosus and gracilis tendons are both tied together with a simple knot. A bottle-neck-like tunnel is created on the femoral side, in which the knot of the tendon loop is firmly secured just proximal to the cortex of the notch. The tibial side was fixed with sutures over a bone bridge

Table 5.1 Fourteen studies and results of material free-graft fixation in one or both sides are listed. Thirteen are press-fit anchored on the femoral side (dark blue). Five use an interference screw (IF) in hybrid fixation at the tibia with patella bone-tendon-bone (BTB). Four use a suture over a bone bridge on the tibia side. One uses a hamstring with a knot in a femoral bottle neck. Five use press-fit fixation (dark blue). Three are "all press-fit" fixation as "all-rounders" with self-adapted bottom to top (BTT) fixation with every graft and the development from (1) Patellar BTB, (2) hamstring to (3) quadriceps tendon shows the curve of evolution; by creating a standard, simplifying the technique, and higher precision in instruments to achieve better results

	Hertel [28]	Gobbi et al. [35]	Biazzo et al. [43]	Felmet	Al-Husseiny and Batterjee [42]	Pavlik et al.	Wipfler et al. [4]	Wipfler et al. [4]	Halder et al. [46]	Felmet al.	Barie et al.	Widuchowski et al. [65]	Akoto et al.	Felmet
Studies with material free and press-fit fixation														
Year	1987–1991	1994–1995	1994–1997	1998–2000	1998–2000	1998–2002	1998–1999	1998–1999		2003–2005	2007–2008		2010	2009–2012
Graft	BTB	BTB	BTB	BTB	BTB	BTB	BTB	Hamstring	BTB	Hamstring	Quadriceps TB	BTB	Quadriceps TB	Quadriceps tendon
Technique femur	Press-fit	Conical press-fit	Press-fit	Press-fit BTT self-adapted	Press-fit	Press-fit	Press-fit	Knot in bottle neck	Press fit	Press-fit BTT self-adapted	Press-fit	Press-fit	Press-fit	Press-fit BTT self-adapted
Tibia	Tibia trough and press-fit	Metal wire over cortical screw	IF screw	Press fit	Screw/staple	IF screw	Bone bridge	Suture bone bridge	Press fit	Press fit	Suture bone bridge	IF screw	Suture bone bridge	<u>*Press-fit*</u>
Years FU	10.7	5 (36–62 mm)	20	10.3 (9.6–10.8 years)	2.4 (22–41 mm)	3 (24–77 m)	8.8	8.8	2.4 (20–40 mm)	7 (5.3–7.5 years)	12.4 (12–14)	15	1	5 (4.1–5.8)
N=	95	93	56	148	42	285	28	25	40	152	106	52	30	97
Age	42	38.2	23 (18–39)	40.2	26 (21–46)	29.1	29.9 (25–55)	34.2 (26–64)	30 (16–54)	37.9	30 (18–45)	28 (16–43)	31 (16–47)	32 (17–46)
IKDC subjective A/B	95%			96%					87.50%	98%		77%	86.10%	94%
IKDC objective A/B	98%			95%						96%			96.70%	96.40%
IKDC total A/B	84%	57%	64%/32%	87%	88%	84%	84%	94.40%		89%	86%			89.20%
KT 1000/ digital Rolimeter, mm	1,8 mm			1.42 mm (±0.88))		1.91 mm (±2.1)			1.3 mm (±2.2)	1.12 mm (±0.72)	1.36 mm (±0.9)		1.6 (±1.1)	1.09 mm (±0.53)

Lachman A 0–2.9 mm	69%	32%	68%	97%	95.20%		95%	91.70%		97%	83%		83%	96.60%
B 3–5.9 mm	15%	43%	32%	3%	4.80%					3%	17%		3.30%	3.40%
Pivot-shift negative	90%	67%		90%						90%			86.70%	91%
Glide	7%	35%		7%						8%				8%
Lysholm	93%					93.5	87.28	91.82			88,5 (±12.7)	86.4		
Tegner activity														
Pre-trauma	6.8			6.9						7.1				6.8
Follow-up	6	7		5			6.2	6.14		5.5	6	6.9	86.7% same as before	5.8
Complications				Tibia loosening 1, femur loosening 1, infection 3, fracture 0	infection 1				Extension deficit 1, tibia fracture 1, patella fracture 1, infection 1	Tibia loosening 1, femur loosening 1, infection 1, fracture 0	Re-rupture 1, extension deficit >5° 1, flexion deficit >5° 1		Extension deficit 1	Tibia loosening 0, femur loosening 0, infection 0, fracture 0
Osteoarthritis femoral-patellar	31%			33%						24%			10%	6%
Osteoarthritis gap increasing	45%	17%		27%						22%				2%

FU follow-up, *TB* tendon-bone, *IKDC* International Knee Documentation Committee

5.3 History of All Press-Fit

The many steps and influences of that time may motivate the reader to derive their own variants.

Felmet was influenced at that time by the usual IF screw made of titanium. Not knowing the work of Hertel and Boszotta, he developed his own patellar BTB "all press-fit" technique in 1995 [36, 37].In the early days he started with wedged bone plugs harvested from of the patellar and tibia head using an oscillating saw, each on the mid third of the patellar tendon (Fig. 5.6). By observation during his surgeries and in native uninjured ACL he learned from the typical behavior of ACL tension from flexion to extension to use this in his later self-adapted graft tension. The bone plug from the tibial tuberosity is press-fit fixed into the tibial tunnel near the joint. On the femoral side the bone plug from the distal patella is pushed deep into the tunnel and the graft is tensioned. A second bone plug fixes near the original insertion (Fig. 5.7). Felmet inserted the graft from distal to proximal and fixed the tibial bone plug first near the joint (contrary to the usual standard implantation). In 120° knee flexion he then tensioned the graft and fixed it with two bone plugs near the joint (Fig. 5.8). Although the graft is tensioned in flexion (regularly ACL is not under tension in 90° knee flexion) the tension increases in extension and so adapts itself correctly and mechanically on the basis of knee function (Fig. 5.9). The self-adapted "bottom-to-top" (BTT) tension with fixation of the graft near the original insertion has been the basis of all press-fit ACL and ligament reconstruction since then (Figs. 5.8 and 5.9).

In 1998, Felmet introduced the diameter of the hollow reamer with different sizes for a precise and reproducible harvest. The diamond hollow reamer worked "wet grinding" with cooling water flow. The bone cylinder of a patellar BTB graft was harvested with two sizes. First, the 9 mm diamond bur removed a small cylinder at a shallow angle from the distal patella. This was inserted with attached ligament into an 11-mm diamond cutter, which harvested the bone cylinder from the tibial tuberosity. The ribbon-like graft mimics the anteromedial (AM) and posterolateral (PL) bundle [38] (Figs. 5.10 and 5.11).

Since 1997, Felmet has also used the QT as a bone tendon graft for revision surgery. From 1998 onward, he used a second bone cylinder for a bone-tendon-bone graft. Today, the QT is mostly used without the patellar bone. Typically, the bone cylinder out of the tibial tunnel is fixed at the femoral end [38] (Fig. 5.12).

A similar method but with top-down fixation was developed later by Huber using an oscillating hollow saw [34]. In parallel, without any knowledge from one another Halder developed his double press-fit fixation with patellar tendon BTB graft commonly fixed and tensioned top-down [46].

In 1997/1998, Felmet used homologous ACL replacement. The graft was harvested from a patella-tendon-tibia head and an all press-fit BTT was implanted (Fig. 5.13). The technique was stopped after three implantations with less anterior stability than autologous grafts. Biological intolerances with the European homologous explants had to our knowledge never been observed.

The late 1990s were the years of robotic surgery and a new era of computer assistance [47–50]. In 1998, Felmet was also involved in developing the use of robotic support in ACL reconstruction. This was a new important step toward a consensus in anatomical ACL insertion. Use of a robot needed CT matching and planning. CASPAR (Computer Assisted Surgical Planning and Robotics) was from OrthoMaquet company in Rastatt, Germany. This robot was used by Prof. Gotzen and Dr. Petermann from the University of Marburg, Germany, and was first used to perform surgery on 28 April 1998 in Rastatt with a diamond grinder from the all press-fit equipment as a further progress toward higher precision (Fig. 5.14). It was not adopted for frequent use, but had been important in finding the way between technically possible and helpful surgery.

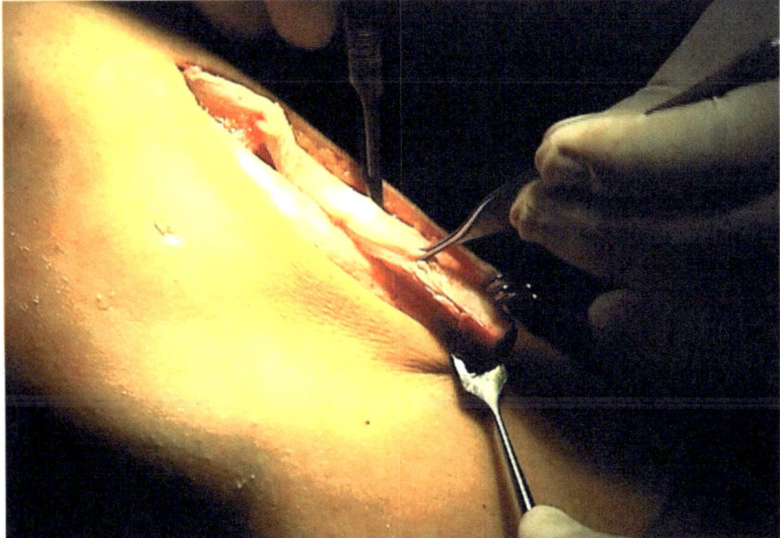

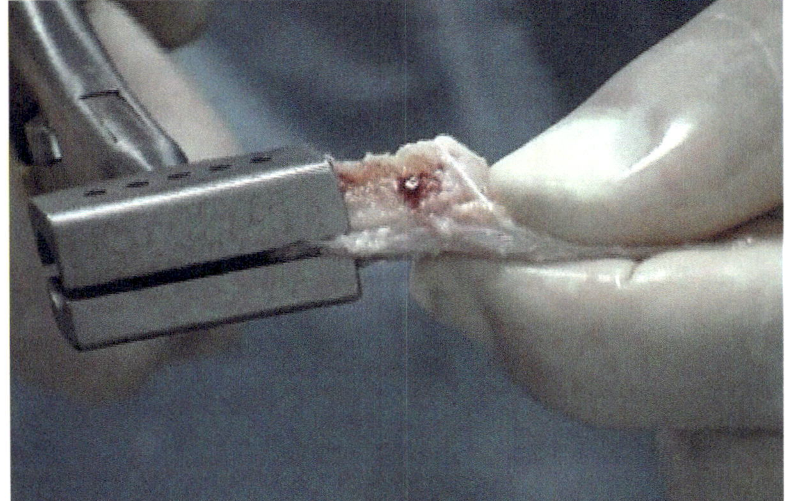

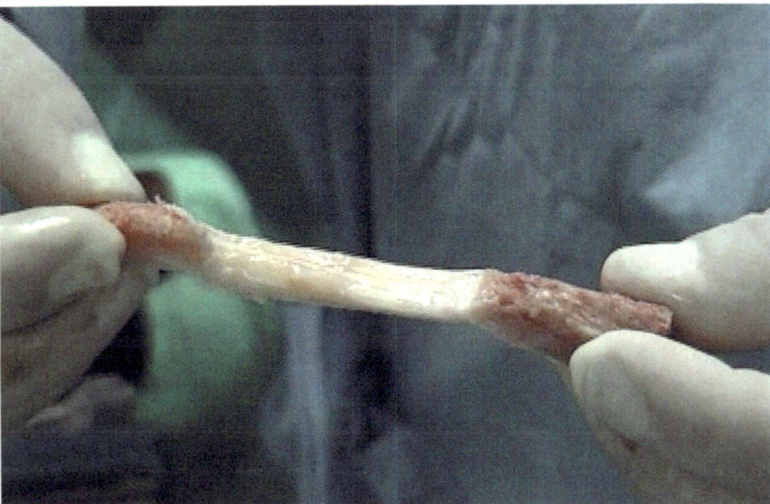

Fig. 5.6 Felmet started in 1995 with wedged bone plugs using an oscillating saw out of the patella and tibial tuberosity each on the more medio-lateral third of the patellar tendon

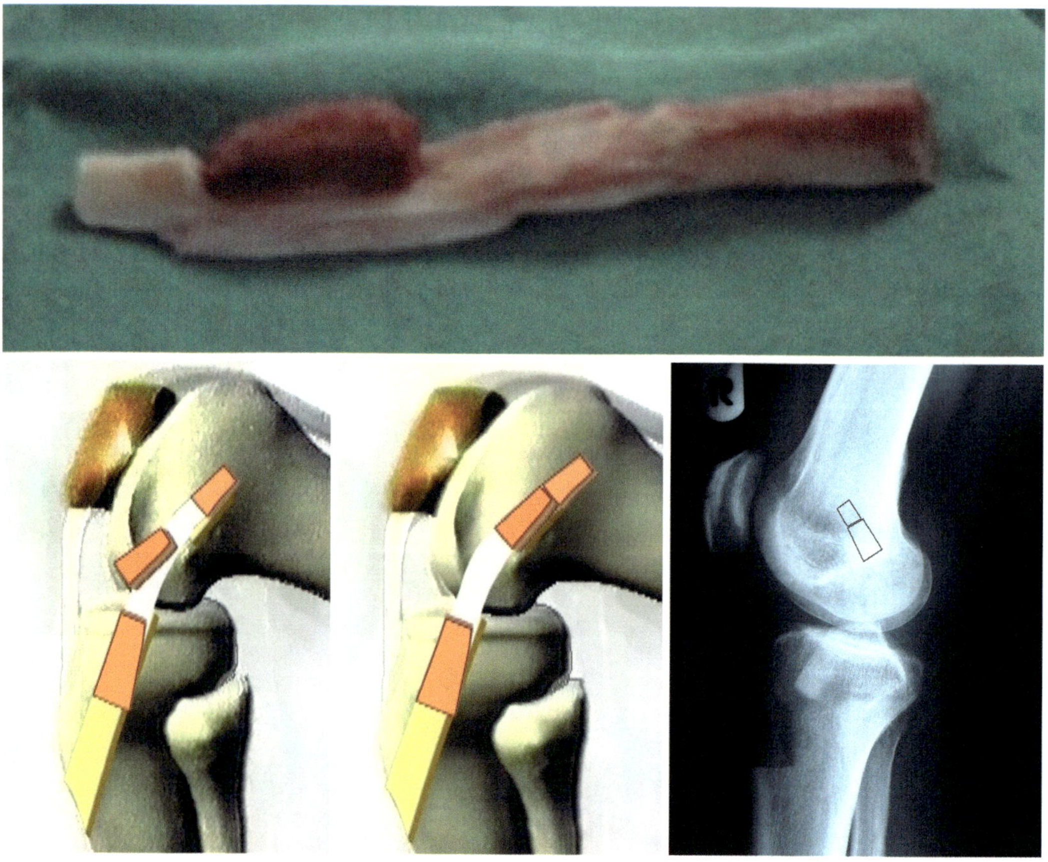

Fig. 5.7 The bone plug from the tibial tuberosity is press-fit fixed in the tibial tunnel near the joint. On the femoral side the bone plug from the distal patella is pushed deep into the tunnel and the graft is tensioned. A second bone plug fixes near the original insertion

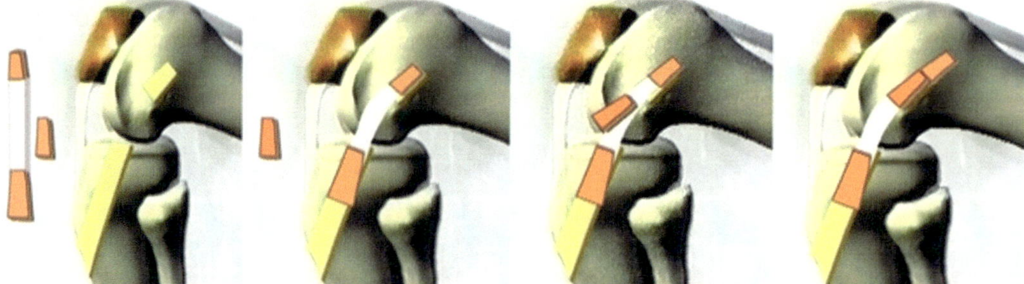

Fig. 5.8 Press-fit fixation of the patellar bone-tendon-bone graft under bottom-to-top fixation: (1) Press-fit fixation of the bone plug in the tibial tunnel near the joint. The tendon-bone graft is pulled into the femoral tunnel and tensioned; (2) fixation in 120° knee flexion with a second bone plug near the original insertion

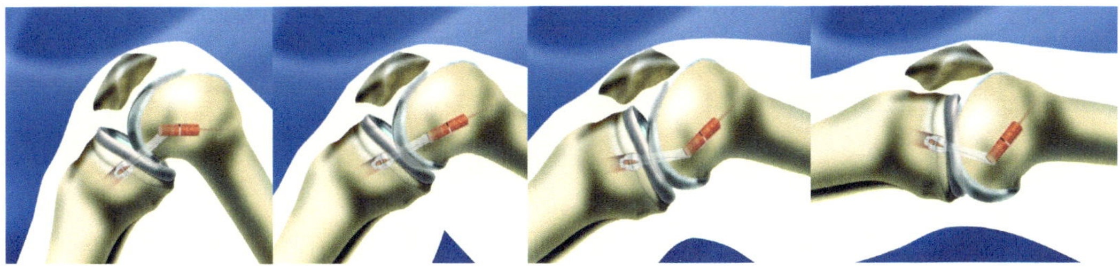

Fig. 5.9 The graft is tensioned in flexion (usually the anterior cruciate ligament is not under tension in 90° knee flexion). The tension increases in extension and adapts correctly and physiologically on the basis of the knee function

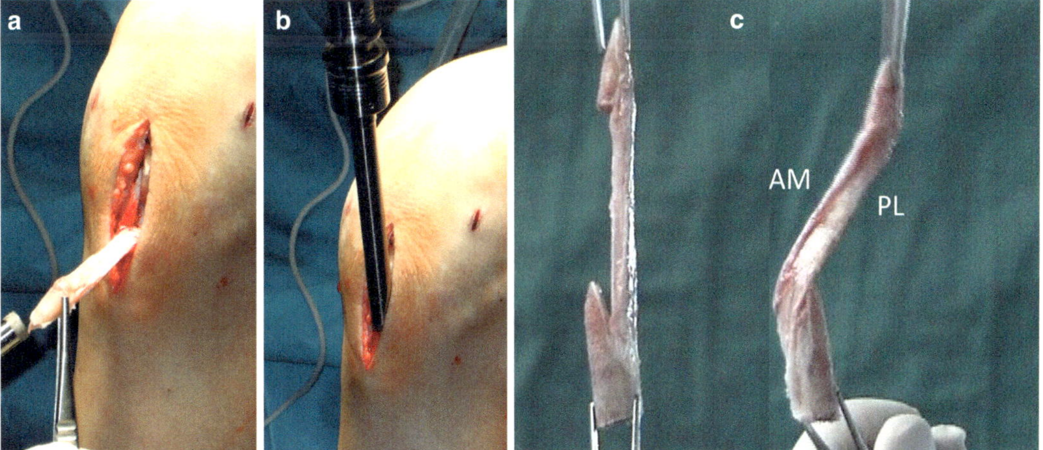

Fig. 5.10 (**a**) A 9-mm hollow miller is inserted in a flat angle over the distal patella. The harvested half cylinder with the central third of the patellar tendon is placed into (**b**) the 11-mm miller and a 2-cm bone cylinder is milled out (**c**, original from 1998). A patellar bone-tendon-bone graft is harvested with a 9- and 10-mm bone cylinder on each side. The ribbon-like graft mimics the anteromedial and posterolateral bundle

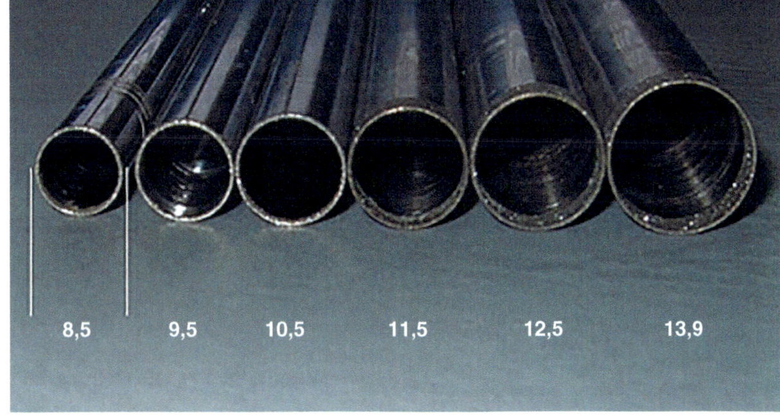

Fig. 5.11 Diamond hollow reamer for anterior cruciate ligament reconstruction and revision work as wet grinding process with water to cool and clean. Diameters range from 8 to 14 mm. Standard used 8–11 mm

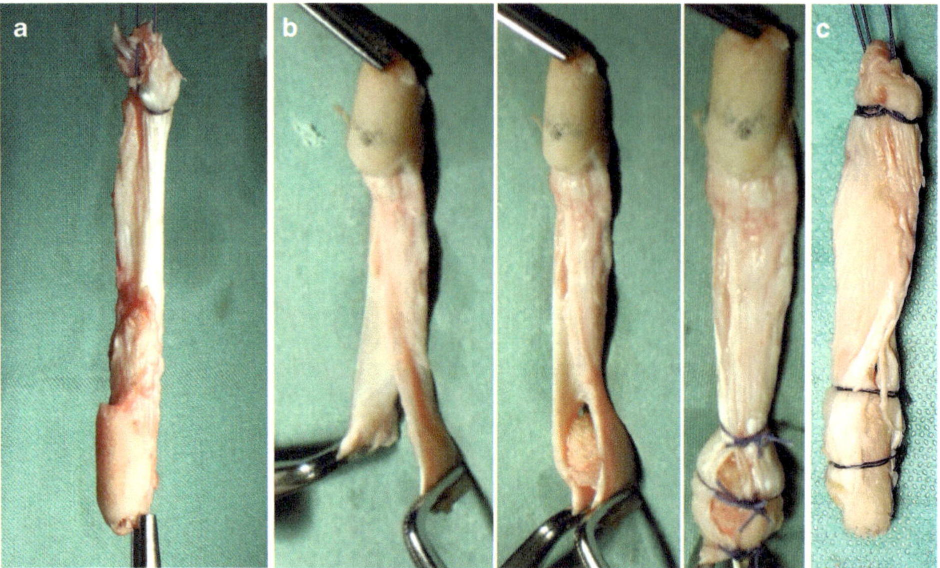

Fig. 5.12 The quadriceps tendon is harvested from the central third and the anterior two thirds of the quadriceps tendon with a width of 8–10 mm and a length of about 70 mm. Adherent on the ligament a "half bone cylinder" can be harvested with a hollow miller (**a**). A 9.4-mm bone cylinder from the tibial head analogous to the hamstring graft can be sutured in the proximal bisected quadriceps tendon for a bone-tendon-bone graft (**b**)—or as our standard today—used in this way while harvested without a patellar bone cylinder (**c**). Implantation follows analogously (Figs. 5.7 and 5.8)

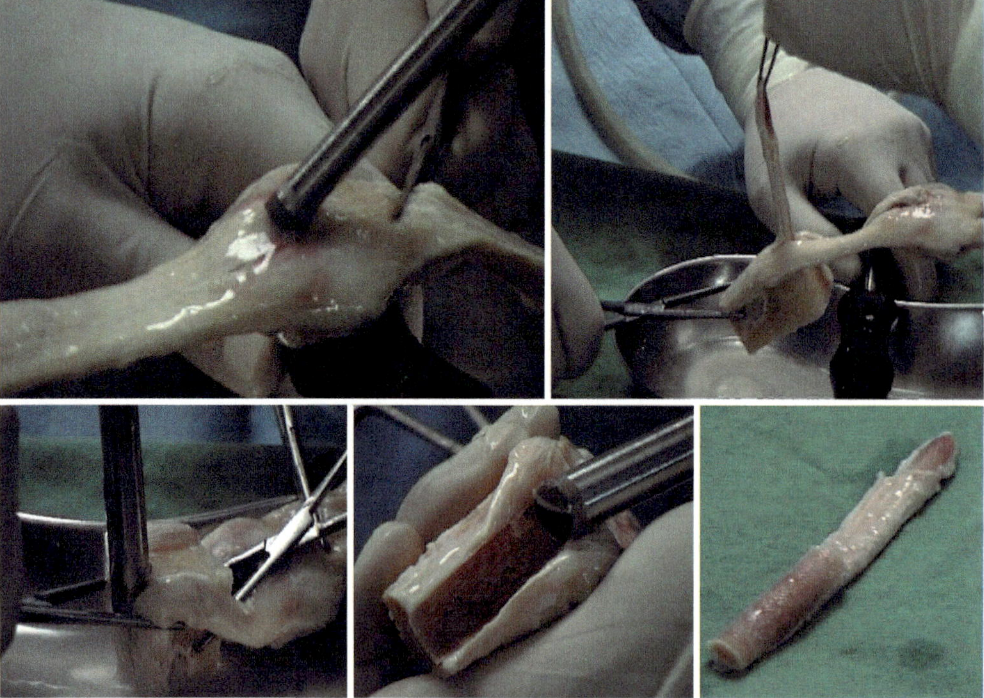

Fig. 5.13 Out of a homologous patella-ligament-tibia a patellar bone-tendon-bone graft was harvested with a diamond hollow reamer and all press-fit in three cases in 1998

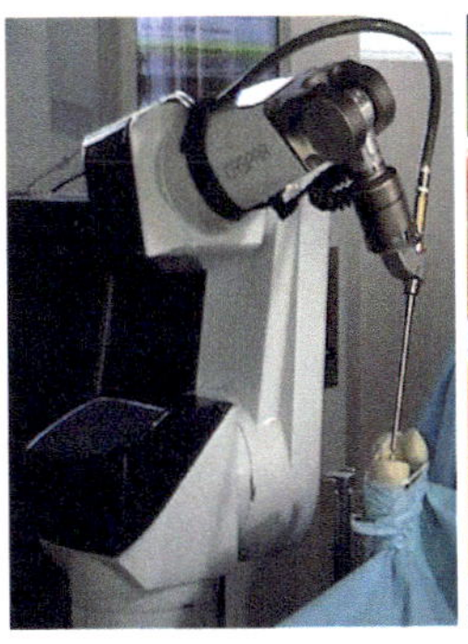
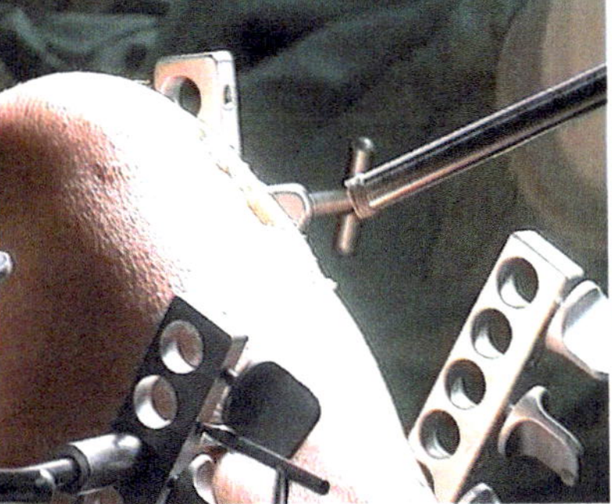
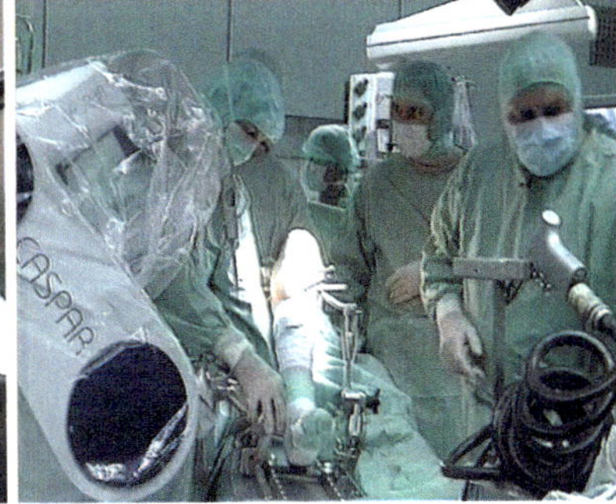

Fig. 5.14 The late 1990s were the time of robotics in surgery. The German Computer Assisted Surgical Planning and Robotics from Orthomaquet, in Rastatt, Germany (CASPAR) requested CT matching and planning for surgery. Prof. Gotzen and Dr. Petermann from the University of Marburg, Germany performed live surgery to a audiance in a theatre on 28 April 1998 in Rastatt with a diamond reamer from Felmets equipment

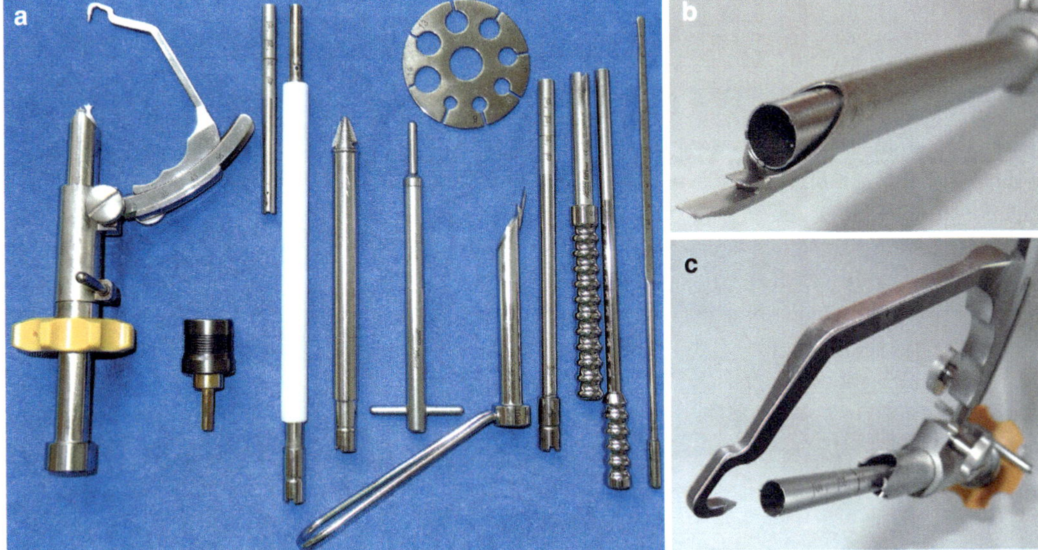

Fig. 5.15 In 2004, Felmet presented his press-fit technique for hamstrings with tubed guiding devices. (**a**) Standard set with 9-mm hollow reamer, femoral and tibial (extender) adapter, universal drilling machine adapter, cone reamer and cone pusher, harvester, applicator, ruler, (**b**) femoral guide, (**c**) tibial guide [39]

In 2004, Felmet presented his press-fit technique for hamstrings with newly developed tubed guiding [39] (Figs. 5.15 and 5.16). The hamstring was quadrupled and a 9-mm bone cylinder from the tibial tunnel was inserted (Fig. 5.17). The bone cylinder had a "bone window" for bone-to-bone healing and to create a C-shape like the original tibial insertion (Fig. 5.18). The graft is proximally inserted into the femoral bone cylinder ribbon like to mimic the bundles [51] (Fig. 5.19).

From 2005, the instruments were manufactured in Germany by Articomed Ltd, with Reinhard Feinmechanik GmbH in Dietzenbach, Germany. Because of hygienic issues, disposable diamond cutters were designed with alpha lock connectors in 2007. Different diameters, each with extractors and applicators and tubed guiding devices where produced. Front ends with stable mechanics for solid bone, aggressive cutting, and less heat for cheap production were postulated.

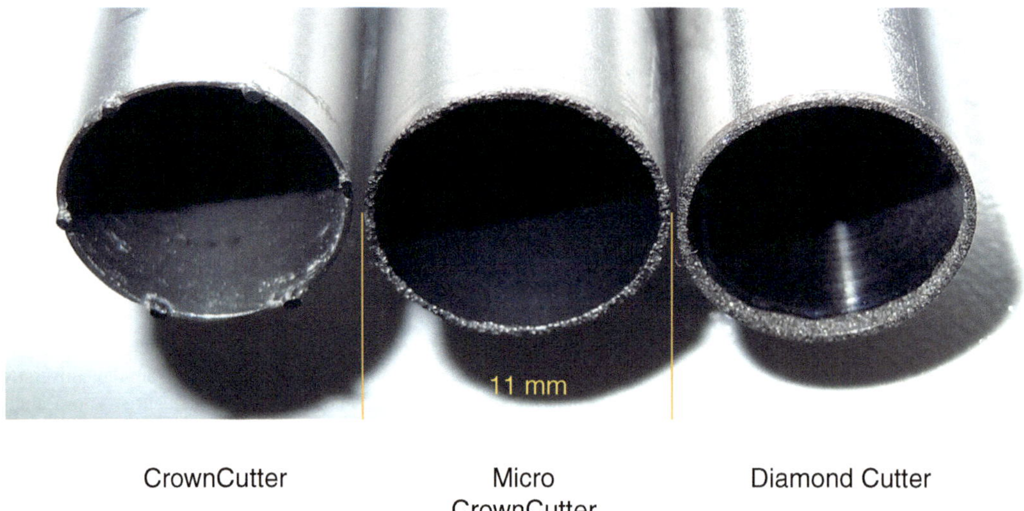

Fig. 5.16 "Crown cutter" and "micro crown cutter" were followed by particularly resistant metal for diamonds in 2010

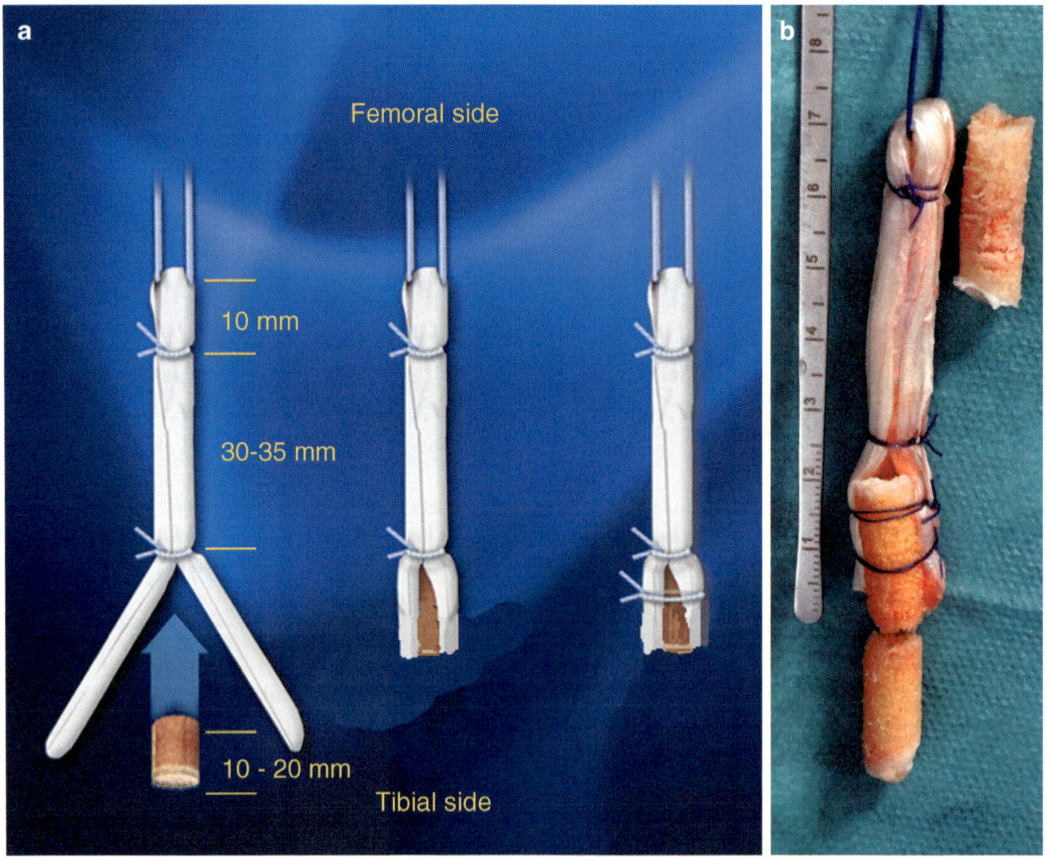

Fig. 5.17 (**a**) A 9.5-mm bone plug from the tibia is inserted into the quadrupled hamstring. The femoral side suture indicates the minimum length in the femoral tunnel. The tibial side sutures keep the tibial bone cylinder (**b**). The bone plugs 9.5 mm in diameter from the tibial and femoral tunnel in position of their later implantation. The "bone window" is for the tibial C-shaped bone to heal

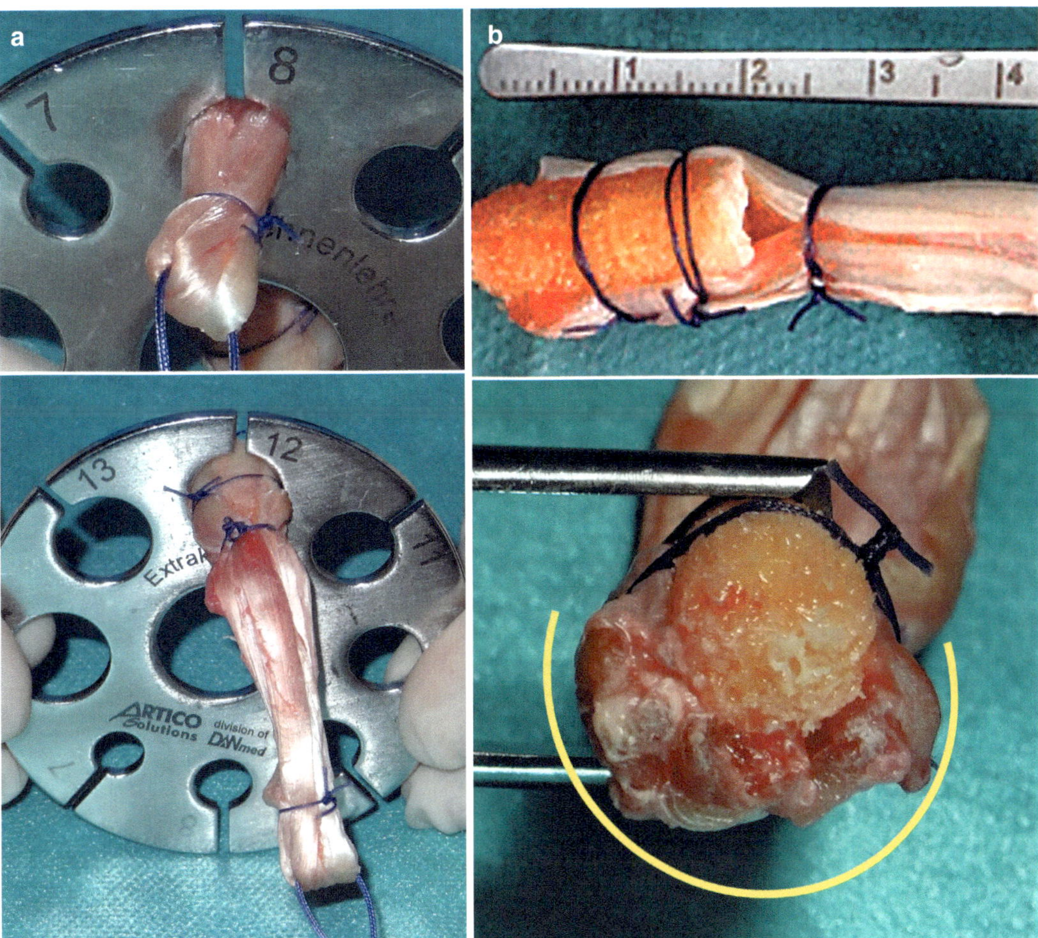

Fig. 5.18 Graft diameter is about 8–9 mm; the tibial diameter with a 9-mm bone cylinder is about 12 mm (**a**). The proximal half of the 9-mm bone cylinder from the tibial tunnel is sutured on the distal graft as a C-shaped tibial side (**b**)

They were implemented in 2010 by a second manufacturer ARTICOsolutions, a division of Dannoritzer Medical Instruments in Tuttlingen, Germany, as the next generation together with the "crown cutter" [52]. The "Micro Crown Cutter" with extra resistant metal was the replacement for the original "Diamond Cutter" (Figs. 5.15 and 5.16). Instruments were interchangeable between the different generations, which eased a switch to the new leading pieces (Table 5.2).

Despite all the efforts, technical improvements, and publications, a resounding success did not materialize. In 2008 and the following years, the first implantations were performed in Poland. High interest and being convinced by the results of the established opinion leader of knee surgeons in Egypt helped to establish all press-fit ACL reconstruction at the Cairo University with Prof. Singergy, Prof. Ezzat Kamel, Prof. Adel Hamid, Prof. Ahmed Abdel Aziz, and in other places (Fig. 5.20). A fruitful input with the experience of excellent surgeons and thousands of ACL reconstructions in Egypt also helped to simplify and optimize the standard of the press-fit fixation with excellent results up to today.

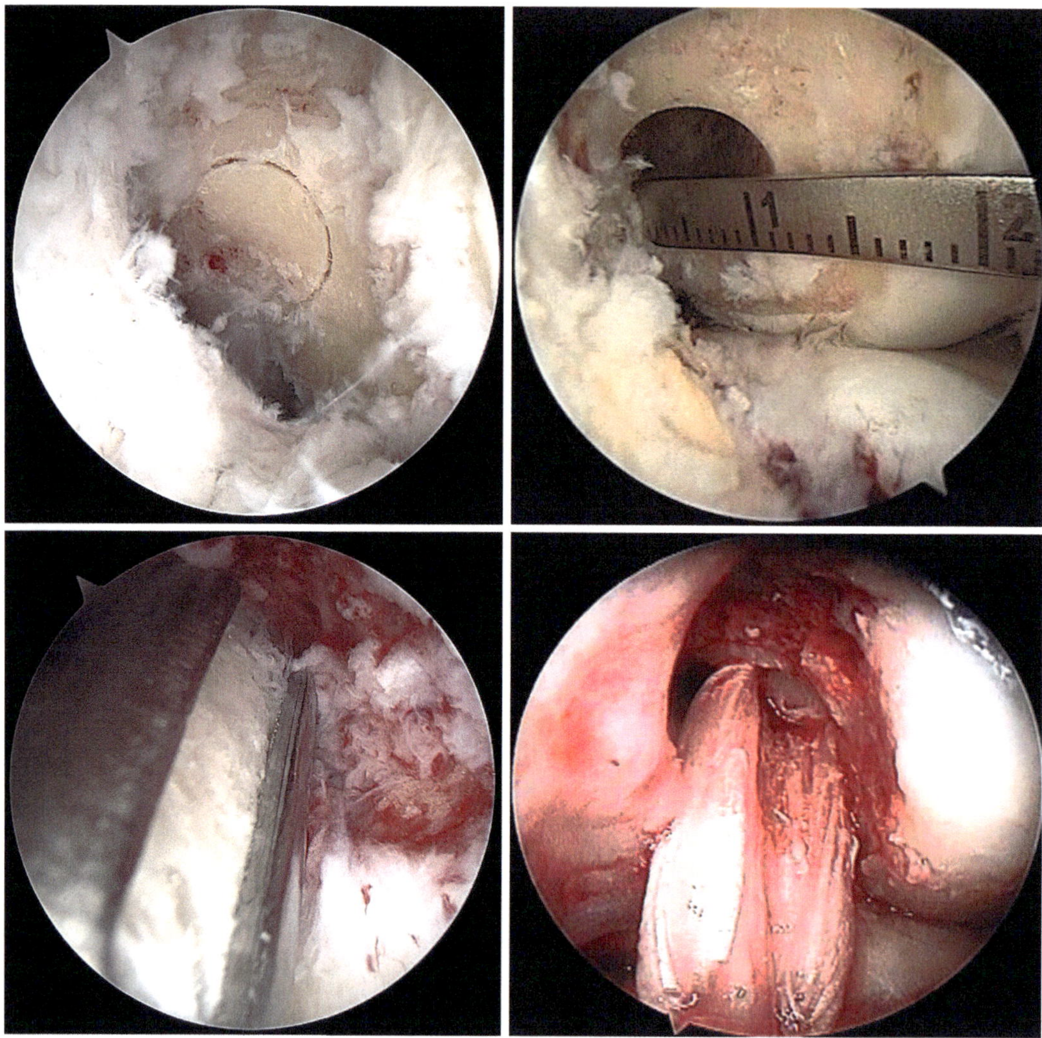

Fig. 5.19 The femoral tunnel is placed at the original insertion and proved after a "probe cutting" through the antero-medial (AM) portal. The tunnel should overlap the intermediate ridge between AM and posterolateral bundle insertion. The individual size here with a 9.5-mm crown cutter is an oval, measured by a ruler of 11 mm. The crescent-shaped femoral insertion mimics the two bundles ribbon like along the intercondylar ridge

Table 5.2 The ideal ACL reconstruction was postulated and could be fulfilled by foreign material free press-fit technique at all points

10 rules were postulated for an ideal ACL reconstruction
1. Fixation near the original insertion
2. Broad proximal ribbon-like insertion to mimic the bundles
3. No foreign material
4. Biological healing by press-fit fixation
5. MRI control without artifacts
6. No enlarged bone defects for ease in revision
7. Primary stability for
8. Fast rehabilitation
9. Secure simple, standardized, reproducible, sustainable surgical technique
10. With low costs

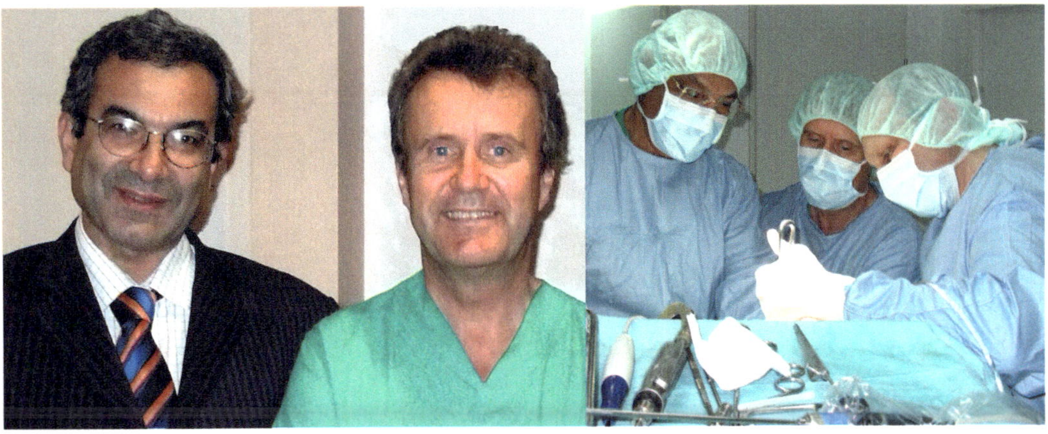

Fig. 5.20 The leading figures in Egypt with Prof. Adel Hamid and Prof. Ezzad Kamel visited the Artico Sports clinic for education in the all press-fit method in 2009. and from left: Prof. Abdel Aziz El Singergy, later head of the Department of Orthopaedics and Traumatology of Cairo University, Egypt; Right hand side in the OR: Prof. Ahmed Abdel Aziz, Gernot Felmet and Alexander Gassert

5.4 "Against the Wind": How to Establish a Scientific Working Group for Foreign Material-Free ACL Replacement

In 2002, a cooperation of the leading German authors of work on foreign material-free and biological ACL reconstruction started. In 2003, a series of annual meetings began in Villingen-Schwenningen/Black Forest and later at the University of Hannover, Germany (Figs. 5.21 and 5.22). A lot of political work had to be done to finally create the AGA Knee Ligament Committee in 2014. In a letter to the AGA Knee Ligament Committee, Felmet summarized in 2017:

> Let me look back over the last 14 years from an idea until today:
> Historically, it was the common idea, fascination, and activity regarding foreign material-free cruciate ligament replacement procedures on the knee that united us:
> Peter Hertel (Berlin), Hans Pässler (Heidelberg), Gernot Felmet (VillingenSchwenningen), and Manfred Bernard (Berlin), as well as Paul Hefner, (Offenburg/Baden-Baden), Harald Boszotta (Eisenstadt, Austria), and many others.
>
> The idea grew to bundle and spread this knowledge (from 2003 onwards). The 'Joint Symposium in Villingen-Schwenningen and in Hannover' had particularly addressed this topic in the following years thanks to the commitment of Peter Hertel and the support of Helmut Lill, further development was achieved for scientific and professional social connections:
> As working group 'Arthroscopic Surgery 22.10.2009 within the DGOU (German Society of Orthopaedic and Traumatology)' established with spezial interest for 'Foreign material-free cruciate ligament reconstruction and biological optimization.' Later, it was because of the support of Harald Boszotta, AGA—Congress President in Vienna 2010 at that time that a transfer to the AGA IFK Committee 'Implant-free cruciate ligament replacement and biological optimization' was possible and subsequently as the official constitution at the AGA Congress in Regensburg in 2011. In 2014, at the AGA Meeting in Innsbruck/Austria, the 'AGA Knee Ligament Committee' was founded.
>
> The Knee Ligament Committee has now positioned itself very positively thanks to its activities. I would like to thank all of you who have contributed to this again very warmly! I have only one wish: 'May the future activities not forget the material-free biological anchoring concepts. No matter how big the conflict of interest is.'
>
> In the long term, it is the compromises of 'doing one thing and not letting others do it,' such as a hybrid system, which many have long been successful at.
>
> Intensive research is still necessary.
>
> The interest of the industry and the conflict for formation of a fair and comprehensive opinion can be lived in this way, wisely, perhaps also in the long term.

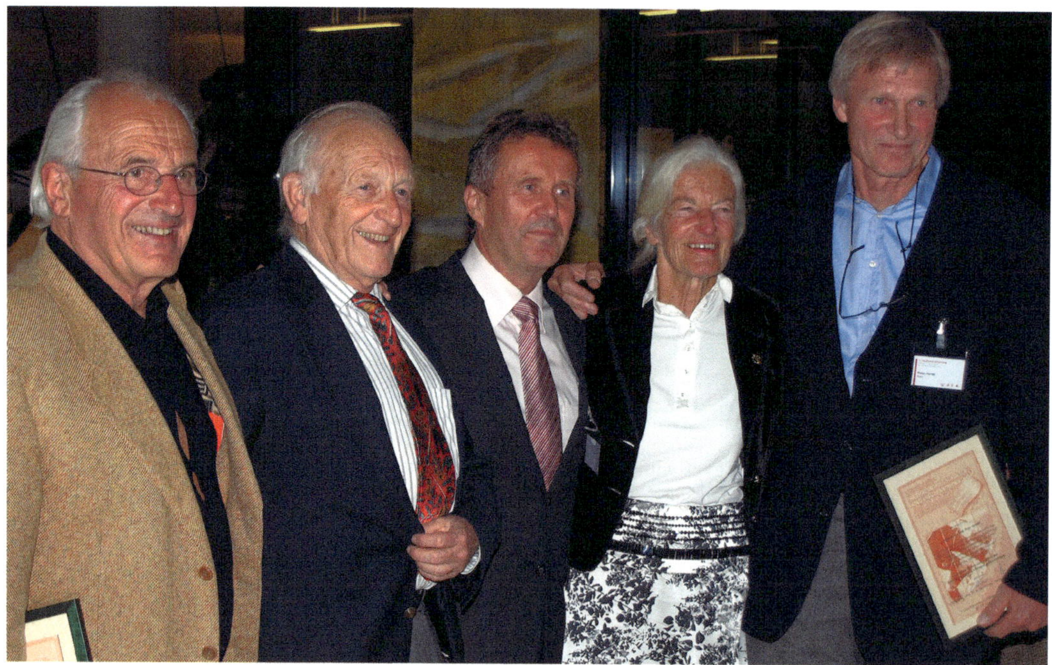

Fig. 5.21 Hans Paessler, Werner Mueller, Gernot Felmet, and Peter Hertel at the "Gelenk-Symposium" in Villingen-Schwenningen, 2009

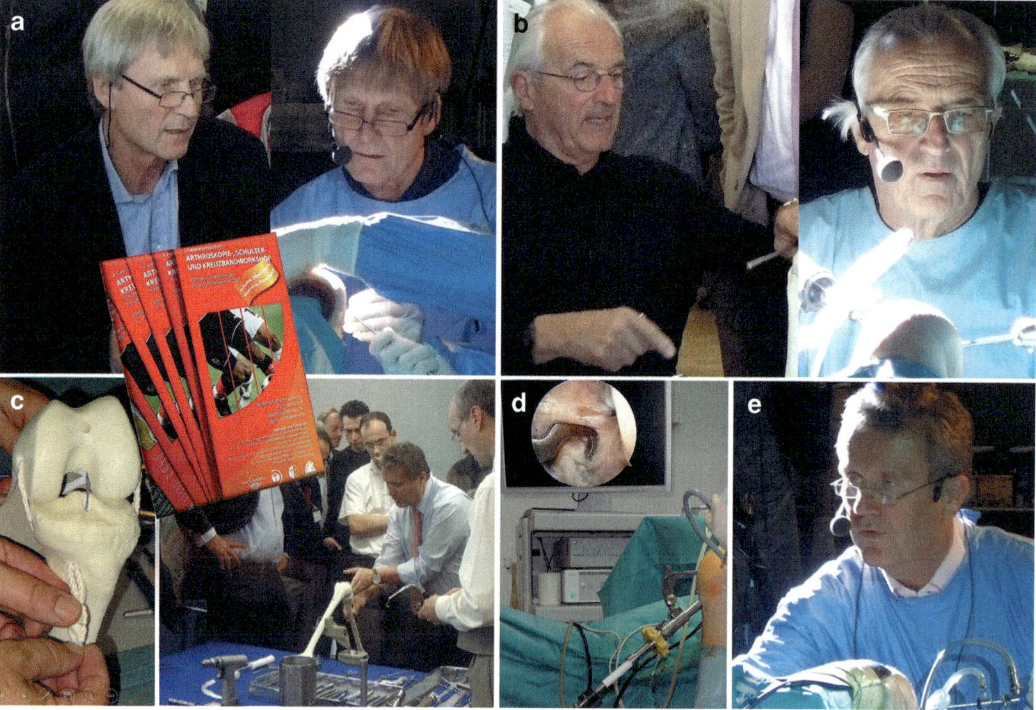

Fig. 5.22 Annual workshops and teaching. (**a**) Peter Hertel, (**b**) Hans Paessler, (**c**, **d**) saw bone and cadaver, (**e**) G. Felmet (pictures 2004 to 2015)

Several brochures and books in the German language were published out of the activities of the Ligament Committee and other committees (http://www.aga-online.ch/komitees).

In 2015, the Biological Ligament and Joint Academy was established to spread and teach among other issues the press-fit fixation technique and biological treatment on joints. It was an activity out of the European Federation of Orthopedic and Sports Traumatology (EFOST). Felmet was president at that time and guided EFOST to the new established European Sports Medicine Associates as a section of the European Society for Sports Traumatology, Knee Surgery and Arthroscopy.

5.5 Stability of Fixation

Biomechanical strength testing of press-fit techniques has been studied in detail by various authors. Most of the work has been done on femoral-sided fixation. Rupp et al. compared femoral press-fit fixation with biodegradable and titanium IF screws in porcine lower limbs. They found significantly higher ultimate loads in screws than in press-fit [53]. Musahl et al. also compared press-fit femoral fixation with IF screw fixation in the hind limbs of Saanen breed goats. In their analysis, no statistical significant difference was found between the two groups based on the cyclic creep tests and uniaxial tensile loading. But they also noted a lower ultimate load for press-fit fixation versus screw fixation. Data from their study supported early functional postoperative rehab regimens but suggested tailoring the rehab protocols to allow bone healing [14]. Seil et al. used a cyclic loading protocol in porcine lower limbs. The press-fit group failed in five specimens [54]. The authors concluded that press-fit fixation is not secure enough for an accelerated rehabilitation protocol.

On the contrary, Lee et al. compared femoral press-fit fixation performed with a 1.4-mm oversized bone plug to IF screw and reported no difference in stiffness and linear load, or failure mode [15]. Kuhne et al. reported an average primary stability amounted to 570 N (±100 N) for the bone-blocking BTB technique, and to 402 N (±79 N) for IF screw fixation [55]. Mayr et al. reported the same fixation properties for a press-fit dowel (slashed circle 7 mm) with a 100-N axial load and IF screw [56].

Authors have also investigated the effect of variables such as loading direction, the length of the bone plug and the method of preparation for the femoral tunnel. Schmidt-Wiethoff measured a failure rate of 333 N for a length of 25 mm and recommended a length of the bone cylinder of 20–30 mm [16]. Pavlik et al. measured an ultimate tensile strength of 534 N at 45° [57] and Seil et al. at an angle of 80° between load axis and tunnel axis with 708 N (±211) [54]. Dargel et al. found a higher fixation quality for a dilated tunnel up to 1 mm and thereby compacting cancellous bone [11]. He also reported comparable failure loads for QT patellar bone and patellar BTB in a cadaveric study. Kilner et al. [31] compared the knot/press-fit technique for hamstrings with the commonly used Endobutton technique and found no difference in anterior tibial translation response to an anterior tibial load. Stiffness of the knot/press-fit complex was found to be 37.8 N/mm, and the load at failure was 540 N, which was comparable with other devices. Similar findings were noted for knot/press-fit hamstrings by Lin et al. [32].

Press-fit tibial fixation has been compared with other commonly used methods. Boszotta et al. showed a significantly higher primary stability of 758 N (range 513–993 N) for press-fit fixation in comparison with IF screw 572 N (range 473–680 N), staple 608.4 N (range 511–727 N), and suture over a bone bridge 304.5 N (range 120–327 N) [58]. Jagodzinski et al. found the highest maximum load to failure for the extra tape fixed press-fit fixation at 970 ± 83 N, followed by IF screw fixation at 544 ± 109 N, and suture press-fit fixation at 402 ± 78 N [59]. In the porcine femur, Ettinger et al. found that a tibial press-fit technique that uses an additional bone block has a better maximum load to failure than an IF screw fixation. But for the bone block fixation-only technique (the author's technique) it was found to be 290 ± 74 N only [60]. The same group investigated tibial posterior cruciate ligament (PCL) fixation. The maximum load to failure was 518 ± 157 N for the hamstring with a knot, 558 ± 119 N for the interference screw, and 620 ± 102 N (541–699 N) for the QT bone block [61]. Arnold et al. found a femoral pull-out of the femoral tunnel with a median ultimate load to failure of 852 N (R = 448–1349 N) [13].

5.6 Techniques for All Press-Fit

5.6.1 Patellar BTB

The use of a diamond wet grinding hollow milling cutter (Surgical Diamond Instruments) since 1998 has given us a reproducible precision of 0.2 mm of the bone dowels for press-fit fixation in different diameters. This was the first time that it was possible to harvest the BTB patellar ligament with different diameters of bone cylinders with a hollow milling cutter system. Currently, we use a sharper crown cutter as a hollow reamer, which produces less heat and has low-priced disposables.

The patellar bone half-cylinder has a diameter of 9 mm. This bone cylinder at the central third of the patellar tendon is inserted into the 11-mm hollow reamer. The complete graft is harvested as a bone cylinder with a diameter of 9 and 11 mm on each side (Fig. 5.10). The tibial 9.5-mm and femoral 9.5-mm tunnels are made with a hollow reamer (Figs. 5.11 and 5.16). K-wire guiding devices can be used with a central adapter. Special guiding devices with tubes for a hollow reamer have been developed for precise and reliable positioning of the tunnels (Fig. 5.15). The femoral guide is placed with the longer tip behind the femoral condyle in 9.30 or 2.30 o'clock positions. The correct position in the original insertion is proved through the anteromedial portal. It should overlap with the intermediate ridge between the AM and PL bundle. Diameter can be measured by a ruler and can be chosen up to 11 mm in larger knees for individual reconstruction [51] (Fig. 5.19). The tibial tube guide is positioned in the original insertion. Depending on the graft size an 8- or 9-mm tibial tunnel is milled.

As opposed to common fixation, the graft is implanted from distal to proximal. We turned the common procedure upside down into the BTT implantation (Fig. 5.8).

BTT Fixation

First, the graft is fixed press-fit with the tibial bone cylinder near the joint beyond the eminentia intercondylaris. At a 120° knee flexion the 9-mm bone cylinder from the patella is inserted with the ligament into the femoral tunnel and pressed in. The bone cylinder from this tunnel fixes the ligament near the joint.

The ligament is tightened in flexion. Mechanically, the ACL is lax in flexion. Extending the knee, the graft has self-adapted tension on the basis of the physiological knee function. Later, the tunnel is closed with the bone cylinder from this tunnel [52] (Figs. 5.9 and 5.17).

5.6.2 Hamstring

Based on this method we developed a technique for a hamstring graft in 2003.

The semitendinosus and gracilis tendons are harvested. For a diameter of about 8 mm and a length of 70 mm the semitendinosus or both tendons are folded three or four times.

The femoral tunnel is drilled with the guiding device in the anatomical insertion for 9 mm. The tibial tunnel is drilled by the tibial guiding device for 9 mm like the femur. Two bone cylinders (femur + tibia) are harvested (Fig. 5.17).

The folded hamstring is marked at the femoral end with a suture at 10 mm (for minimum depth in the femoral tunnel). At a distance of 3–4 cm a bone cylinder from the tibial tunnel 10–20 mm long is sutured into the graft in a C-shape (Figs. 5.17 and 5.18).

In a BTT fixation, the graft is inserted from distal to proximal and is first fixed directly under the tibial plateau press fit with the 11-mm bone cylinder. The proximal graft is pulled into the femoral tunnel and fixed with the 9-mm bone cylinder (harvested from this tunnel) in 120° knee flexion. The intermediate ridge has to be covered.

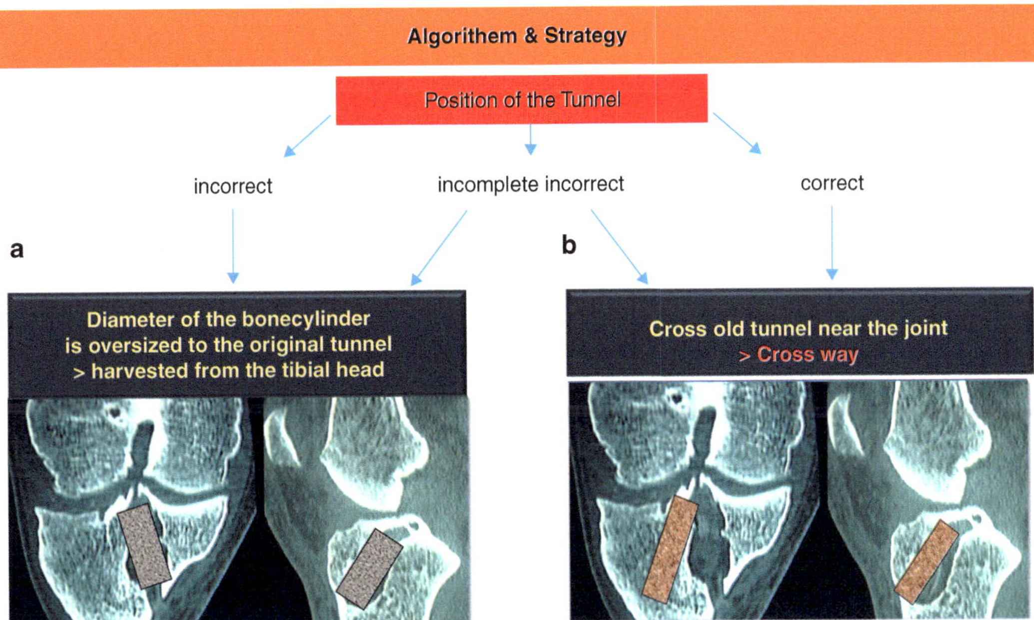

Fig. 5.23 The strategy in revision offers in plan (**a**) the use of an oversized bone cylinder from the tibial head only—in a diameter "plus 1 mm" of the old tunnel—to fix the graft and close the defect in one step. Plan (**b**) uses the "crossway" as a tunnel parallel to the first tunnel

The press-fit fixation with the bone cylinder forms a crescent shape to imitate the AM and PL bundle [51] (Fig. 5.19). The ligament is now tightened in knee flexion. Extending the knee, the graft has self-adapted tension in each fiber. The tunnel is closed with the bone cylinder from this tunnel (Fig. 5.17).

Similar principles can be applied for PCL reconstruction using a press-fit hamstring autograft (Fig. 5.23). A secondary fixation in the manner of a suture over a cortical bridge can be used if the bone quality is debatable.

5.6.3 Quadriceps Tendon

The QT was used in the past for revision cases. Today, we use it in primary ACL reconstruction. The mid-third of the QT is harvested at 10–12 mm in width, 4–5 mm in thickness and 80 mm in length. An attempt is made not to open the knee joint. A half bone cylinder can be harvested with a hollow reamer (crown cutter, micro crown cutter, or diamond miller) from the proximal patella connected to the tendon. The bone cylinder can be harvested with an inclined cut from distally onto the QT. Alternatively, the prepared QT third is inserted into the hollow miller and the cut is made from proximally. To receive a BTB graft an 9- to 11-mm bone cylinder is harvested, usually from the tibial tunnel, and sutured in the bifurcated proximal QT analogous to the preparation of the hamstring. This can be helpful in revisions. In primary reconstruction we prefer the free QT graft without patellar bone—secondarily armed with the 9-mm bone cylinder from the tibial head (Fig. 5.12). Implantation is done in the BTT fixation with self-adapted tensioning (Figs. 5.8 and 5.9).

5.6.4 Revision

Bone plug fixation is easy in revision—sometimes in a single step. After re-rupture of a press-fit ACL reconstruction with any common graft a second reconstruction can be performed with the remaining graft on this side using the same tech-

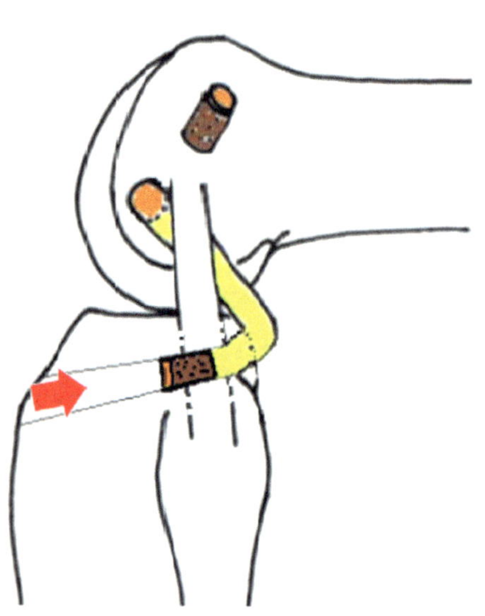

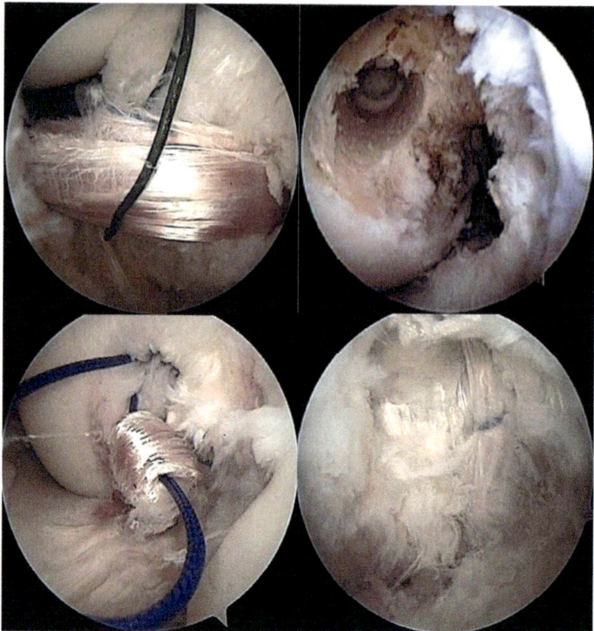

Fig. 5.24 The posterior cruciate ligament is reconstructed with a hamstring prepared with the bone dowel from the tibial tunnel (Fig. 5.5) and fixed press-fit at the posterior tibial head. The graft is implanted through a tibial tunnel, cached and pulled forward into the anteromedial tunnel und fixed with a bone cylinder. A suture over a bone bridge at the medial femoral condyle is necessary

nique [62]. Adapted from the tunnel size different diameters of bone cylinders can be harvested (Figs. 5.11, 5.15, and 5.16). Different sizes of cortical-cancellous bone cylinders have been harvested from the tibial head and sutured to the tibial side of the graft. Therewith, the enlarged tunnel is closed and the graft is fixed in one stage. The femoral tunnel fixation is treated in the same way (Fig. 5.24). The "cross way" uses a new tunnel (e.g., with the patellar BTB graft through the harvesting defect at the tibial tubercle) while crossing the old tunnel only at the joint line of the plateau [62] (Fig. 5.24). A single-stage revision with 10-mm cylindrical bone allografts in a press-fit construct in combination with the ACL graft is reported [63]. Because of some compromises of the tunnel position, today we tend to use two stages. The hollow reamer eases the cleaning of the previous tunnels and saves bone. The applicator in different sizes fills the tunnels with autologous or homologous bone chips. After 3–4 months the bone stock quality is stable enough for an all press-fit ligament reconstruction without compromises.

5.6.5 Other Ligaments Reconstruction

Reconstruction of the PCL, lateral collateral ligament (LCL), medial collateral ligament (MCL) and medial patellar femoral ligament (MPFL) reconstruction are performed using the same method of a ligament–bone plug press-fit fixation. Because of lower bone stability it is helpful to add a suture over a bone bridge on the femoral side of fixation (Figs. 5.23, 5.25, 5.26, and 5.27).

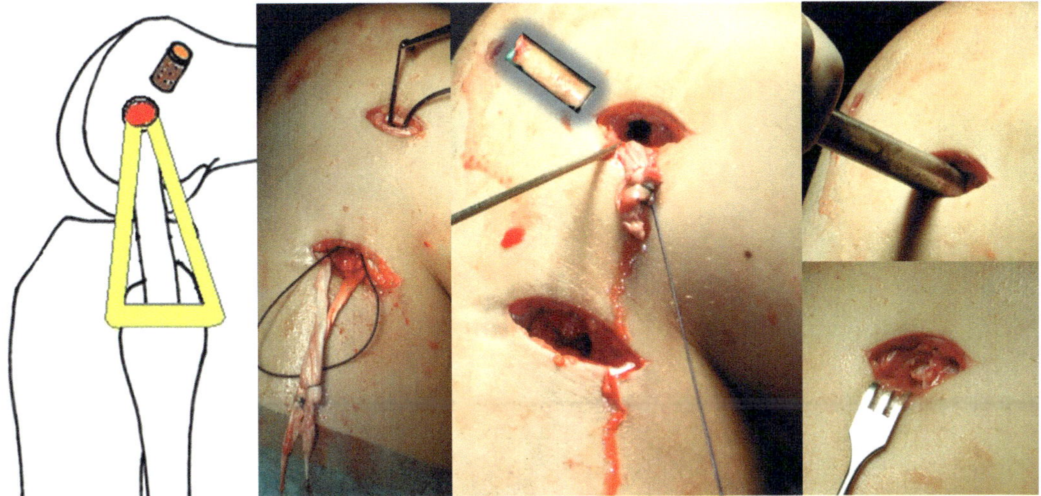

Fig. 5.25 A hamstring tendon is guided through a tunnel of the proximal fibular head and fixed press-fit in femoral anchorage with the bone dowel from this tunnel. A suture over a bone bridge at the medial femoral condyle is necessary

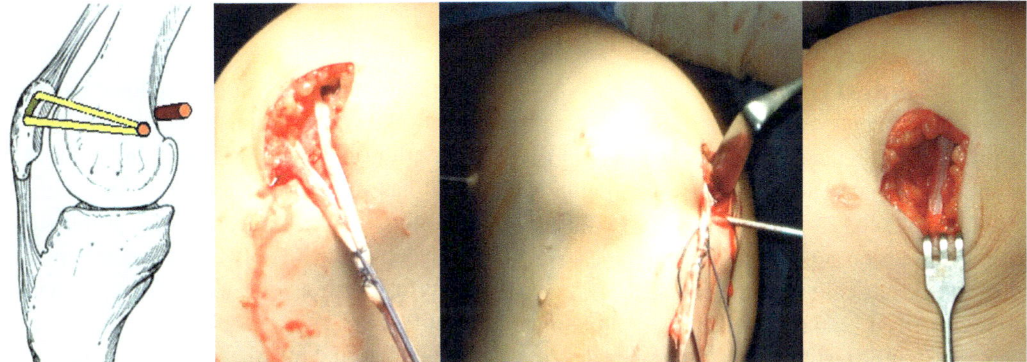

Fig. 5.26 In a right knee: a hamstring tendon is guided through a tunnel of the medial patella and fixed press-fit in a femoral anatomical anchorage with the bone dowel from this tunnel. The analogous lateral quadriceps tendon can be used (Fig. 5.28). A suture over a bone bridge at the lateral femoral condyle is necessary

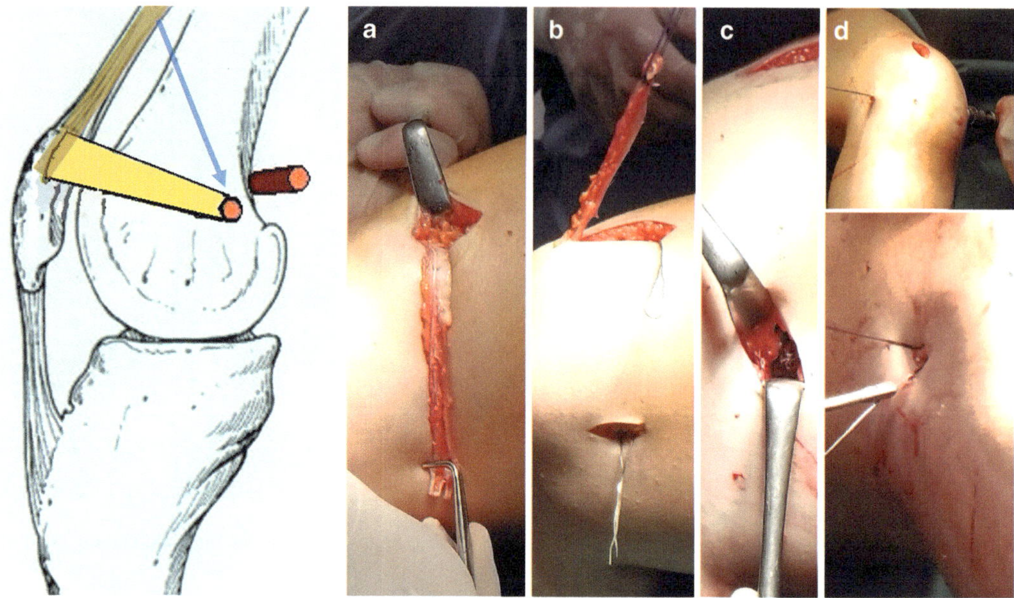

Fig. 5.27 In a right knee. (**a**) The lateral quadriceps tendon is separated approximately 90 mm in length and two thirds of the height and 10 mm in width. Adherent on the medial patella the skin is tunneled under with sutures (**b**) and the tendon is fixed press-fit in the anatomical femoral anchorage with the bone dowel from this tunnel (**c**). A suture over a bone bridge is necessary at the lateral femoral condyle (**d**)

5.7 Clinical Outcome

Twelve studies report a total of 1096 individuals with foreign material-free press-fit fixation [1–4, 8, 34, 35, 42, 46, 52, 64, 65] (Table 5.1). Results overall have been good to excellent. Four cases of bone block loosening without clinical relevance were described [2, 52]. Patellar-femoral crepitus was noted in 10–40% cases. Long-term radiological signs of osteoarthritis were observed in 17–45%, more commonly in patients who had concomitant partial meniscectomy [1–3, 35, 52].

5.8 What We Learned

For accelerated rehabilitation, the initial fixation strength should be strong enough to counteract these resultant forces. Full extension of the knee by contraction of the quadriceps muscle has been shown to produce forces up to 200 N on the ACL graft [45]. Press-fit fixation for hamstrings on both sides has a stability of about 300 N at the tibial anchorage [60]. Early functional rehabilitation is followed in the postoperative period. The lower graft stability of the hamstring in the first 6 weeks has to be respected [66]. Free range of movement is allowed from day 1 in individuals with good bone quality. In cases where bone quality is questionable, we limit extension/flexion in 0–20–90 for 3 weeks in a brace. A brace then is suggested for week 4–6 after surgery. Full weight-bearing is possible at the 1-week if there is no contraindikation. We have shown positive effects of aquasprint [67] and proprioceptive vibration training on the quadriceps muscle [68]. Proprioceptive vibration training (PowerPlate, etc.) is used after 3 weeks postoperatively twice a week. We suggest undertaking clinical measurements of anterior stability with tools such as the Articometer, a digital Rolimeter, and muscle function tests after 3 months [67–70].

Most biomechanical studies are performed on porcine, bovine, or human cadavers, which exhibit different osseous properties. Pigs or goats have thick, non-elastic cortical bone but no cancellous bone. Human bone cylinder has stiff cortical and elastic cancellous bone. The behavior of viscoelastic strain and deformation can be observed in the freshly harvested cortical-cancellous bone cylinder. Cancellous bone swells after harvesting and an increase in bone diameter is noted when it is ready to be impacted into the tunnel. A similar viscoelastic deformity is working after fixing the press-fit graft inside the tunnel—this will mean that the fixation quality is higher after implantation. This is supported by clinical results with an excellent performance [2, 3, 52].

Direct bone contact is necessary for secure biological integration of the press-fit fixation, which takes around 4–6 weeks [16, 66]. It contributes to rapid and stable graft healing. If bone contact is lacking, atrophy of the tibial bone cylinder can be observed. This technique also involves fixation of the graft close to the tunnel entrance. It has multiple advantages. It avoids the "bungee effect," whereby the graft moves longitudinally within the tunnel because fixation is away from the tunnel entrance. It also prevents synovial fluid from entering the tunnel, hence, avoiding the possibly negative effects of cytokines [71]. A broad anatomical femoral insertion with autogenous bone plugs inserted near the cortex seems to improve rotational stability [51, 72, 73]. Individual follow-up demonstrates a flat femoral insertion along the posterior femoral cortex and a C-shaped ribbon like tibial insertion on digital volume tomography (DVT), a multislice computed tomography device, a two cone-beam CT (CBCT) device [74–77], MRI controls, and in re-rupture with arthroscopy (Figs. 5.28, 5.29, 5.30, and 5.31). Tunnel widening is mostly observed in combination with a high-volume, large-diameter graft, but is not usually widened near the joint. Bone cylinders are partially absorbed. This obviously follows Wolff's law of no force input at the deeper graft.

As with other fixation methods, press-fit fixation is adaptable to different graft types with good results [78] (Table 5.1). All press-fit fixation shows good results with patellar BTB at 10 years' follow-up. Better results with hamstrings and QTs might be achieved by a learning curve and the evolution of instruments and methods (Table 5.1). The latest reports of press-fit hamstring versus QT demonstrated similar stability and muscle strength to the uninjured side [5, 6, 9, 79]. In a 10-year prospective analysis no significant difference in stability was observed between press-fit QT versus patellar BTB [7].

There are two main issues, which makes revision ACL reconstruction quite challenging, i.e., removal of the primary fixation device and dealing with dilated tunnels. With press-fit fixation, both these issues are not seen. If tunnel widening is encountered, different diameter harvesters can be very useful. A larger bone cylinder can be harvested from the tibia and the dilated tunnel can be obliterated, making it possible to perform the procedure in single stage. A cross tunnel technique joining the old tibial tunnel has also been described [62] (Fig. 5.23).

A limitation of this technique is the technically demanding nature of the procedure as tunnel size mismatch can lead to inadequate fixation and hence risk of failure. Use of different sized reamers and tunnel compaction has made the procedure more precise and reproducible. Another problem is inadequate fixation in patients with osteoporotic bone, where secondary fixation might be required. The bone stock should be restored with autologous or homologous cancellous bone chips and a two-stage procedure is recommended. (See also Chap. 7.)

The knowledge of hollow reamers and press-fit fixation is transferred to the PCL (Fig. 5.24), the LCL (Fig. 5.25), the MCL and the MPFL with hamstring (Fig. 5.26), and the medial third of the QT (Fig. 5.27). Bone dowels harvested out of the tunnels are used for fixing the graft in a press-fit manner. Sutures over a bone bridge are suggested at anchorage in the mid or anterior femoral condyle because of soft bone and lower primary press-fit bone cylinder stability. Anatomical correct insertion mostly allows a self-adapted tension of the graft.

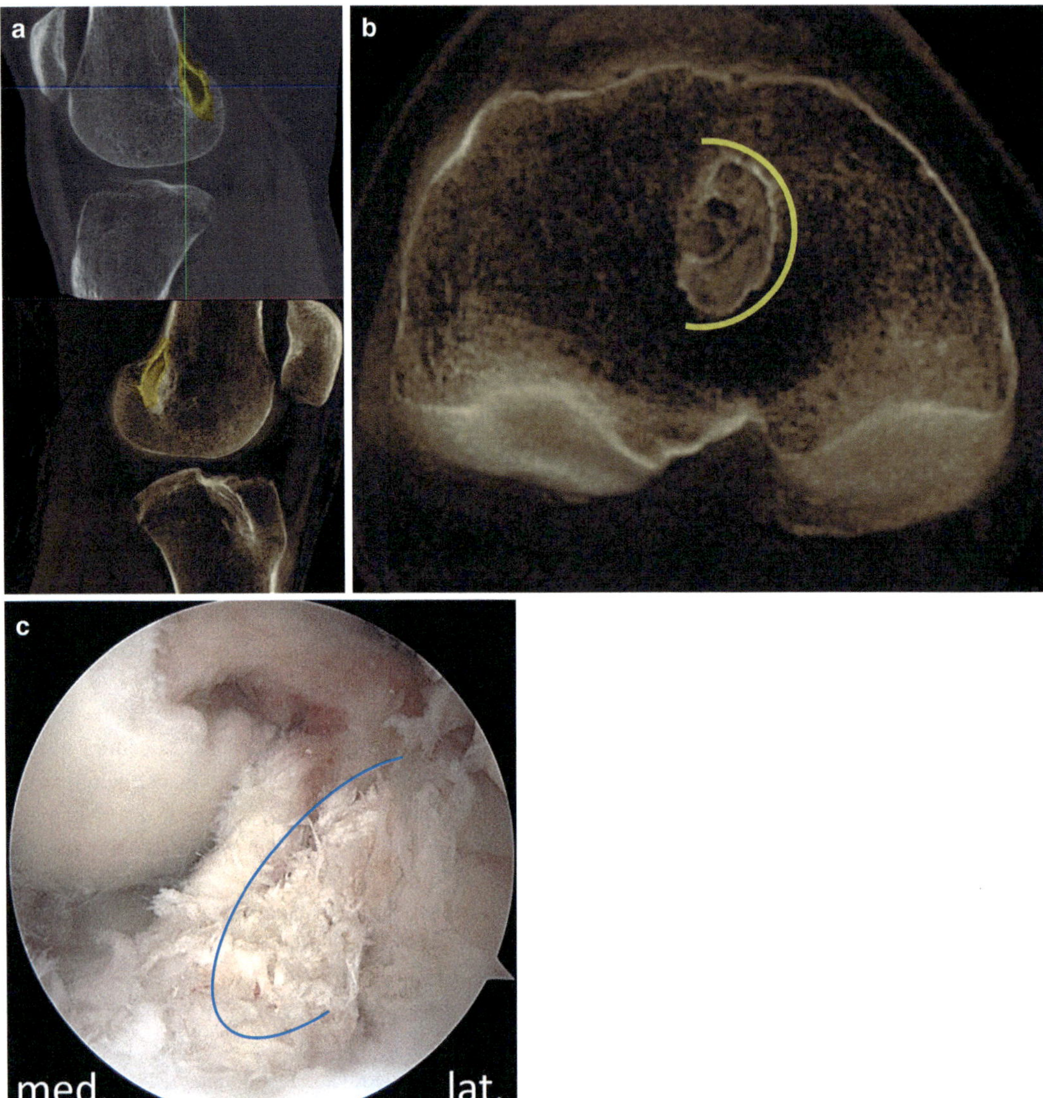

Fig. 5.28 (**a**) Digital volume tomography (DVT) after 2 years in a left knee, 46 years of age, female: anatomical foot print on the femoral side with ribbon-like insertion along the intercondylar ridge (**a**). (**b**) On the tibia a C-shaped insertion of the all press-fit fixed 8-mm quadrupled hamstring, as Smigielski and Siebold found [80–82]. DVT is a multislice computed tomography device, two cone-beam CT device [74–77]. (**c**) Re-rupture after 9 months in high-velocity skiing downhill, 43 years, male (left knee). Ribbon-like C-shaped footprint after resection of the stump (blue line)

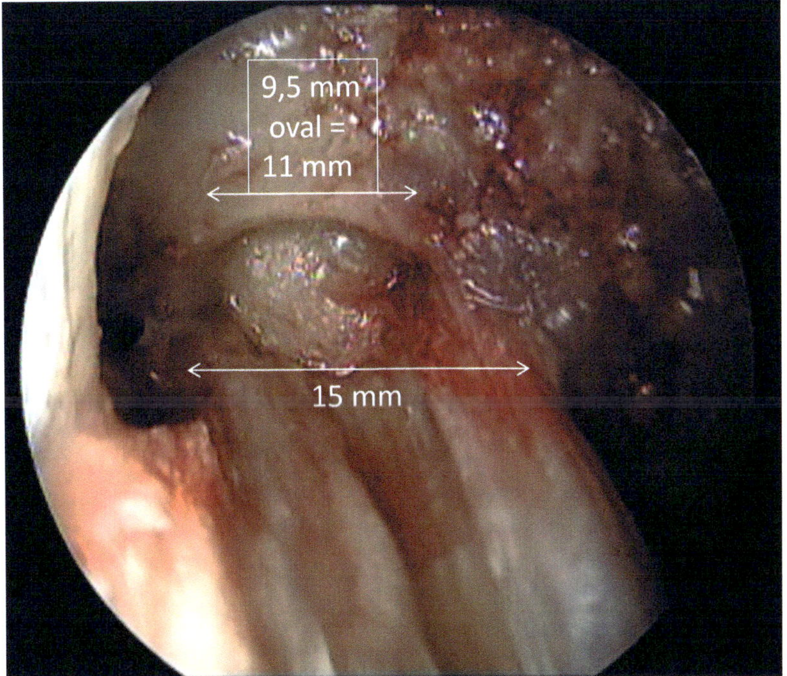

Fig. 5.29 The femoral insertion in an approximately 9.5-mm tunnel in reality gets as an oval a diameter of 11 mm. The graft itself has a width of about 15 mm, ribbon like [51]

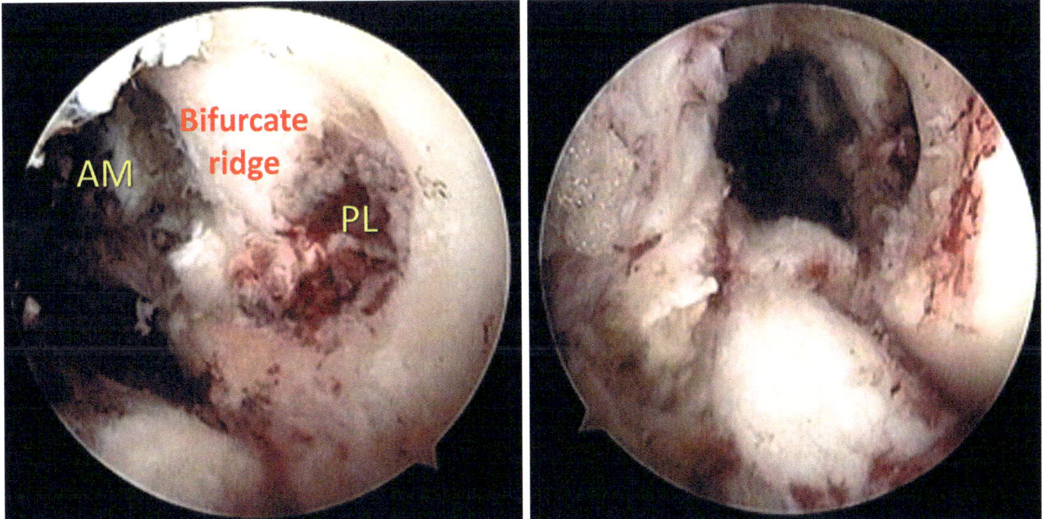

Fig. 5.30 Anatomical reorganization after 7 months with 8-mm hamstring: a re-rupture after 7 months showed an insertion of the two bundles in between a new bifurcate ridge under the intercondylar ridge [51]

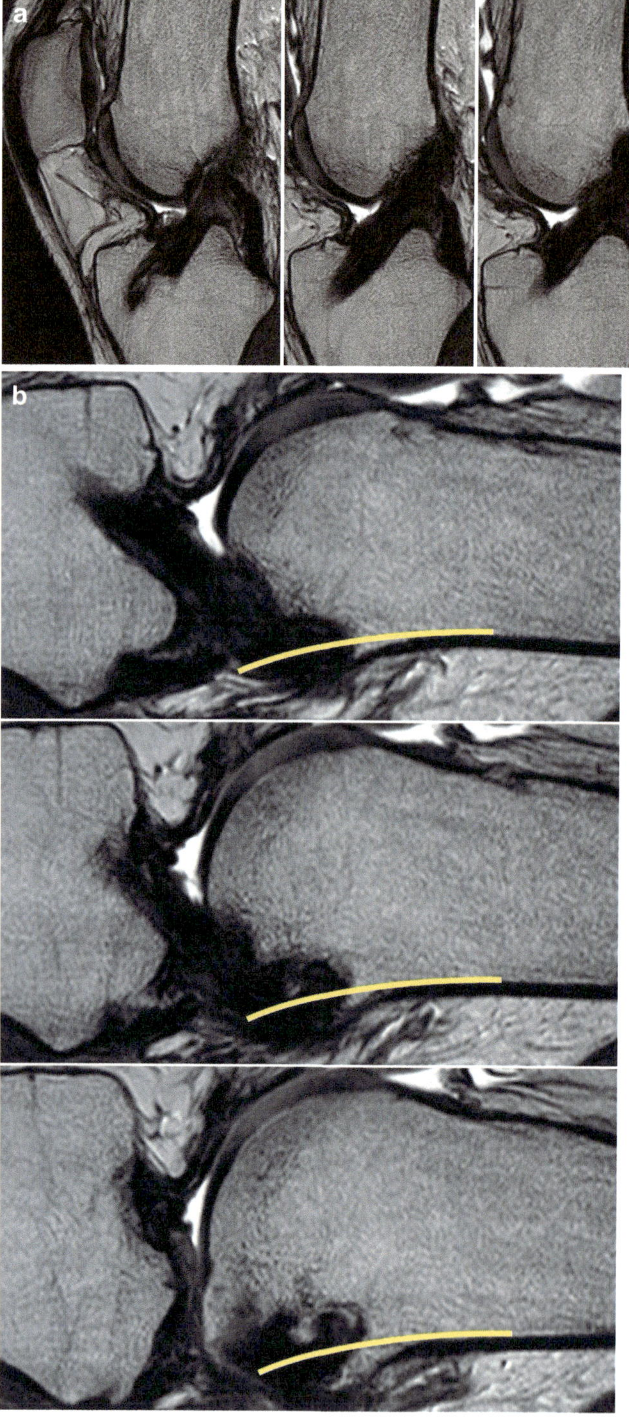

Fig. 5.31 (**a**) MRI 24 months after hamstring all press-fit fixation (28 years/male soccer player) with an anatomically reinsertion and fixation near the joint on both sides and excellent stability. (**b**) MRI 24 months after hamstring all press-fit fixation (28 years/male soccer player) with a direct insertion of the ribbon-like anterior cruciate ligament fibers in continuity with the posterior femoral cortex, as Smigielski described [82]

5.9 Conclusion

All press-fit fixation has been established for more than 25 years. Much input has been given to the methodology of ACL replacement in other techniques such as fixation near the joint at the original insertion with ribbon-like anatomical reconstruction of all grafts. It provides undisturbed bone-to-bone healing and avoids any problems associated with hardware fixation, such as graft laceration, biocompatibility, biodegradability, and local reactions leading tunnel enlargement. BTT is a trademark of biomechanical self-adapted tensioning of the graft. Ease of revision to restore the bone stock with hollow reamers and applicators save time and money. A growing number of sports trauma and re-ruptures place high financial pressure on health care systems and insurance schemes. An incentive by a German insurance company has been given as a higher financial rating of 10% of biological fixation since 2015. Knee surgeons should understand the principles of techniques that make implants in ligament surgery non-essential.

Pros

Biological approach

- Anatomical and individual insertion
- Ribbon like
- No implant-related complications
- Cost effective
- Decreased risk of tunnel widening
- No signal interference during follow-up MRI
- Relatively less challenging revision reconstruction
- Short learning curve

Cons

Modified rehabilitation in osteopenic bone and need for secondary fixation in the PCL, LCL, and MPFL.

References

1. Hertel P, Behrend H, Cierpinski T, Musahl V, Widjaja G. ACL reconstruction using bone-patellar tendon-bone press-fit fixation: 10-year clinical results. Knee Surg Sports Traumatol Arthrosc. 2005;13(4):248–55.
2. Felmet G. Implant-free press-fit fixation for bone-patellar tendon-bone ACL reconstruction: 10-year results. Arch Orthop Trauma Surg. 2010;130(8):985–92.
3. Felmet G. Implant-free anterior cruciate ligament reconstruction with diamond instruments. A biological and anatomic method for every ligament transplantation. Unfallchirurg. 2010;113(8):621–8.
4. Wipfler B, Donner S, Zechmann CM, Springer J, Siebold R, Paessler HH. Anterior cruciate ligament reconstruction using patellar tendon versus hamstring tendon: a prospective comparative study with 9-year follow-up. Arthroscopy. 2011;27(5):653–65.
5. Horstmann H, Felmet G, Tegtbur U, Krettek C, Jagodzinski M. Influence on graft choice between hamstring and quadriceps tendon on muscle function in implant free ACL reconstruction. DKOU; 28 October–31, 2014, Berlin.
6. Horstmann H, et al. Quadriceps and hamstring tendon autografts in ACL reconstruction yield comparably good results in a prospective, randomized controlled trial. Arch Orthop Trauma Surg. 2022;142(2):281–9.
7. Barie AHJ, Streich NA. Implant-free replacement of the anterior cruciate ligament – quadriceps tendon versus patellar tendon – long-term results of a prospective randomized clinical study. Knee Surg Sports Traumatol Arthrosc. 2012;20(1):34.
8. Akoto R, Hoeher J. Anterior cruciate ligament (ACL) reconstruction with quadriceps tendon autograft and press-fit fixation using an anteromedial portal technique. BMC Musculoskelet Disord. 2012;13:161.
9. Akoto R, Albers M, Balke M, Bouillon B, Hoher J. ACL reconstruction with quadriceps tendon graft and press-fit fixation versus quadruple hamstring graft and interference screw fixation – a matched pair analysis after one year follow up. BMC Musculoskelet Disord. 2019;20(1):109.
10. Dargel J, Schmidt-Wiethoff R, Schmidt J, Koebke J. Histomorphology and microradiography of quadriceps tendon-patellar bone grafts in press-fit anterior cruciate ligament reconstruction. J Orthop Res. 2005;23(5):1206–10.
11. Dargel J, Schmidt-Wiethoff R, Bruggemann GP, Koebke J. The effect of bone tunnel dilation versus extraction drilling on the initial fixation strength of press-fit anterior cruciate ligament reconstruction. Arch Orthop Trauma Surg. 2007;127(9):801–7.
12. Barie A, Kopf M, Jaber A, Moradi B, Schmitt H, Huber J, et al. Long-term follow-up after anterior cruciate ligament reconstruction using a press-fit quadriceps tendon–patellar bone autograft. BMC Musculoskelet Disord. 2018;19(1):368.
13. Arnold MP, Burger LD, Wirz D, Goepfert B, Hirschmann MT. The biomechanical strength of a hardware-free femoral press-fit method for ACL bone-tendon-bone graft fixation. Knee Surg Sports Traumatol Arthrosc. 2017;25(4):1234–40.
14. Musahl V, Abramowitch SD, Gabriel MT, Debski RE, Hertel P, Fu FH, et al. Tensile properties of an anterior

cruciate ligament graft after bone-patellar tendon-bone press-fit fixation. Knee Surg Sports Traumatol Arthrosc. 2003;11(2):68–74.
15. Lee MC, Jo H, Bae TS, Jang JD, Seong SC. Analysis of initial fixation strength of press-fit fixation technique in anterior cruciate ligament reconstruction. A comparative study with titanium and bioabsorbable interference screw using porcine lower limb. Knee Surg Sports Traumatol Arthrosc. 2003;11(2):91–8.
16. Schmidt-Wiethoff R, Dargel J, Gerstner M, Schneider T, Koebke J. Bone plug length and loading angle determine the primary stability of patellar tendon-bone grafts in press-fit ACL reconstruction. Knee Surg Sports Traumatol Arthrosc. 2006;14(2):108–11.
17. Dargel J, Schmidt-Wiethoff R, Schneider T, Bruggemann GP, Koebke J. Biomechanical testing of quadriceps tendon-patellar bone grafts: an alternative graft source for press-fit anterior cruciate ligament reconstruction? Arch Orthop Trauma Surg. 2006;126(4):265–70.
18. Geiges B, von Falck C, Knobloch K, Haasper C, Meller R, Krettek C, et al. Biodegradable screw versus a press-fit bone plug fixation for ACL reconstruction: a prospective randomized study. Unfallchirurg. 2013;116(2):109–17.
19. Jones KG. Reconstruction of the anterior cruciate ligament. A technique using the central one-third of the patellar ligament. J Bone Joint Surg Am. 1963;45:925–32.
20. Clancy WG, Nelson DA, Reider B, Narechania RG. Anterior cruciate ligament reconstruction using one-third of the patellar ligament, augmented by extra-articular tendon transfers. J Bone Joint Surg Am. 1982;64(3):352–9.
21. Creenshaw AH. Campbells's operative orthopaedics. Mosby, St. Louis – Washington D.C. – Toronto; 1987, pp. 2263–417.
22. Brückner H. A new method for plastic surgery of cruciate ligaments. Z Alle Gebiete Oper Medizen. 1966;37(9):413–4.
23. Passler HH. History of implant-free anterior cruciate ligament reconstruction. Unfallchirurg. 2010;113(7):524–31.
24. Hertel P. Anatomic reconstruction of the ACL: a new technique for ACL replacement. 4th ESSKA Congress; Stockholm, 1990.
25. Felmet G, Soni A, Becker R, Musahl V. Press-fit ACL reconstruction. In: Controversies in the technical aspects of ACL reconstruction: an evidence-based medicine approach. Cham: Springer; 2017. p. 247–61.
26. Hertel P, Behrend H. Implant-free anterior cruciate ligament reconstruction with the patella ligament and press-fit double bundle technique. Unfallchirurg. 2010;113(7):540–8.
27. Hertel P. Specific techniques in recent knee ligament surgery. Editions Scientifiques et Medicales Elsevier SAS (Paris) Surgical Techniques in Orthopaedics and Traumatology. 2001;55-530-C-10, 2000, 8 p.
28. Hertel P. Technique of an open ACL reconstruction with autologous patella tendon. Arthroskopie. 1997;10:240–5.
29. Bernard M, Hertel P, Hornung H, Cierpinski T. Femoral insertion of the ACL. Radiographic quadrant method. Am J Knee Surg. 1997;10(1):14–21. discussion 22
30. Wuchech HB. ACL reconstruction with frontosagittal approach. 6th Congress AGA – Society for Arthroscopy and Joint Surgery (German speaking Association for Arthroskopy) in Lucerne (Switzerland) 13–14 October 1989; Lucerne (Switzerland).
31. Boszotta H. Arthroscopic anterior cruciate ligament reconstruction using a patellar tendon graft in press-fit technique: surgical technique and follow-up. Arthroscopy. 1997;13(3):332–9.
32. Boszotta H. Arthroscopic reconstruction of anterior cruciate ligament using BTB patellar ligament in the press-fit technique. Surg Technol Int. 2003;11:249–53.
33. Boszotta H. Implant-free replacement of the anterior cruciate ligament with the double bundle technique: a modification of Passler's operation technique. Unfallchirurg. 2010;113(7):549–54.
34. Barie A, Kargus S, Huber J, Schmitt H, Streich NA. Anterior cruciate ligament reconstruction using quadriceps tendon autograft and press-fit fixation. Unfallchirurg. 2010;113(8):629–34.
35. Gobbi A, Diara A, Mahajan S, Zanazzo M, Tuy B. Patellar tendon anterior cruciate ligament reconstruction with conical press-fit femoral fixation: 5-year results in athletes population. Knee Surg Sports Traumatol Arthrosc. 2002;10(2):73–9.
36. Felmet G. [ACL Reconstruction with the central third of the patellar ligament and simultanous proximal and distal press fit fixation, ALL PRESS FIT] In: AGA, editor. 14 Kongress der deutschsprachigen Arbeitsgemeinschaft für Arthroskopie AGA; October 3rd and 4th 1997 Berlin, 1997.
37. Felmet G. ALL-PRESS-FIT, a new surgical method with femoral and tibial press fit fixation. Arthroskopie. 1999;12:299–304.
38. Felmet G. ACL reconstruction with proximal and distal press fit fixation (ALL PRESS FIT) with SDI (surgical diamond instrument) instruments. Osteosynthese Int. 2000;8:173–4.
39. Felmet G. [ALL PRESS FIT, a near the origin ACL reconstruction with demitendinosus and gracilis tendon, a new surgical technique] 21 Kongress der deutschsprachigen Arbeitsgemeinschaft für Arthroskopie (AGA); 1–2 October 2004, Lucerne, Switzerland. 2004.
40. Paessler HH, Mastrokalos DS. Anterior cruciate ligament reconstruction using semitendinosus and gracilis tendons, bone patellar tendon, or quadriceps tendon-graft with press-fit fixation without hardware. A new and innovative procedure. Orthop Clin North Am. 2003;34(1):49–64.
41. Liu YJ, Li ZL, Wang ZG, Wang Y, Zhou M, Wang AY, et al. The clinical application and biomechanical study of reconstruction of anterior and posterior cruciate ligament with hamstring tendons knot implant fixation. Zhonghua Wai Ke Za Zhi. 2005;43(4):239–42.

42. Al-Husseiny M, Batterjee K. Press-fit fixation in reconstruction of anterior cruciate ligament, using bone-patellar tendon-bone graft. Knee Surg Sports Traumatol Arthrosc. 2004;12(2):104–9.
43. Biazzo A, Manzotti A, Motavalli K, Confalonieri N. Femoral press-fit fixation versus interference screw fixation in anterior cruciate ligament reconstruction with bone-patellar tendon-bone autograft: 20-year follow-up. J Clin Orthop Trauma. 2018;9(2):116–20.
44. Forkel P, Petersen W. Anatomic reconstruction of the anterior cruciate ligament with the autologous quadriceps tendon. Primary and revision surgery. Oper Orthop Traumatol. 2014;26(1):30–42.
45. Zink EJ, Trumper RV, Smidt CR, Rice EL, Reiser RF. Gender comparison of knee strength recovery following ACL reconstruction with contralateral patellar tendon graft. Biomed Sci Instrum. 2005;41:323–8.
46. Halder AM, Ludwig S, Neumann W. Arthroscopic anterior cruciate ligament reconstruction using the double press-fit technique: an alternative to interference screw fixation. Arthroscopy. 2002;18(9):974–82.
47. Mauch F, Apic G, Becker U, Bauer G. Differences in the placement of the tibial tunnel during reconstruction of the anterior cruciate ligament with and without computer-assisted navigation. Am J Sports Med. 2007;35(11):1824–32.
48. Klos TV, Habets RJ, Banks AZ, Banks SA, Devilee RJ, Cook FF. Computer assistance in arthroscopic anterior cruciate ligament reconstruction. Clin Orthop Relat Res. 1998;354:65–9.
49. Zaffagnini S, Klos TV, Bignozzi S. Computer-assisted anterior cruciate ligament reconstruction: an evidence-based approach of the first 15 years. Arthroscopy. 2010;26(4):546–54.
50. Zaffagnini S, Urrizola F, Signorelli C, Grassi A, Di Sarsina TR, Lucidi GA, et al. Current use of navigation system in ACL surgery: a historical review. Knee Surg Sports Traumatol Arthrosc. 2016;24(11):3396–409.
51. Felmet G. Anatomic double bundle single tunnel foreign material free ACL-reconstruction – a technical note. Muscles Ligaments Tendons J. 2011;1(4):148–52.
52. Felmet G. Foreign material-free ACL reconstruction with hollow miller: a biological and anatomic method for every ligament. Tech Orthop. 2013;28(2):166–75.
53. Rupp S, Krauss PW, Fritsch EW. Fixation strength of a biodegradable interference screw and a press-fit technique in anterior cruciate ligament reconstruction with a BPTB graft. Arthroscopy. 1997;13(1):61–5.
54. Seil R, Rupp S, Krauss PW, Benz A, Kohn DM. Comparison of initial fixation strength between biodegradable and metallic interference screws and a press-fit fixation technique in a porcine model. Am J Sports Med. 1998;26(6):815–9.
55. Kuhne JH, Fottner M, Plitz W. Experimental stability of a new implant-free fixation technique in ACL replacement. Unfallchirurg. 1999;102(10):791–6.
56. Mayr HO, Beck T, Hube R, Jager A, von Eisenhart-Rothe R, Bernstein A, et al. Axial load in case of press-fit fixation of the ACL graft – a fundamental study. Z Orthop Grenzgeb. 2005;143(5):556–60.
57. Pavlik A, Hidas P, Czigany T, Berkes I. Biomechanical evaluation of press-fit femoral fixation technique in ACL reconstruction. Knee Surg Sports Traumatol Arthrosc. 2004;12(6):528–33.
58. Boszotta H, Anderl W. Primary stability with tibial press-fit fixation of patellar ligament graft: an experimental study in ovine knees. Arthroscopy. 2001;17(9):963–70.
59. Jagodzinski M, Scheunemann K, Knobloch K, Albrecht K, Krettek C, Hurschler C, et al. Tibial press-fit fixation of the hamstring tendons for ACL-reconstruction. Knee Surg Sports Traumatol Arthrosc. 2006;14(12):1281–7.
60. Ettinger M, Liodakis E, Haasper C, Hurschler C, Breitmeier D, Krettek C, et al. Tibial press-fit fixation of flexor tendons for reconstruction of the anterior cruciate ligament. Unfallchirurg. 2012;115(9):811–5.
61. Ettinger M, Wehrhahn T, Petri M, Liodakis E, Olender G, Albrecht UV, et al. The fixation strength of tibial PCL press-fit reconstructions. Knee Surg Sports Traumatol Arthrosc. 2012;20(2):308–14.
62. Felmet G. [ACL revision material free in a single step]. 25th annual meeting of GOTS; 18–20 June 2010; Munich, Germany. 2010.
63. Demyttenaere J, Claes S, Bellemans J. One-stage revision anterior cruciate ligament reconstruction in cases with excessive tunnel osteolysis. Results of a new technique using impaction bone grafting. Knee. 2018;25(6):1308–17.
64. Pavlik A, Hidas P, Tallay A, Toman J, Berkes I. Femoral press-fit fixation technique in anterior cruciate ligament reconstruction using bone-patellar tendon-bone graft: a prospective clinical evaluation of 285 patients. Am J Sports Med. 2006;34(2):220–5.
65. Widuchowski W, Widuchowska M, Koczy B, Dragan S, Czamara A, Tomaszewski W, et al. Femoral press-fit fixation in ACL reconstruction using bone-patellar tendon-bone autograft: results at 15 years follow-up. BMC Musculoskelet Disord. 2012;13:115.
66. Tomita F, Yasuda K, Mikami S, Sakai T, Yamazaki S, Tohyama H. Comparisons of intraosseous graft healing between the doubled flexor tendon graft and the bone-patellar tendon-bone graft in anterior cruciate ligament reconstruction. Arthroscopy. 2001;17(5):461–76.
67. Felmet G. In: Frenzel G, Wuschech H, editors. "Aquasprint" in the early functional rehabilitation program after ACL reconstruction. Berlin: Kongress Compact Verlag; 2002. p. 188–96.
68. Felmet G. [The significance of proprioceptive vibration training in postoperative treatment after ACL reconstruction]. DGOOC; 19.–24. October 2004; Berlin.
69. Krautter A, Rohnstock LM, Zhao Z, Felmet G. Instrumented arthrometry of the anterior cruciate ligament. A comparison. Biomed Tech. 2012;57:4299.
70. Runer A, et al. The evaluation of Rolimeter, KLT, KiRA and KT-1000 arthrometer in healthy individuals shows acceptable intra-rater but poor inter-rater reliability in the measurement of anterior tibial knee translation. Knee Surg Sports Traumatol Arthrosc. 2021.

71. Cameron M, Buchgraber A, Passler H, Vogt M, Thonar E, Fu F, et al. The natural history of the anterior cruciate ligament-deficient knee. Changes in synovial fluid cytokine and keratan sulfate concentrations. Am J Sports Med. 1997;25(6):751–4.
72. Jarvela T, Moisala AS, Sihvonen R, Jarvela S, Kannus P, Jarvinen M. Double-bundle anterior cruciate ligament reconstruction using hamstring autografts and bioabsorbable interference screw fixation: prospective, randomized, clinical study with 2-year results. Am J Sports Med. 2008;36(2):290–7.
73. Muneta T. Twenty-year experience of a double-bundle anterior cruciate ligament reconstruction. Clin Orthop Surg. 2015;7(2):143–51.
74. Koivisto J, Kiljunen T, Kadesjo N, Shi XQ, Wolff J. Effective radiation dose of a MSCT, two CBCT and one conventional radiography device in the ankle region. J Foot Ankle Res. 2015;8:8.
75. Koivisto J, Kiljunen T, Wolff J, Kortesniemi M. Assessment of effective radiation dose of an extremity CBCT, MSCT and conventional X-ray for knee area using MOSFET dosemeters. Radiat Prot Dosim. 2013;157(4):515–24.
76. Koivisto J, van Eijnatten M, Kiljunen T, Shi XQ, Wolff J. Effective radiation dose in the wrist resulting from a radiographic device, two CBCT devices and one MSCT device: a comparative study. Radiat Prot Dosim. 2018;179(1):58–68.
77. Pallaver A, Honigmann P. The role of cone-beam computed tomography (CBCT) scan for detection and follow-up of traumatic wrist pathologies. J Hand Surg Am. 2019;44(12):1081–7.
78. Chmielnicki M, Siebert W, Prokop A. Foreign material-free anterior cruciate ligament repair with hamstring graft, Felmet technique. Z Orthop Unfall. 2018;156(2):223–5.
79. Mouarbes D, Menetrey J, Marot V, Courtot L, Berard E, Cavaignac E. Anterior cruciate ligament reconstruction: a systematic review and meta-analysis of outcomes for quadriceps tendon autograft versus bone-patellar tendon-bone and hamstring-tendon autografts. Am J Sports Med. 2019;47(14):3531–40.
80. Siebold R, Schuhmacher P, Fernandez F, Śmigielski R, Fink C, Brehmer A, Kirsch J. Erratum to: Flat midsubstance of the anterior cruciate ligament with tibial "C"-shaped insertion site. Knee Surg Sports Traumatol Arthrosc. 2016;24(9):3046. https://doi.org/10.1007/s00167-014-3230-z. Erratum for: Knee Surg Sports Traumatol Arthrosc. 2015 Nov;23(11):3136–42. PMID: 25149644; PMCID: PMC6828258.
81. Siebold R, Schuhmacher P, Fernandez F, Smigielski R, Fink C, Brehmer A, et al. Flat midsubstance of the anterior cruciate ligament with tibial "C"-shaped insertion site. Knee Surg Sports Traumatol Arthrosc. 2015;23(11):3136–42.
82. Smigielski R, Zdanowicz U, Drwiega M, Ciszek B, Ciszkowska-Lyson B, Siebold R. Ribbon like appearance of the midsubstance fibres of the anterior cruciate ligament close to its femoral insertion site: a cadaveric study including 111 knees. Knee Surg Sports Traumatol Arthrosc. 2015;23(11):3143–50.

6 ACL All Press-Fit: A Surgical Guide Step by Step

This chapter is a guide to foreign material-free anterior cruciate ligament (ACL) reconstruction with bone dowels with "all press-fit" fixation with a checklist of:

- Indication,
- Symptoms,
- Preoperative and clinical assessment,
- Management in the operating room and
- First postoperative treatment [1–7].

1. Hamstring
2. Quadriceps tendon
3. Patellar bone-tendon-bone (BTB)

6.1 Hamstring "All Press-Fit" Fixation with Bone Dowels

6.1.1 Indications

Reconstruction of a complete tear of the anterior cruciate ligament (ACL) is indicated in:

- Patients under 25 years of age (children 12 years, favoured with hamstring) to prevent the occurrence of secondary meniscal tears, which are a causal factor of later degeneration
- Patients wishing to return to full pivoting activities
- Patients over 40 years old when the attempt at proprioceptive rehabilitation failed to stabilize the knee
- Patients complaining of functional pivoting instability regardless of age
- Patients with unicondylar replacement

6.1.2 Preoperative Assessment

6.1.2.1 Clinical Assessment

Basic Signs of ACL Tear

Patients describe feeling a popping from the injured knee while twisting the knee and immediate instability. The knee quickly becomes swollen—or not. Pain is variable. Examination assesses the amount of swelling, location of the pain. Both can limit the range of motion. The examiner undertakes gentle manipulation with the Lachman at 30° of flexion, anterior drawer at 90° of flexion and the pivot shift test on the patient supine, comparing with the opposite side. The Rolimeter or ArticoMeter (digital Rolimeter) is helpful for greater precision.

Further Physical Assessment

- Investigate the posterior laxity and posterior drawer (posterior cruciate ligament, PCL).
- Investigate frontal laxity in extension. If present, this could indicate an additional peripheral ligamentous lesion.

G. Felmet, *Press-Fit Fixation of the Knee Ligaments*, https://doi.org/10.1007/978-3-031-11906-4_6

- Investigate the presence of pain at the joint line, which could indicate a meniscal tear.
- The presence of lateral pain is often related to the bony impact.

6.1.2.2 Imaging Assessment

Radiographs, Computed Tomography (CT), Digital Volume Tomography (DVT)
DVT is a multislice computed tomography (MSCT) device, two cone-beam CT (CBCT) device [8–11].

Anteroposterior and lateral views detect possible avulsion of the ACL at the tibial level or a partial fracture of the lateral aspect of the tibial plateau (Segond's fracture). This fracture is an indirect sign of an ACL tear.

Magnetic Resonance Imaging (MRI)
MRI is useful for detecting associated lesions, although this should be delayed until swelling has partially resolved to improve image contrast.

A delay is also useful as some lesions heal spontaneously.

Direct ACL tears are visible as disorganisation of the ligament fibres.

Be aware of indirect signs of ACL tear: bone bruising in the lateral compartment.

Curved appearance of the PCL.

Check menisci and cartilage.

6.1.3 Timing of Surgery

Surgery takes place once inflammation around the knee has mostly resolved.

The patient must display good quadriceps strength and coordination.

The knee joint must be essentially pain free and be able to flex actively to at least 120°.

6.1.4 Surgical Preparation

6.1.4.1 Surgical Equipment

- Entire arthroscopic ACL set includes tibial and femoral tubed guides for hollow reamer or for K-wires with a central guide for hollow reamer crown cutter, micro crown cutter or diamond hollow reamer with a diameter of 8–11 mm (Figs. 6.1 and 6.2)

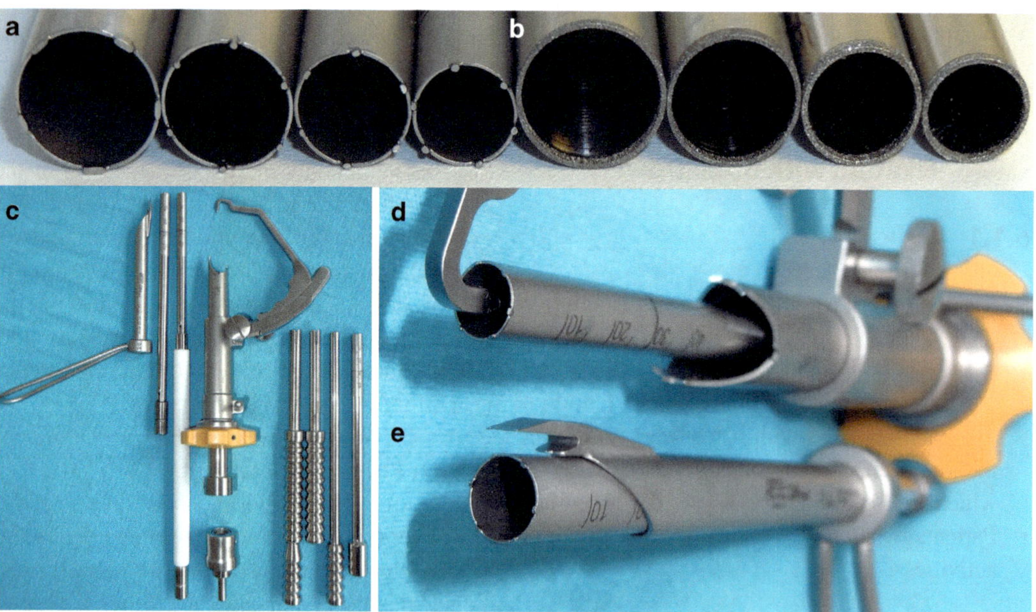

Fig. 6.1 Hollow reamer as a crown cutter (**a**) and a micro crown cutter (**b**) with diameter 8–11 mm. Basic set from left: guiding devices, hollow reamer for tibia and femur 9 mm, universal adapter for drilling machine, applicator and harvester (**c**). Tubed guiding devices: for the tibia (**d**) and the femur (**e**)

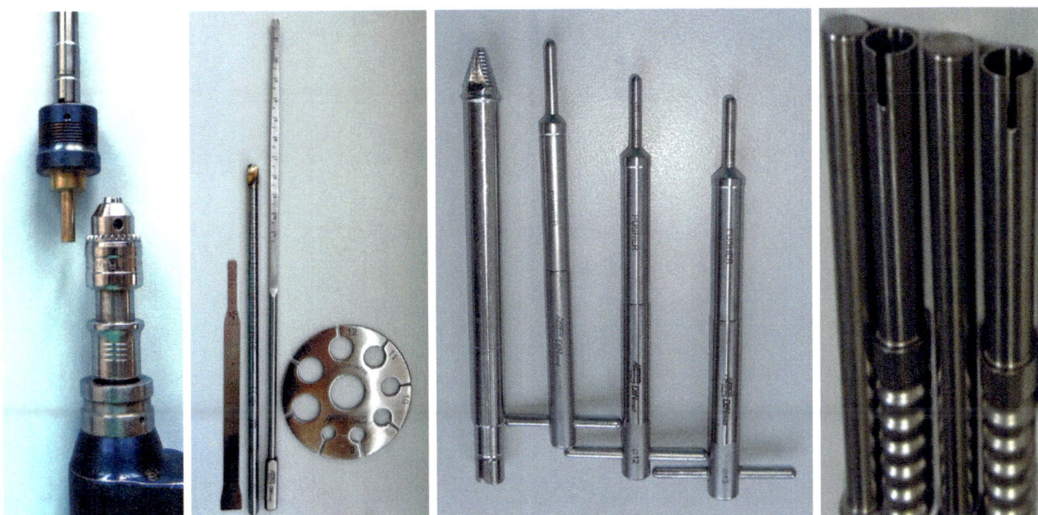

Fig. 6.2 Universal adapter, meter and calibrating devices, cone reamer and cone pusher, applicator and pusher

- Harvester, applicator and pusher with a diameter of 8–11 mm
- Cone reamer and cone pusher 11 mm
- Graft calibrating devices
- Universal hollow reamer adapter
- Drill with Jacobs connector
- Two Kantrowitz clamps
- Hamstring tendon stripper
- Sutures
- USP 5, 90 cm to pull in the graft folded at the femoral end
- USP 2/0 DS 25 for sutures on the graft and periosteum
- USP 3/0 DS 24 for sub- and intracutaneous suture
- USP 1, HRT 37 (non-traumatic) 90 cm, 2× for pull (for quadriceps/patellar tendon only)
- Complete arthroscopic set with a shaver
- Curette
- An arthroscopy pump is not used routinely

6.1.4.2 Equipment Positioning

The arthroscopic tower faces the surgeon on the opposite side of the table at the level of patient's shoulder.

6.1.4.3 Patient Positioning

Lay the patient supine with the knee flexed at 90°, stabilized in a leg holder.

Ensure that the knee can be mobilized from full extension up to 120° flexion.

A tourniquet is applied to the upper thigh.

6.1.4.4 Further Preparation

Transplantation of material justifies antibiotic prophylaxis.

6.1.4.5 Arthroscopic Cleaning

Portals

Place anterolateral and anteromedial portals for scope insertion (Fig. 6.3).

The high anterolateral portal should be placed 2 cm above the lateral joint line and 1 cm lateral to the margin of the patellar tendon at the soft spot.

The anteromedial portal should be placed opposite, 1 cm above the lateral joint line and 1 cm lateral to the margin of the patella tendon and should be checked by inserting a needle under scope control.

Assess by inspection and probing the menisci, cartilage and ligaments.

Remove the ACL Stump and Leave a Smal Rest at the Tibial Insertion

Clean the axial aspect of the lateral condyle with a shaver until the periosteum is visible, with the

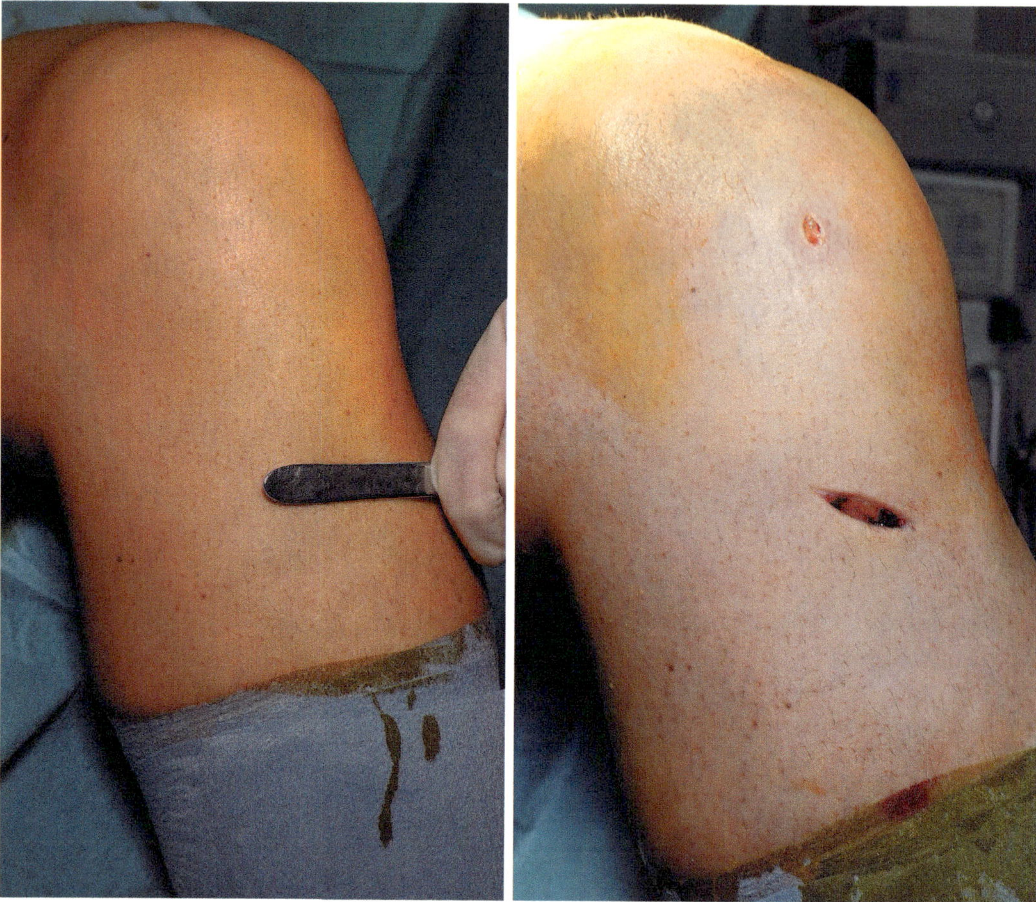

Fig. 6.3 Line underneath the tibial tuberosity (left). Arthroscopic portals and medial including hamstring portals

posterolateral capsular recess just behind (Fig. 6.4).

Clean the PCL by sliding a basket forceps between the two cruciate ligaments.

Finally, clean the tibial ACL footprint with the shaver and leave a remnant for later biological reattachment to the graft.

6.1.5 Surgical Technique

6.1.5.1 Harvesting Hamstring Graft

Inflate the tourniquet to 350 mmHg. Exsanguinate the limb before making the first incision.

Skin incision is about 2 cm, slightly angulated opposite the tibial tubercle, midway between the tubercle and the posterior edge of the tibia parallel over the hamstrings.

Palpate the pes anserinus; the gracilis tendon and deeper the semitendinosus tendon will be felt as the sartorius thins out well proximal to its insertion.

Attempt to identify the saphenous nerve.

Make an incision directly over and in line with the gracilis tendon.

Open the tendon sheath and release adhesions and fibrous extensions that attach to the sheath.

Pes anserinus is exposed through a short vertical incision.

Mobilize with Kantrowitz clamps and pull the deeper semitendinosus anteriorly and harvest with a tendon stripper (Fig. 6.5).

It can be necessary to add the gracilis tendon, achieving an 8-mm tripled or quadrupled graft 7 cm long.

Residual muscle is removed.

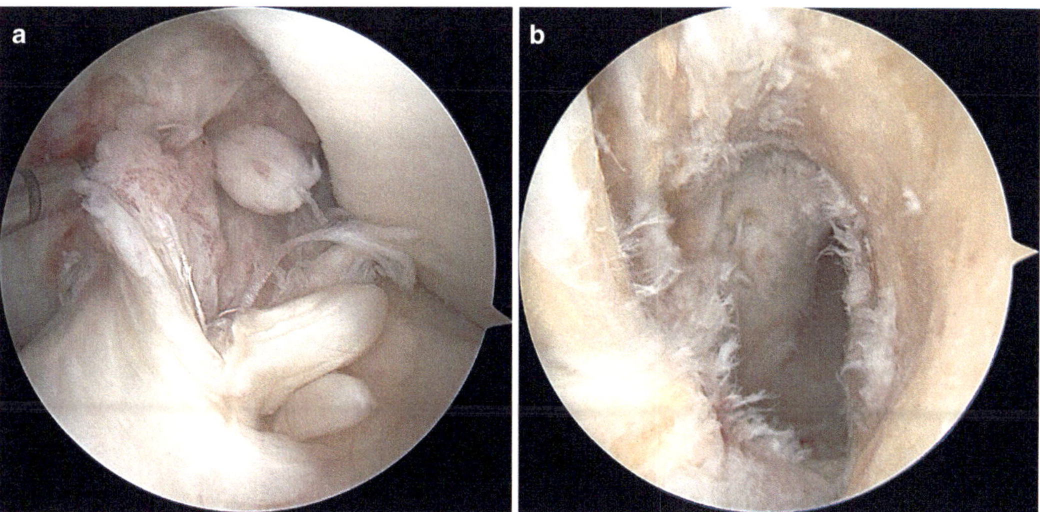

Fig. 6.4 (**a**, **b**) Preparing the posterior notch

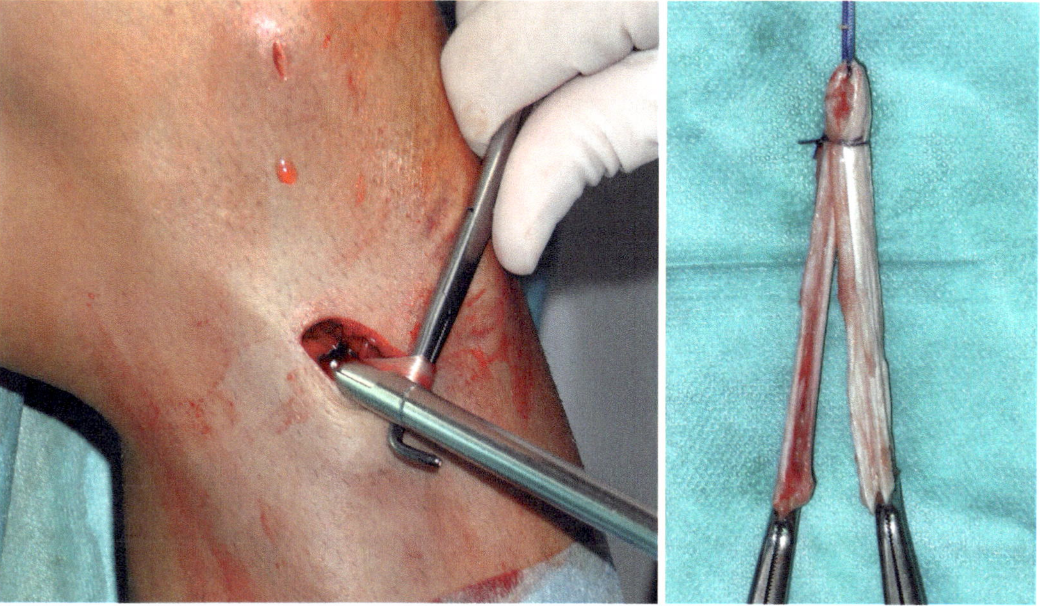

Fig. 6.5 Hamstring harvested with tendon stripper, semitendinosus tendon folded four times and fixed with Kantrowitz clamps

The tendon should be placed in a moistened sponge or saline.

6.1.5.2 Performing Tunnels

Femoral Tunnel

Standard diameter for thc fcmoral tunnel in adults is the 9-mm hollow reamer.

Choose the 9-mm femoral guide.

The long tip is in contact behind the posterior lateral condyle.

The short tip controls the posterior 1-mm bone bridge of the tunnel to prevent a blowout.

Position the femoral guide in 120° knee flexion.

Insert the 9-mm hollow reamer and make a 1-mm incision with the hollow reamer to mark the tunnel position.

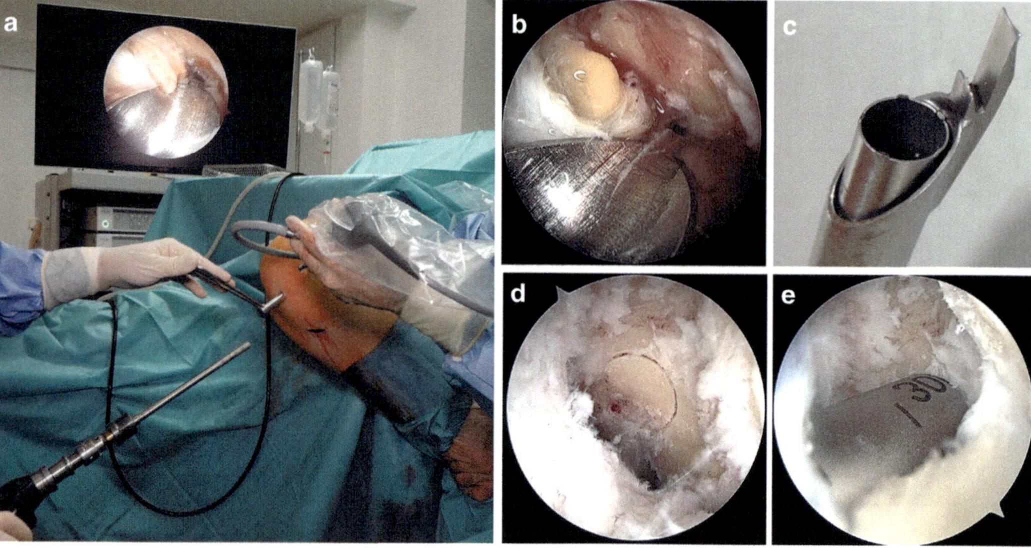

Fig. 6.6 Femoral guide in 120° knee flexion (**a**) positioned with its tip at the posterior lateral notch (**b**, **c**); print foot marked over the bifurcate ridge near the intermediate ridge (**d**); 9-mm hollow reamer and harvester harvest a 30 mm bone dowel (**e**)

Remove the reamer and guide and control arthroscopically through the anteromedial portal the position of the tunnel (find the bifurcate ridge in the middle of the mark).

In this step the position can be corrected (Fig. 6.6).

Insert the hollow reamer (in 120° knee flexion) and mill to a depth of 30 mm.

Remove the hollow reamer.

Insert the 9-mm extractor in 120° knee flexion and push it to the 30-mm mark.

Insert the small rod into the end of the connector for a T-handle.

Rotate for 180° clockwise and pull it out.

Push the bone cylinder out of the harvester.

Check the 30-mm-deep socket and an oval width of about 11 mm (Fig. 6.7).

Tibial Tunnel

- Flex the knee to 90° and insert the tibial tubed guide into the medial portal (Fig. 6.8).
- Set the angle of the tibial tubed guide to 25°.
- Centre the tip of the tibial guide so that the intra-articular guide pin enters the joint just anterior to the PCL (Fig. 6.8).
- Position the tubed guide and fix it on the tibia with its sharp ends (use correct side left/right up) (Figs. 6.1 and 6.8).
- Insert the 9-mm hollow reamer with the extension into the tibial tube guide (Fig. 6.8).
- To get the central position of the tunnel under the guide:
  - In a left knee turn the motor to the right side (Fig. 6.8).
  - In a right knee turn the motor to the left side.
- Run the motor on maximum.
- Carefully touch the bone.
- Pull back and prove your position.
- Drill through the tibial head and control the hollow reamer inside the joint arthroscopically.
- Open the fixation of the guide taking care not to harm the tip of the guide inside the joint (Fig. 6.8).
- Drill the complete bone cylinder and harvest it inside the hollow reamer and pull it out.
- Remove the tibial guide.
- Disconnect the hollow teamer from the extension and push out the bone cylinder with a

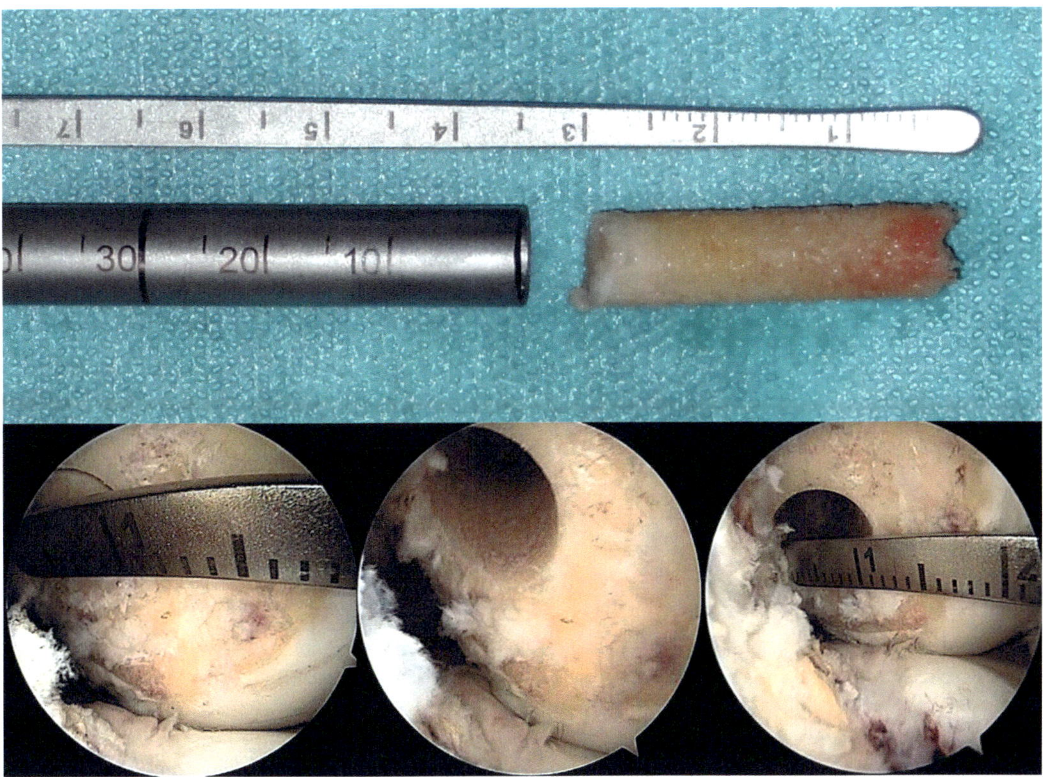

Fig. 6.7 Harvest a 30-mm long bone cylinder with the extractor. Here with a 9-mm diameter. Because of the oval insertion the width is about 11 mm. Check the size

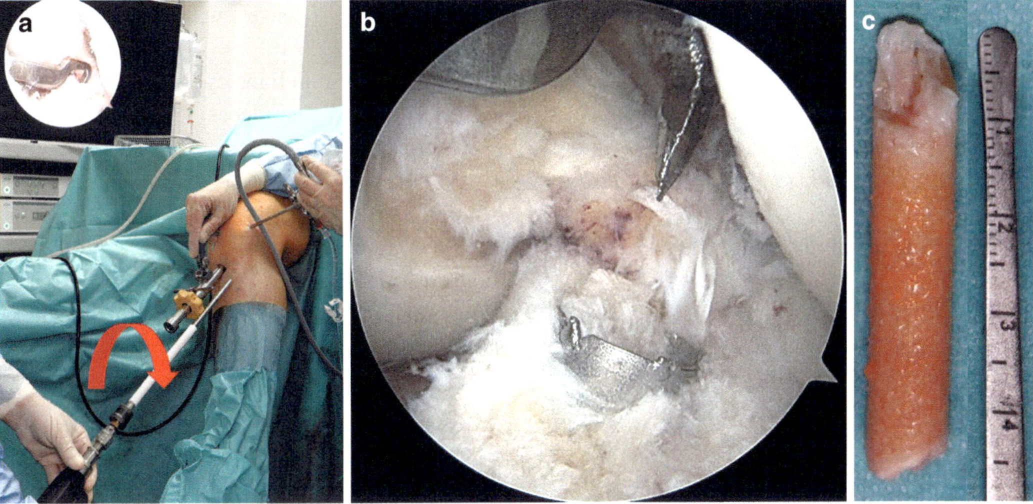

Fig. 6.8 Position the tibial guide anterior to the posterior cruciate ligament (**a**, **b**), mill a 9-mm diameter tunnel and harvest an approximately 40-mm-long bone cylinder (**c**). Caveat: to reproduce the central position of the tunnel under the guide: In *left knee* (as here) turn the motor to the *right hand* > red arrow (**a**). In a *right knee* turn the motor to the *left hand*

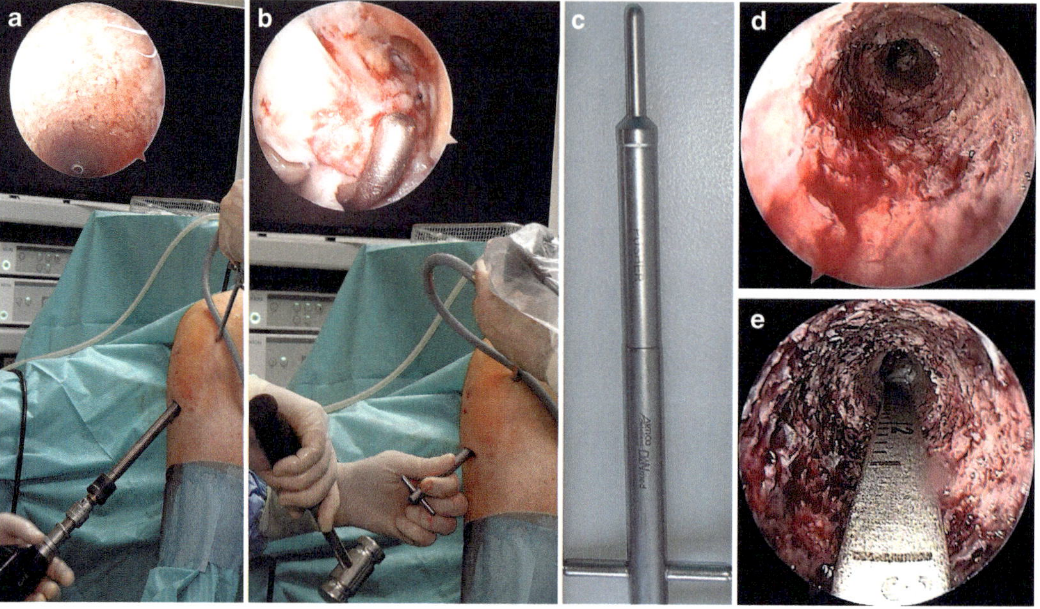

Fig. 6.9 Enlarge the distal tibial tunnel to the bottleneck with a cone reamer (**a**) and a cone pusher (**b**, **c**) depending on the tibial slice of the graft with a diameter from 11 to 13 mm. Check the bottle neck with a distance of about 2 cm under the tiabia plateau (**d**, **e**)

small pusher and harvest an approximately 40-mm-long bone cylinder (Fig. 6.8c).

- To ease implantation of the graft:
  - Connect the cone reamer and open the distal entrance of the tibial tunnel.
  - Take the 11-mm cone pusher and enlarge the distal tibial tunnel like a bottle neck until you see the tip of the control pin (Fig. 6.9).
  - The bottle neck (9 mm in diameter) now has a length of approximately 20 mm for press-fit fixation (Fig. 6.9).

6.1.5.3 Prepare the Graft

Take the semitendinosus tendon twice and double it to quadrupled over the no. 5 thread to an approximately 70-mm-long graft and a diameter of 8–9 mm (Fig. 6.10).

Fix each of the two leaves with a Kantrowitz clamp (Fig. 6.10a).

Check the diameter (Fig. 6.11).

If necessary add the gracilis tendon.

Mark approximately 10 mm from the top with a USP 2/0 suture (minimum length for fixation in the femoral tunnel) (Fig. 6.10).

Place the first sack suture 35 mm lower.

Open the two leaves with both Kantrowitz clamps.

Divide the 9-mm bone cylinder from the tibial tunnel into two equal pieces.

Insert the proximal bone cylinder.

Fix the bone cylinder with two circulated sutures.

Place them to open a bone window for bone-to-bone contact healing (Fig. 6.10). This bone surface is later positioned to the lateral side to mimic the C-shaped tibial insertion (Fig. 6.11).

6.1.5.4 Passage of the Graft

Measure the length of the tibial tunnel with the ruler (Fig. 6.9).

Pass the threads through the tibial tunnel and pull them inside out of the anteromedial portal.

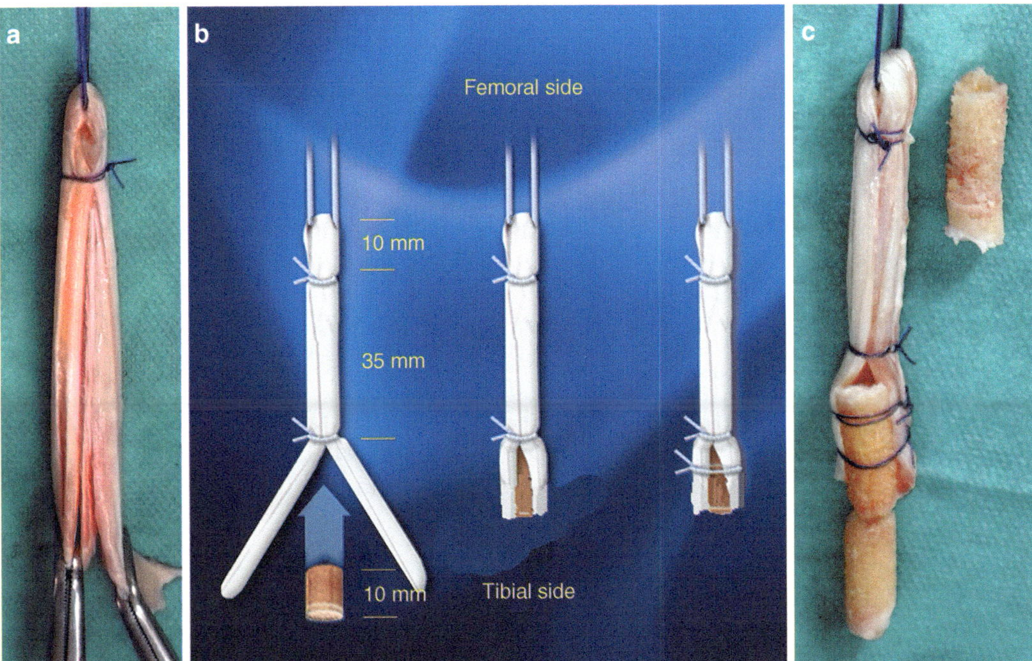

Fig. 6.10 The semitendinosus tendon is taken twice and doubled to quadrupled over the no. 5 thread to an approximately 70-mm-long graft with a diameter of 8–9 mm (**a**). Each leaf is fixed with a Kantrowitz clamp (**a**). Mark approximately 10 mm from the top with a USP 2/0 suture (minimum length for fixation in the femoral tunnel) (**a**, **b**). Place the first sack suture 35 mm lower. Open the two leaves with both Kantrowitz clamps (**b**). Divide the 9-mm bone cylinder from the tibial tunnel into two equal pieces. Insert the proximal bone cylinder. Fix the bone cylinder with two circular sutures (**b**, **c**)

Insert and drill the pull-out-pin through the anteromedial portal in 120° knee flexion through the femoral tunnel.

Insert the thread through the eye of the pull-out pin linked to the graft and pull it out.

Fix the thread with a clamp.

Pull the graft inside the tunnel while pushing the tibial bone cylinder into the tibial tunnel (Fig. 6.12).

Check the position of the tibial fixation nearest the plateau.

6.1.5.5 Fixation and Tensioning of the Graft

Tibial Fixation

Fixation is performed with the complete passage of the graft.

The C-shaped open bone of the graft (Fig. 6.11) is rotated laterally (Fig. 6.12) to mimic the anatomical tibial insertion.

As the graft is drawn in on the threads, the transplant is simultaneously driven into the tibial canal to below the tibial plateau.

The tibial fixation is press-fit with an oversize of 2–3 mm at the 9-mm bottle neck (Fig. 6.12).

The correct position of the graft can be checked by the depth of the distal tunnel compared with the length of the rest of the tibial bone cylinder (Figs. 6.10, 6.11, and 6.12).

Femoral Fixation

Take the bone cylinder from the femoral tunnel 30 mm in length.

Cut it into two pieces.

Push the cancellous bone cylinder into the 9-mm applicator.

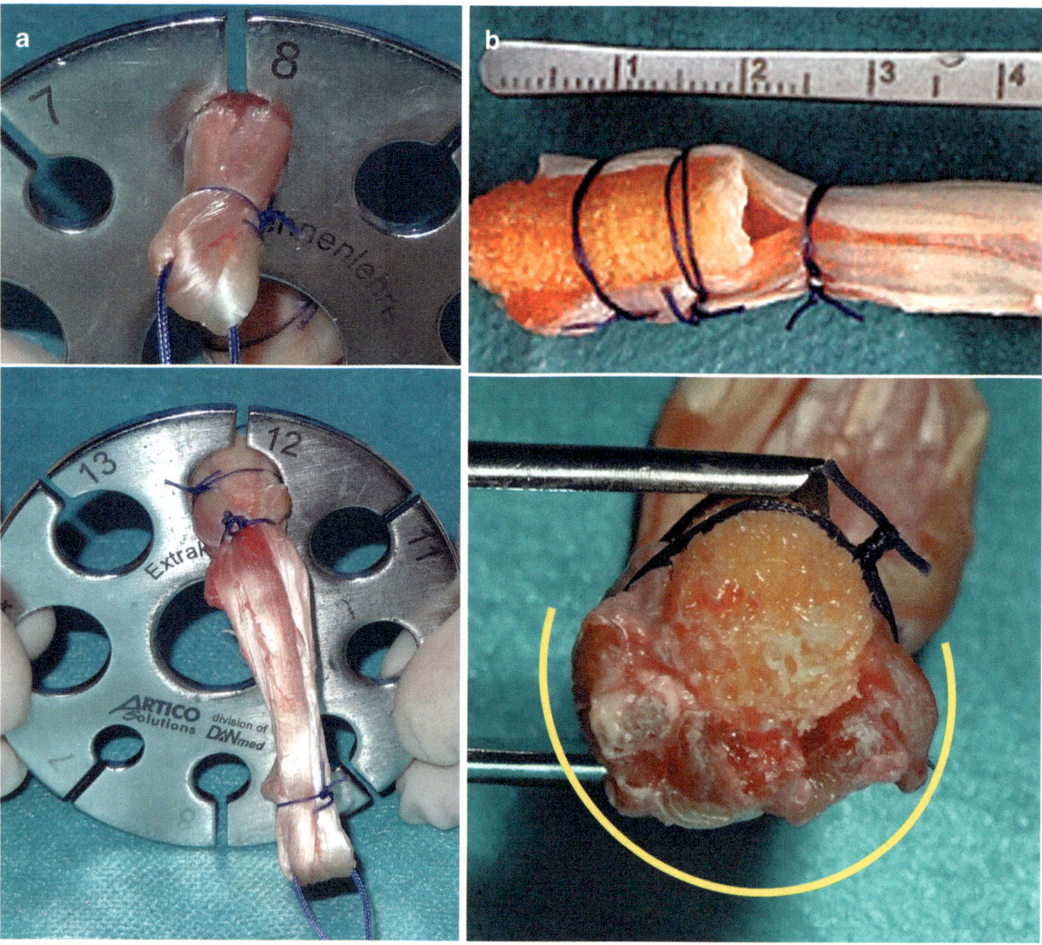

Fig. 6.11 Prepared graft with bone cylinder from the tibial and femoral tunnel. Size and diameters of the graft on the femoral (8 mm) and tibial (12 mm) ends (**a**). The tibial side has an open bone window and a C-shaped graft (**b**)

Insert the applicator with pusher through the anteromedial portal to the femoral tunnel (Fig. 6.13). Control the bone cylinder through the small slot of the applicator (Fig. 6.13).

In 120° knee flexion pull on the thread and simultaneously push the bone cylinder parallel to the graft inside the tunnel.

A crescent-shaped insertion appears ribbon like to mimic the anteromedial and posterolateral bundle (Fig. 6.13).

Go back to flexion.

Pull strong on the thread.

The graft tensions a little.

Push the second bone cylinder into the applicator with cortical bone end first.

Insert the applicator with pusher through the anteromedial portal to the femoral tunnel again.

Control the bone cylinder through the small slot at the side again.

In 120° knee flexion push the bone cylinder parallel to the graft inside the tunnel.

A crescent-shaped insertion appears with the mimic of the two bundles (Fig. 6.13).

Push the cortical bone a little deeper than the surface of the notch.

Extend the knee.

The graft will have self-adapted tensioning in extension in a “bottom-to-top” fixation (Fig. 6.14).

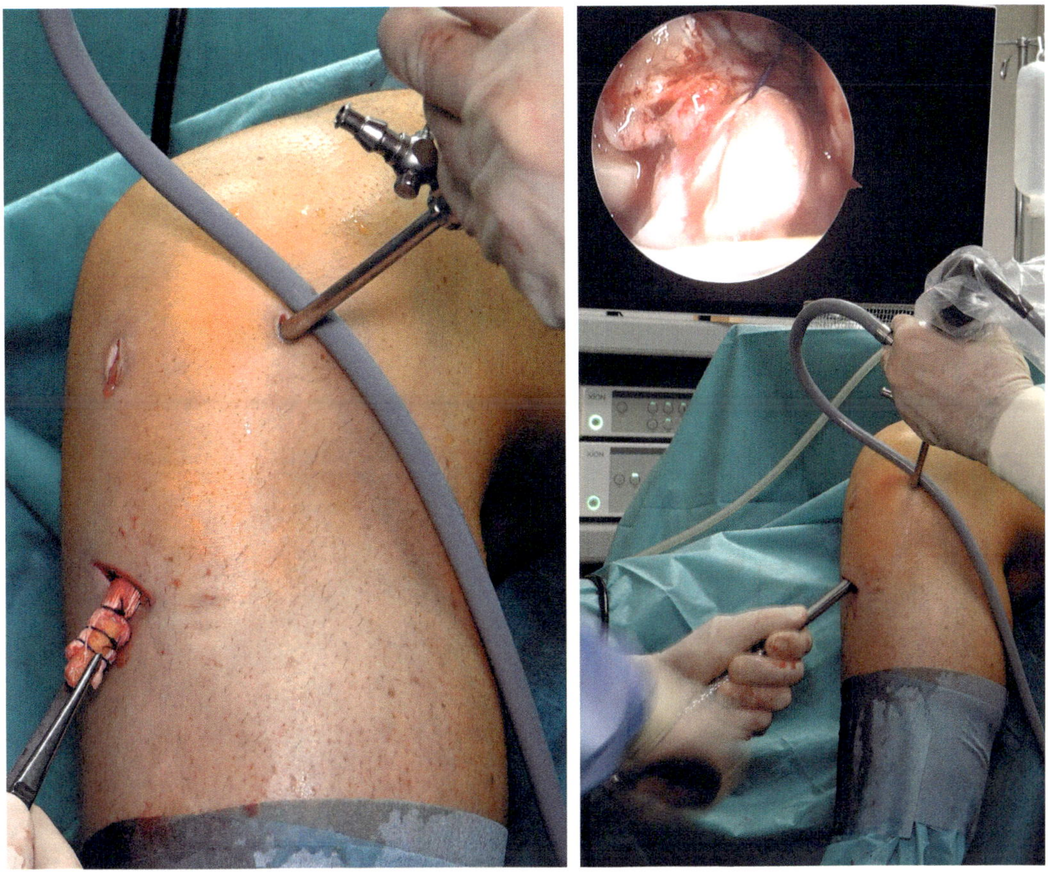

Fig. 6.12 Pull threads through the tunnel and passage the graft. The open bone window of the tibial graft is rotated to the lateral side for the C-shaped ribbon-like insertion at the tibia side. Pull the graft into the tunnel and simultaneously push the tibial bone cylinder up to the plateau (left)

While performing the first extension slight motion at the tibial graft can be observed.

Check stability.

Go back to flexion. Pull strong on the thread again.

Pull out the thread.

6.1.5.6 Reverse to the Established Procedure: "Bottom-to-Top" Fixation Is a "Self-Adapted Tensioning" Based on the Geometry of the Knee

The graft is pulled inside through the tibial tunnel "bottom to top":

1. The bone cylinder is fixed press-fit in the tibial tunnel near the joint.
2. The graft is pulled into the femoral tunnel while the tibial bone cylinder is pushed under the tibial plateau near the original insertion.
3. Now the graft is fixed under tension with a bone cylinder in flexion.
4. The graft is a little overstretched now because the ACL is usually lax in flexion.
5. The graft achieves "self-adapted tensioning" by extending the knee completely (Fig. 6.14).

6.1.5.7 Possible Peri-operative Complications

- Femoral and/or tibial fixation is not stable: limit extension in 20° knee flexion in a brace for 4 weeks postoperatively (Table 6.2).

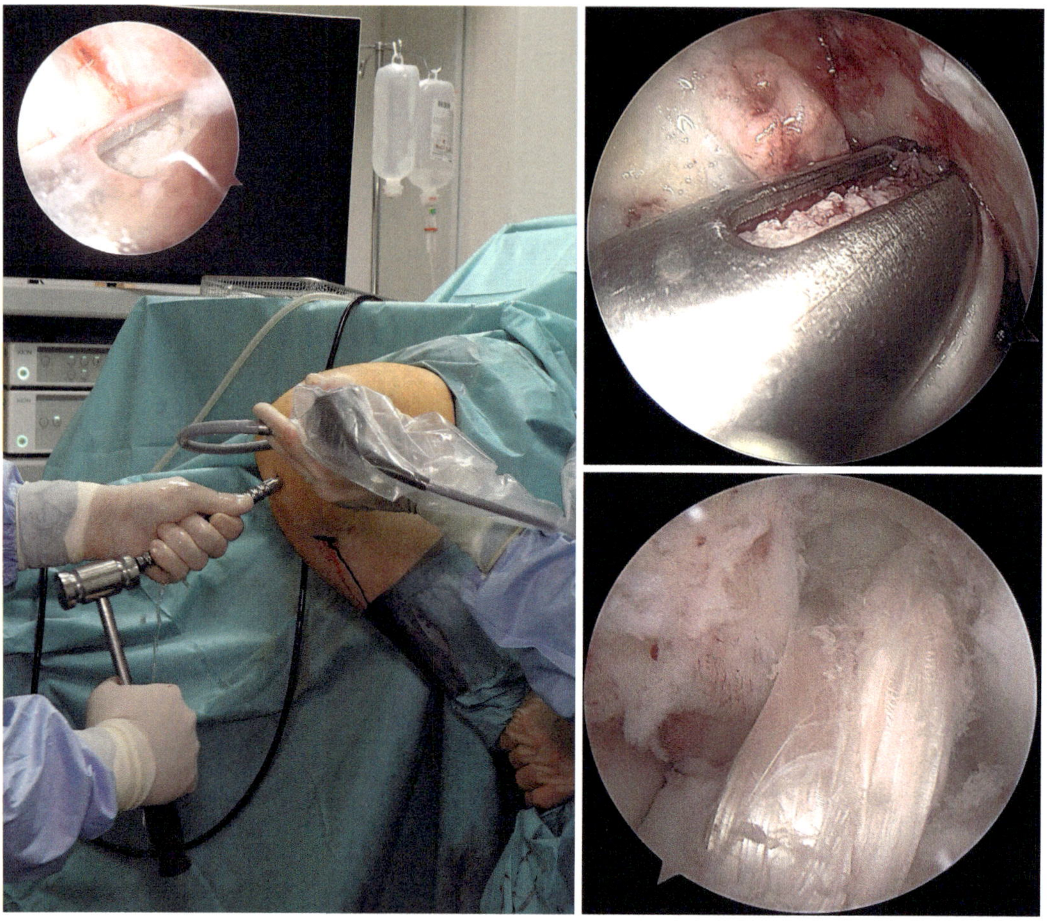

Fig. 6.13 In 120° knee flexion the femoral bone cylinder inside the applicator is pushed into the femoral tunnel to fix the graft press-fit in a crescent-shaped, ribbon-like insertion to mimic the anteromedial and posterolateral bundle

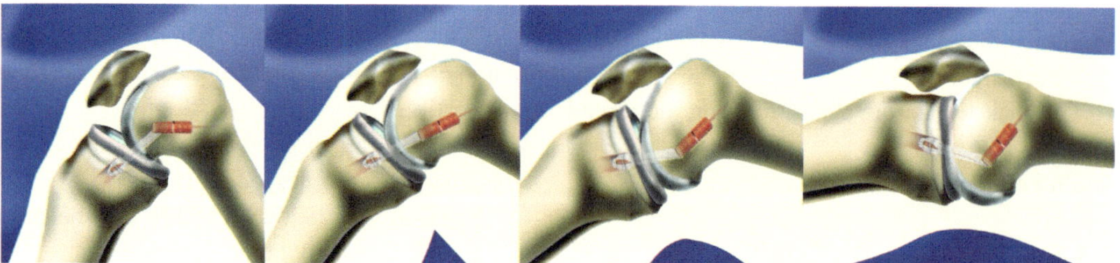

Fig. 6.14 The graft is fixed bottom-to-top and tensioned in flexion (left). By the geometry and the fixed and tensioned graft in flexion a self-adapted tensioning is achieved from flexion to extension (left to right)

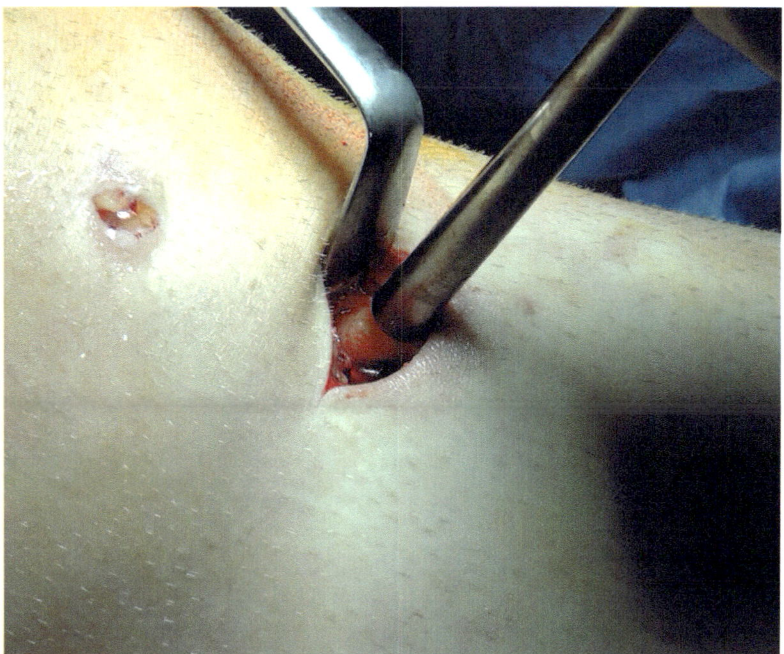

Fig. 6.15 Close the tibial tunnel with the rest of the tibial bone cylinder

- Femoral posterior blow out: if possible vary to a more high noon position for another femoral tunnel.
- Tibial fixation is unstable: push the cylinder into the tibial tunnel and fix it with a K-wire as a cross-pin for 4–6 weeks; then remove.
- Osteoporotic bone/revision surgery: threads on the femoral and tibial sides can each be fixed over a small bone bridge outside the tunnels at the medial tibia and lateral femoral condyle.

6.1.5.8 Closure

Reinsert the rest of the bone cylinders into the tibial tunnel (Fig. 6.15).

Close the peritendon over the tibial tunnel with an absorbable suture.

Close the subcutaneous and skin layers in a standard fashion.

Apply a simple dressing.

Apply a flexed knee splint for 1–2 days maximum.

Plain radiograph control on the same day (Fig. 6.26) or DVT, a MSCT device, two CBCT device [8–11], for correct position of the bone dowels (Figs. 6.27, 6.28, and 6.29).

Use MRI in other questions regarding the graft, e.g. capsule, menisci, cartilage, bone etc. (Fig. 6.30).

6.1.5.9 Postoperative Course

Medications: pain killer, non-steroidal anti-inflammatory drugs (NSAIDs), prevention of deep vein thrombosis.

- In stable fixation extension is allowed: rehabilitation programme plan A is suggested (Table 6.1)
- In osteoporotic or unstable fixation extension should be limited to 20° for 2–4 weeks postoperatively: rehabilitation programme plan B is suggested (Table 6.2).

Full load.

Immediate mobilization without limitation.

Isometric quadriceps contractions and co-contraction with ischiocrural muscles.

At home a brace is used for the first few days in order to become familiar with it.

The brace can be discarded once quadriceps strength is sufficient to walk outside after 3–6 weeks.

Table 6.1 Rehabilitation plan A is suggested in stable fixation (without further damage, which requires a different programme). Complete extension is allowed and a systematic step-by-step program is possible. Some suggestions of exercises and equipment are made. Aqua-sprint can be performed as an adult in 50- to 70-cm-deep water [12] as proprioceptive vibration training [13]

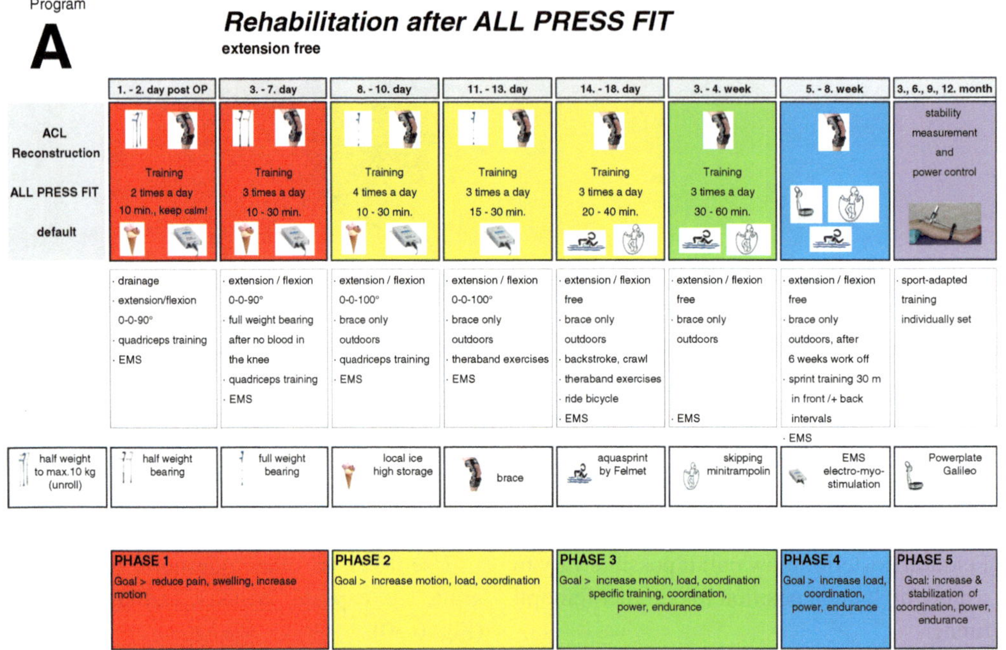

Program **A**

Rehabilitation after ALL PRESS FIT

extension free

	1. - 2. day post OP	3. - 7. day	8. - 10. day	11. - 13. day	14. - 18. day	3. - 4. week	5. - 8. week	3., 6., 9., 12. month
ACL Reconstruction ALL PRESS FIT default	Training 2 times a day 10 min., keep calm!	Training 3 times a day 10 - 30 min.	Training 4 times a day 10 - 30 min.	Training 3 times a day 15 - 30 min.	Training 3 times a day 20 - 40 min.	Training 3 times a day 30 - 60 min.		stability measurement and power control
	· drainage · extension/flexion 0-0-90° · quadriceps training · EMS	· extension / flexion 0-0-90° · full weight bearing after no blood in the knee · quadriceps training · EMS	· extension / flexion 0-0-100° · brace only outdoors · quadriceps training · EMS	· extension / flexion 0-0-100° · brace only outdoors · theraband exercises · EMS	· extension / flexion free · brace only outdoors · backstroke, crawl · theraband exercises · ride bicycle · EMS	· extension / flexion free · brace only outdoors · EMS	· extension / flexion free · brace only outdoors, after 6 weeks work off · sprint training 30 m in front /+ back intervals · EMS	· sport-adapted training individually set

half weight to max.10 kg (unroll)	half weight bearing	full weight bearing	local ice high storage	brace	aquasprint by Felmet	skipping minitrampolin	EMS electro-myo-stimulation	Powerplate Galileo

PHASE 1	PHASE 2	PHASE 3	PHASE 4	PHASE 5
Goal > reduce pain, swelling, increase motion	Goal > increase motion, load, coordination	Goal > increase motion, load, coordination specific training, coordination, power, endurance	Goal > increase load, coordination, power, endurance	Goal: increase & stabilization of coordination, power, endurance

Table 6.2 Rehabilitation plan B is suggested in osteoporotic or unstable fixation (without further damage, which requires a different programme). Complete extension is not allowed for 2–4 weeks to distress the ACL. An adapted systematic step-by-step programme is set. Some suggestions of exercises and equipment are made. Aqua-sprint can be performed as an adult in 50- to 70-cm-deep water [12] as proprioceptive vibration training [13]

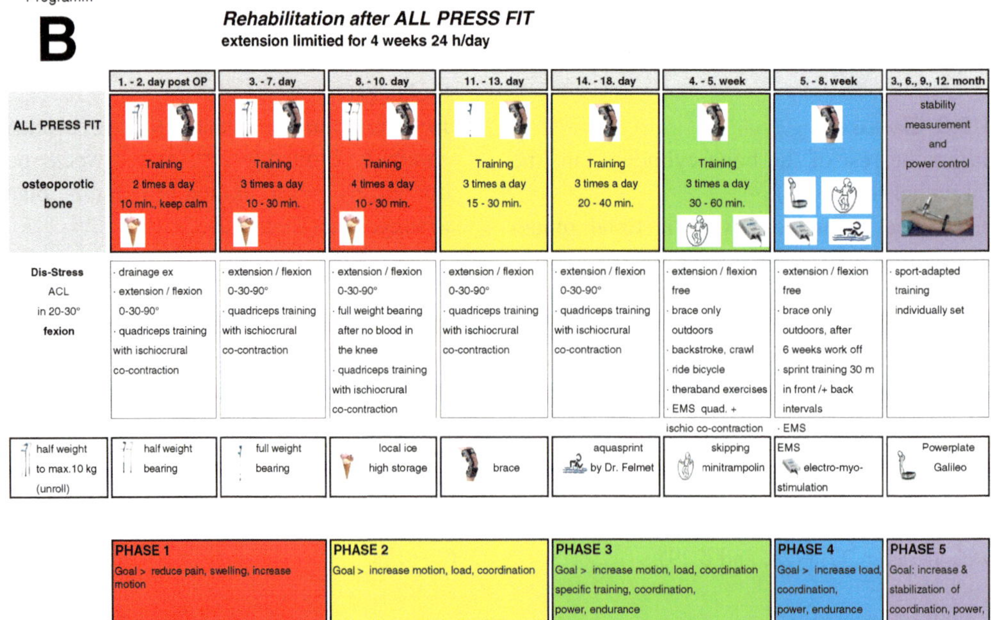

Programm **B**

Rehabilitation after ALL PRESS FIT

extension limitied for 4 weeks 24 h/day

	1. - 2. day post OP	3. - 7. day	8. - 10. day	11. - 13. day	14. - 18. day	4. - 5. week	5. - 8. week	3., 6., 9., 12. month
ALL PRESS FIT osteoporotic bone	Training 2 times a day 10 min., keep calm	Training 3 times a day 10 - 30 min.	Training 4 times a day 10 - 30 min.	Training 3 times a day 15 - 30 min.	Training 3 times a day 20 - 40 min.	Training 3 times a day 30 - 60 min.		stability measurement and power control
Dis-Stress ACL in 20-30° **fexion**	· drainage ex · extension / flexion 0-30-90° · quadriceps training with ischiocrural co-contraction	· extension / flexion 0-30-90° · quadriceps training with ischiocrural co-contraction	· extension / flexion 0-30-90° · full weight bearing after no blood in the knee · quadriceps training with ischiocrural co-contraction	· extension / flexion 0-30-90° · quadriceps training with ischiocrural co-contraction	· extension / flexion 0-30-90° · quadriceps training with ischiocrural co-contraction	· extension / flexion free · brace only outdoors · backstroke, crawl · ride bicycle · theraband exercises · EMS quad. + ischio co-contraction	· extension / flexion free · brace only outdoors, after 6 weeks work off · sprint training 30 m in front /+ back intervals · EMS	· sport-adapted training individually set

half weight to max.10 kg (unroll)	half weight bearing	full weight bearing	local ice high storage	brace	aquasprint by Dr. Felmet	skipping minitrampolin	EMS electro-myo-stimulation	Powerplate Galileo

PHASE 1	PHASE 2	PHASE 3	PHASE 4	PHASE 5
Goal > reduce pain, swelling, increase motion	Goal > increase motion, load, coordination	Goal > increase motion, load, coordination specific training, coordination, power, endurance	Goal > increase load, coordination, power, endurance	Goal: increase & stabilization of coordination, power, endurance

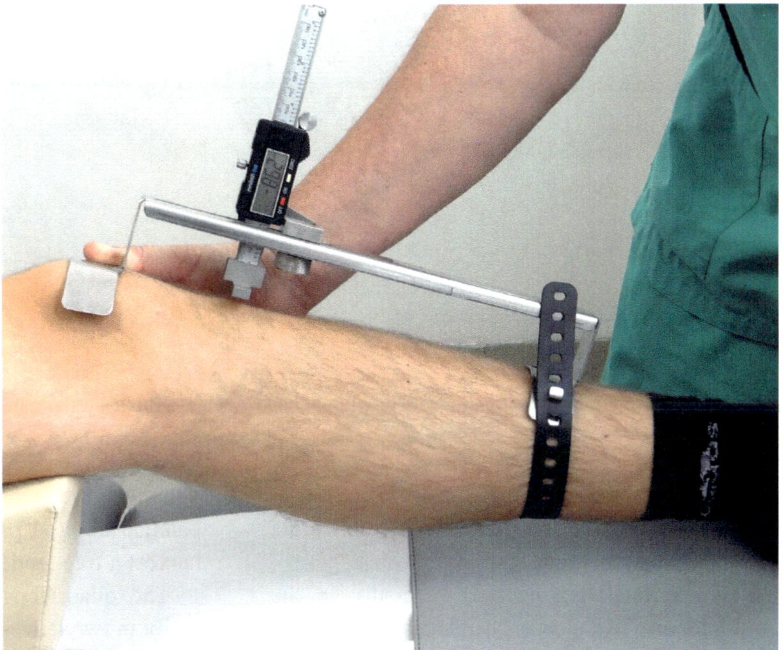

Fig. 6.16 ArticoMeter (digital Rolimeter) and muscle function tests follow 3, 6, 9 and 12 months after surgery [14, 15]

Outpatient controls at 3, 6, 9 and 12 months with

- ACL ArticoMeter (digital Rolimeter) measurement in Lachman position (Fig. 6.16)
- Clinical and muscle function tests for quadriceps and ischiocrural muscle and
- Isometric power measurement

6.1.5.10 Early-Phase Postoperative Complications

- Swelling
- Stiffness in flexion and/or extension
- Saphenous nerve damage
- Thrombosis
- Atrophy of the muscles

6.2 Quadriceps Tendon-Bone or BTB Fixation with Bone Dowels "All Press-Fit"

6.2.1 Surgical Preparation

6.2.1.1 Surgical Equipment

- Crown cutter, micro crown cutter or diamond hollow reamer in diameter 8–11 mm with guiding devices described for hamstrings (Fig. 6.1)
- Quadriceps tendon harvester (helpful supplemet)
- Sutures
- 2× USP 1, HRT 37 (non-traumatic) 90 cm, to pull in the graft sutured onto the femoral end
- or
- 1× USP 5, 90 cm to pull in the graft onto the femoral end with a patellar bone cylinder
- 1× USP 2/0 DS 25 75 cm for sutures on the peritendineum and periosteum
- 1× USP 3/0 DS 24 75 cm for sub- and intracutaneous suture
- Complete arthroscopic set with a shaver
- Curette
- An arthroscopy pump is used routinely

Equipment, positioning and arthroscopic management as described above for the hamstring.

6.2.2 Surgical Technique

6.2.2.1 Harvesting Tendon-Bone Graft

Inflate the tourniquet to 350 mmHg.

Exsanguinate the limb before making the first incision.

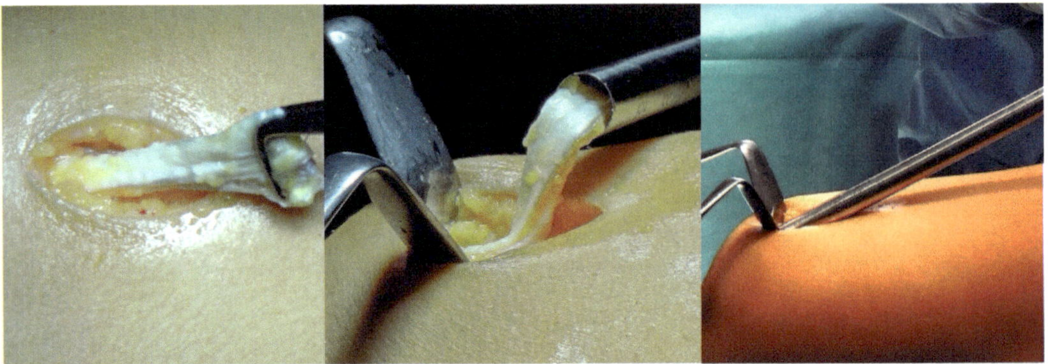

Fig. 6.17 Harvest quadriceps tendon with or without bone cylinder from the proximal patella using the hollow reamer (from left to right)

Make a vertical skin incision from the tip of the proximal patella for about 3–4 cm above the middle of the quadriceps tendon.

The peritendon is incised vertically in the mid-line, and two sleeves are detached from the tendon at its lateral and medial margins.

With the same blade, mark the limit of the bone cylinder on the proximal patella aligned on the tendon (Fig. 6.17).

Using an no. 10 blade, the middle third of the tendon with a width of about 10–12 mm is incompletely incised longitudinally, separating carefully with three quarters of the calibre from the quadriceps tendon with a thickness of about 4–5 mm.

Separate with a small pean clamp the three quarters of the tendon on a minimum length of 70 mm.

If possible keep the internal synovium and joint closed.

Alternatively, a *quadriceps tendon harvester* can be used in the same way.

6.2.2.2 Graft with Patellar Bone Cylinder (A) or Without (B)

A. Carefully cut the tendon proximally with a horizontal incision.

   Push the tendon into a 9-mm hollow reamer

   Position the hollow reamer horizontally and cut a bone half cylinder from the proximal patella (Fig. 6.17).

B. Separate the tendon carefully from the patella, taking a part of the periosteum, and harvest a free tendon.

   The quadriceps tendon separates proximally in two leaves (Fig. 6.18a).

6.2.2.3 Performing Tunnels

See above as for the hamstring (Figs. 6.6, 6.7, 6.8, and 6.9).

6.2.2.4 Prepare the Graft

Analogous hamstring (Figs. 6.10 and 6.11).

A. Fix the bone cylinder with a Kocher clamp and press a hole with a sharp cloth clamp through the bone or use a drill.

   Pull a no. 2 thread into this hole (Fig. 6.18d).

B. Fix two no. 0 sutures on the patellar side end of the quadriceps tendon with Krackow stitches (Fig. 6.18a–c).

   Open the two leaves and stabilize with two Kantrowitz clamps.

   Cut the tibial 9-mm bone cylinder and insert the proximal one with the cortical side down into the two leaves (Fig. 6.18a).

   Fix the bone cylinder with two sutures around the bone dowel and keep a bone window for bone-to-bone contact healing inside the tunnel open (analogous to preparation of the hamstring) (Fig. 6.18b).

   Use A for a BTB graft in the same way, arming the two leaves with a bone cylinder (use different diameters for osteoporotic bone or revision surgery) (Fig. 6.18c, d).

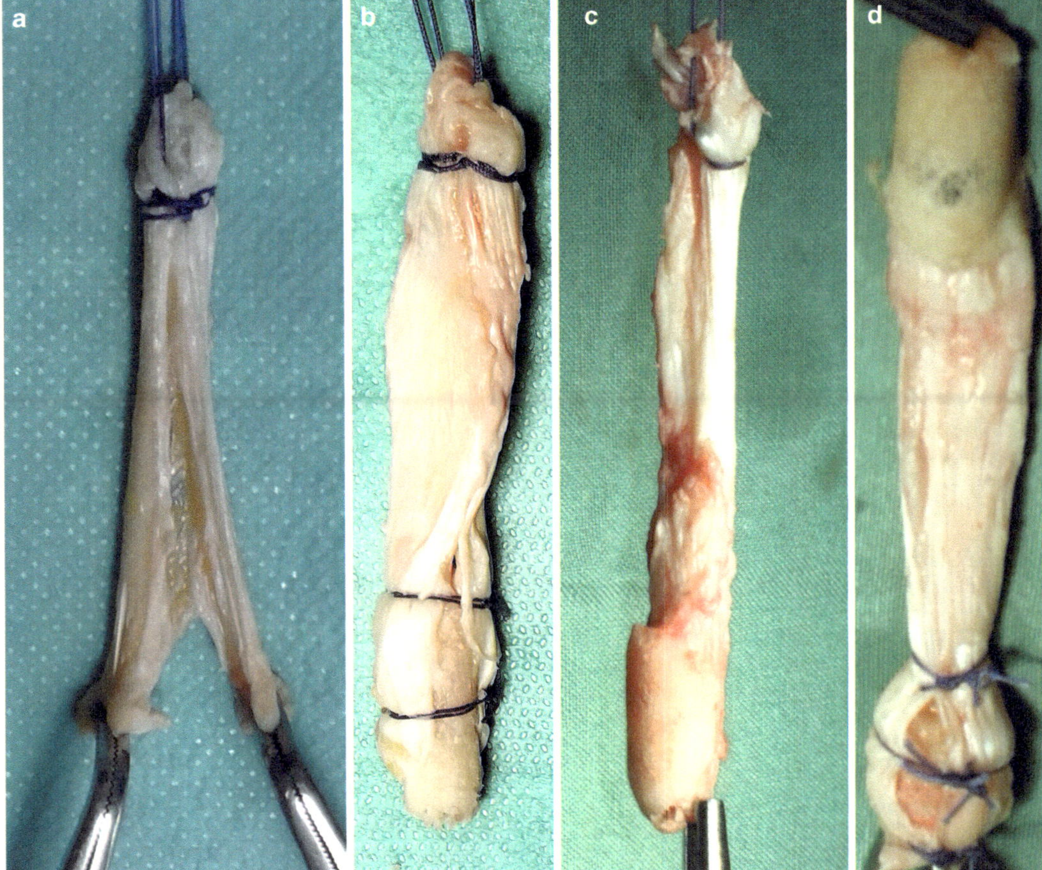

Fig. 6.18 Variation of quadriceps tendon. (**a**) Use two Krackow stitches on the patella side end and (**b**) insert a 10-mm bone cylinder from the tibial tunnel between the two sleeves and circulate and fix it with two sutures (analogous to the hamstring). (**c**) Use the bone cylinder from the proximal patella and (**d**) create a bone-tendon-bone graft with a bone cylinder from the tibial tunnel as in (**a**) and (**b**)

6.2.2.5 Passage of the Graft

Measure the length of your tibial tunnel with a ruler (Fig. 6.9).

For BTB Graft

Pass the threads through the tibial tunnel and pull them inside out of the anteromedial portal (Fig. 6.19).

Insert and drill the pull-out pin through the anteromedial portal in 120° flexion through the femoral tunnel.

Insert the thread through the eye linked to the smaller patellar bone block/or graft and pull it out through the femoral tunnel.

Fix the thread with a clamp and pull the small cylinder into the tibial tunnel.

Pull the graft inside while simultaneously pushing the tibial bone cylinder into the tibial tunnel (Fig. 6.19).

Push the small bone into the femoral tunnel.

Than go back and push the tibial bone cylinder up to the plateau.

Alternate with the femoral cylinder.

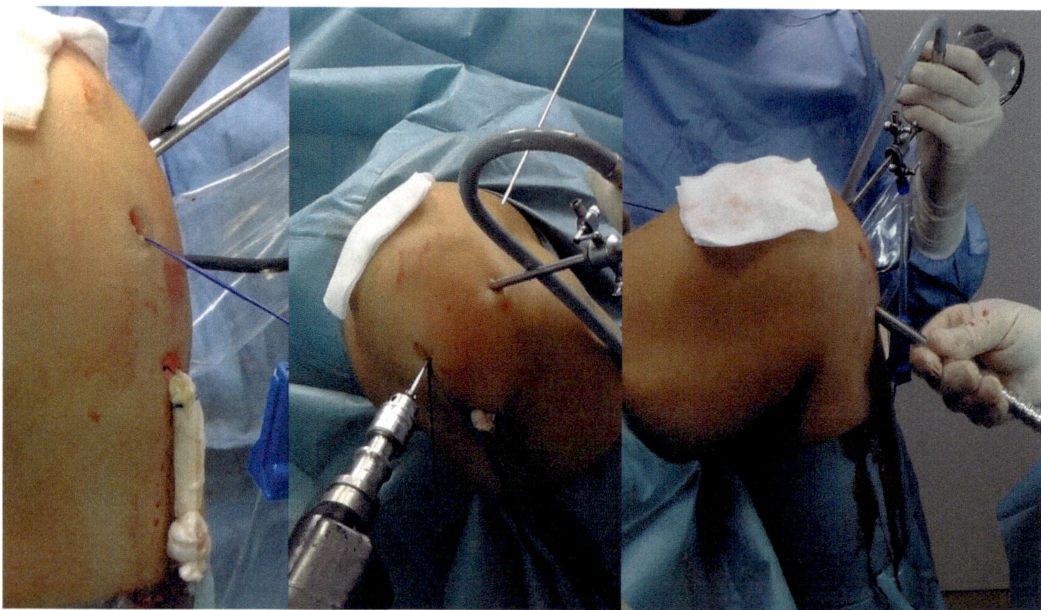

Fig. 6.19 Passage of the quadriceps tendon-bone graft. From left to right: lead the threads through the tibial tunnel out of the anteromedial portal. Insert the pull-out pin over the anteromedial portal into the femoral tunnel and pull the threads and the graft into both tunnels. Pull and simultaneously push the tibial graft with the bone cylinder into the tunnel. Analogous to the hamstring

6.2.2.6 Fixation of the Graft

Analogous to the hamstring (Figs. 6.12, 6.13, and 6.14).

Reverse to the established procedure: "Bottom-to-Top" fixation is a "Self-Adapted Tensioning" based on the geometry of the knee.

See also Sect. 6.3.2.5.

Tibial Fixation

Fixation is performed with the complete passage of the graft.

The tibial bone cylinder (9 + 3 mm of the graft) is pushed and fixed press-fit near the joint analogous hamstring.

The correct position can be controlled by the length of the tunnel minus the length of the bone cylinder = depth of the tibial tunnel after implantation.

Femoral Fixation

Take the bone cylinder from the femoral tunnel with a length of 30 mm.

Cut it into two pieces.

In the case of a **BTB graft**:

- Pull and push the small bone cylinder deep into the femoral tunnel in 120° flexion.
- Insert the cortical–cancellous bone cylinder into the 9-mm applicator.
- Insert the applicator with pusher through the anteromedial portal to the femoral tunnel.
- Check the bone cylinder through the small window at the side of the applicator.
- In maximum knee flexion pull on the thread and simultaneously push the bone cylinder inside the tunnel.
- A crescent-shaped insertion appears ribbon like (Fig. 6.20).
- Extend the knee. The graft will be in self-adapted tensioning in extension in a "bottom-to-top" fixation (Fig. 6.14).
- Push the cortical bone a little deeper into the notch.

In the case of a **tendon bone graft**:

- Analogous to the hamstring (Figs. 6.12 and 6.13).
- Fixation is performed with the complete passage of the graft.
- The tibial bone cylinder (9 + 3 mm of the graft) is pushed and fixed press-fit near the joint analogous hamstring.

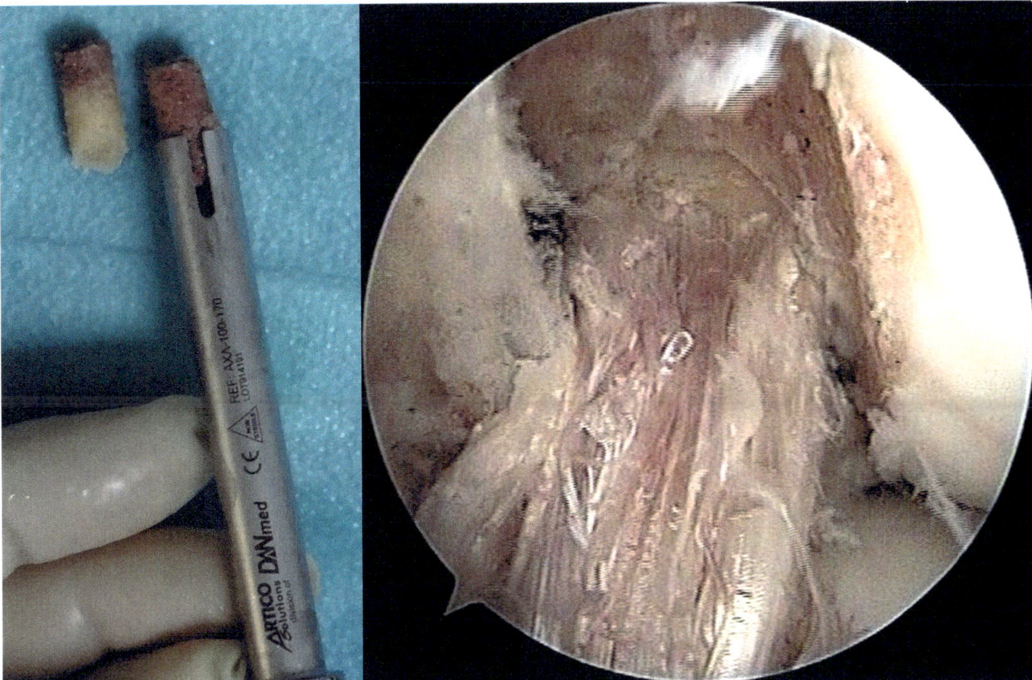

Fig. 6.20 Femoral fixation of ribbon-like, crescent-shaped insertion of 12 mm width to mimic the anteromedial and posterolateral bundle

- The correct position of the graft can be checked by the depth of the distal tunnel compared with the length of the rest of the tibial bone cylinder (Fig. 6.9).
- Check stability.
- Go back to flexion. Pull the threads again and cut them.

6.2.2.7 Possible Peri-operative Complications

- Femoral /and or tibial fixation is not stable: limit extension in 20° knee flexion in a brace for 4 weeks postoperatively (Table 6.2).
- Femoral posterior blow out: if possible variation to a more high noon position for another femoral tunnel.
- Tibial fixation is unstable: push the cylinder into the tibial tunnel and fix it with a K-wire as a cross-pin for 4–6 weeks, then remove.
- Osteoporotic bone/revision surgery: threads on the femoral and tibial side can be fixed each over a small bone bridge outside the tunnels at the medial tibia and lateral femoral condyle.

6.2.2.8 Closure

Close the peritendon over the tendon defect with an absorbable suture.

Close the subcutaneous and skin layers in a standard fashion.

Intra-articular drainage.

Simple dressing.

Apply a flexed knee splint for 1–2 days maximum.

Plain radiograph control on the same day (Fig. 6.26) or DVT, MSCT device, CBCT device [8–11], for correct position of the bone dowels (Figs. 6.27 and 6.28).

MRI in other questions of the graft, e.g. capsule, menisci, cartilage, bone, etc. (Fig. 6.30).

6.2.2.9 Post-operative Course

As for the hamstring.

6.3 ACL Reconstruction with Patella BTB or TB with Bone Dowels "All Press-Fit"

6.3.1 Surgical Preparation

6.3.1.1 Surgical Equipment

- Crown cutter, micro crown cutter or diamond hollow reamer in diameter 8–11 mm with guiding devices described for hamstring (Fig. 6.1).
- Oscillating saw.
- Sutures:
  - 2× USP 1, HRT 37 (non-traumatic) 90 cm, to pull in the graft sutured on the femoral end
  - or
  - 1× USP 5, 90 cm to pull in the graft on the femoral end with patellar bone cylinder
  - 1× USP 2/0 DS 25 75 cm for sutures on the peritendineum and periosteum
  - 1× USP 3/0 DS 24 75 cm for sub- and intracutaneous suture
- Complete arthroscopic set with a shaver
- Curette
- An arthroscopy pump is used routinely

Equipment, positioning and arthroscopic management as described above for the hamstring.

6.3.2 Surgical Technique

6.3.2.1 Harvesting Bone-Tendon-Bone Graft

Inflate the tourniquet to 350 mmHg. Exsanguinate the limb before making the first incision.

Make a vertical skin incision at the lateral border or central of the patellar tendon from the distal tip of the patella down to the tibial tubercle.

The peritendon is incised vertically in the mid-line, and two sleeves are detached from the tendon at its lateral and medial margins.

With the same blade, mark the limits of both bone blocks on the patella and the tibial tubercle.

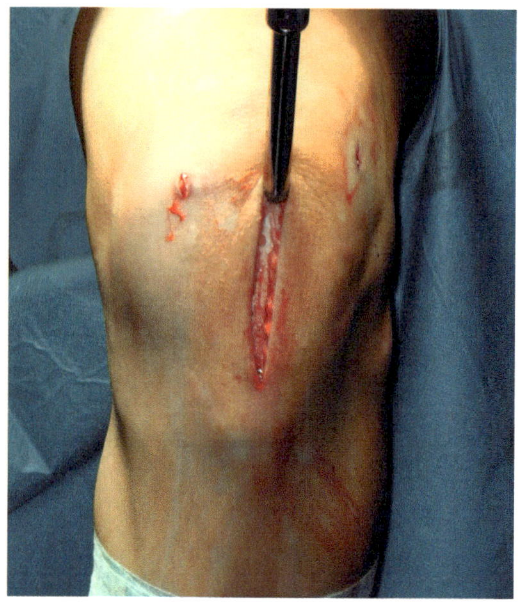

Fig. 6.21 After preparation of the patellar tendon, insert the 9-mm hollow reamer on the distal patella at a flat angle of about 30° to harvest an approximately 10- to 12-mm-long half-cylinder on this patellar tendon end

Drill a 2.7-mm hole in the centre of the tibial bone block before excising, as they are more stable in situ.

Incise the tibial tubercle with the oscillating saw for a 2-cm tibial bone cylinder.

For **BTB**: the 9- or 10-mm diameter hollow reamer is positioned on the distal third of the patella and a half cylinder is harvested (Fig. 6.21).

Using an no. 10 blade, the middle third of the tendon is harvested longitudinally, separating it carefully from the fat pad.

For **tendon-bone**: the proximal tendon is harvested, including the periosteum of the adjacent distal patella.

To excise the tibial bone cylinder use a small oscillating saw and make a 2-cm horizontal cut at the tibial tubercle.

Push the middle third of the tendon (without or with patellar bone cylinder) inside the 11-mm hollow reamer (Fig. 6.22).

Mill the 11-mm hollow reamer to the 2-cm bone incision and harvest the graft.

Release the hollow reamer from the drill and push the (B)TB graft with a long pusher out of the reamer (Fig. 6.23).

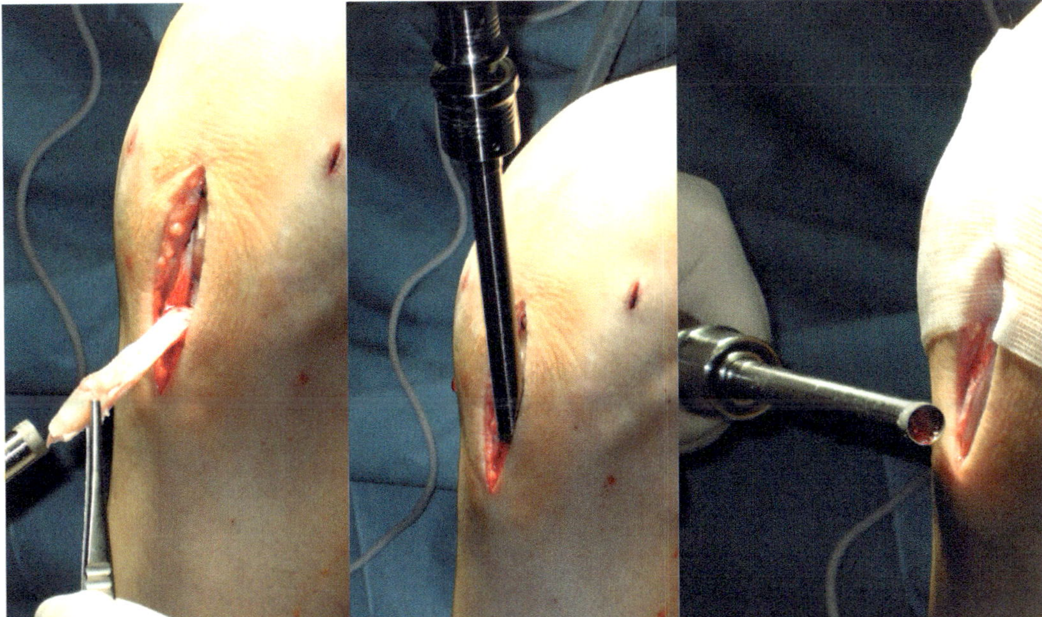

Fig. 6.22 Push the middle third of the patellar tendon into the 11-mm hollow reamer (left), insert the 11-mm hollow reamer over the tibial tuberosity and cut a 10- to 15-mm bone cylinder. Incise this point with an oscillating saw first (middle). Tilt the reamer and harvest the bone-tendon-bone graft (right)

Reshape the bone blocks into cubes with a rongeur.

Pass USP 5 decimal suture through the drill hole in the smaller bone cylinder (normally the patellar bone cylinder)—or fix two USP 1 decimal sutures at the proximal tendon (patella side) with Krackow stitches.

6.3.2.2 Performing Tunnels

Femoral Tunnel

See above as for the hamstring (Figs. 6.6, 6.7, 6.8, and 6.9).

Tibial Tunnel

- Flex the knee to 90° and insert the tibial tubed guide into the medial portal.
- Set the angle of the tibial tubed guide to 25°.
- Centre the tip of the tibial guide so that the intra-articular guide pin enters the joint just anterior to the PCL.
- Fix the guide directly into the **tibial tubercle defect** from the harvested BTB graft (Fig. 6.24, right).
- or
- Move the skin medially for an anatomical standard entrance of the tibial tunnel.
- Fix the guide to the medial cortex, about 20 mm above the pes anserinus (use the correct side left/right up) (Fig. 6.24, left).
- Prepare the tibial tunnel with 9-mm hollow reamer as for the *hamstring* (Figs. 6.6, 6.7, 6.8, and 6.9).

6.3.2.3 Passage of the Graft

As for the quadriceps tendon (Fig. 6.18).

6.3.2.4 Fixation of the Graft

Analogous to the hamstring (Figs. 6.12 and 6.13).

Reverse to the established procedure: "Bottom-to-Top" fixation is "Self-Adapted Tensioning" based on the geometry of the knee.

Tibial Fixation

Fixation is performed with the complete passage of the graft.

The tibial bone cylinder (11 mm) is pushed and fixed press-fit with an oversize of 2 mm in the 9-mm bottle neck of the tibial tunnel near the

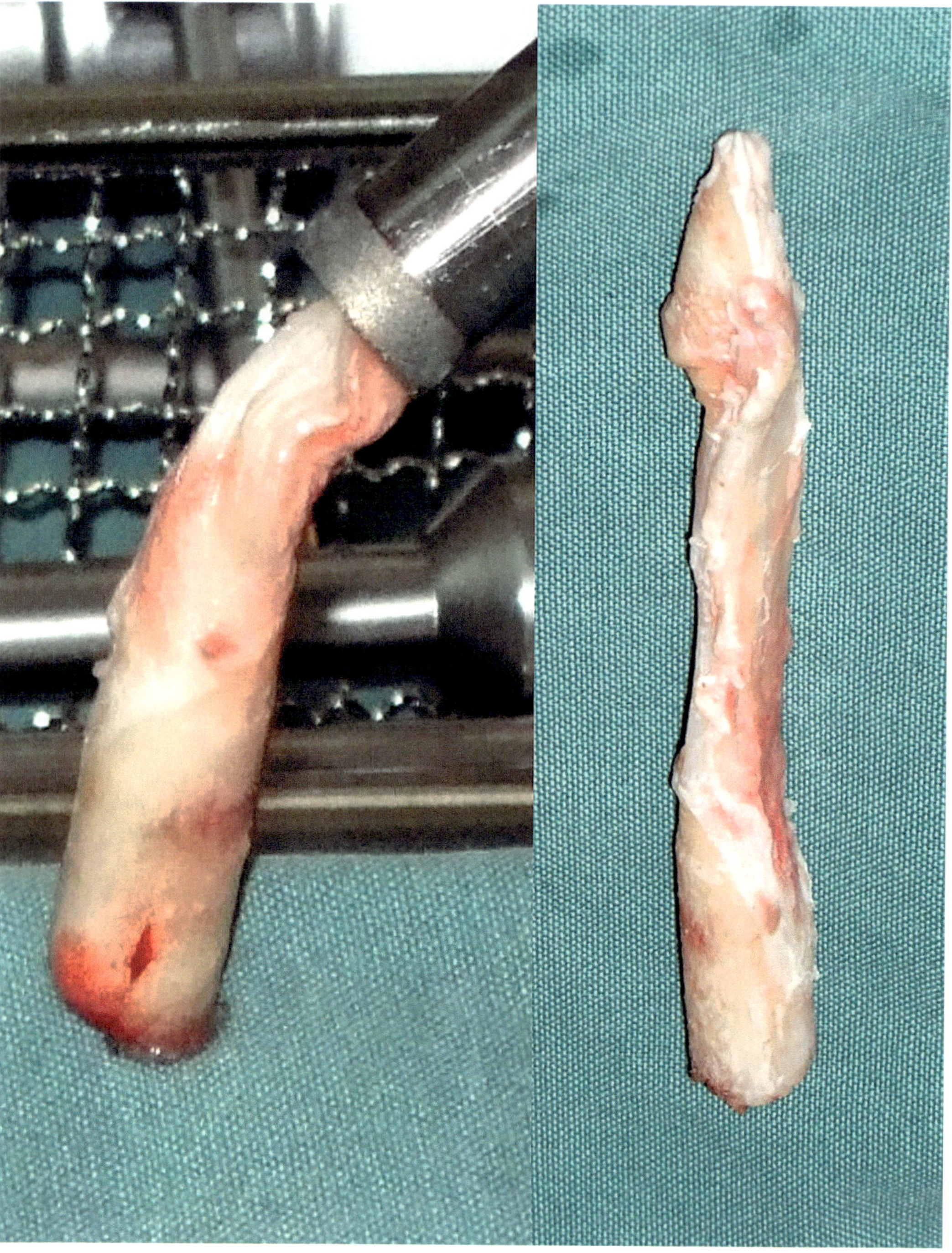

Fig. 6.23 Push the bone-tendon-bone graft out of the hollow reamer

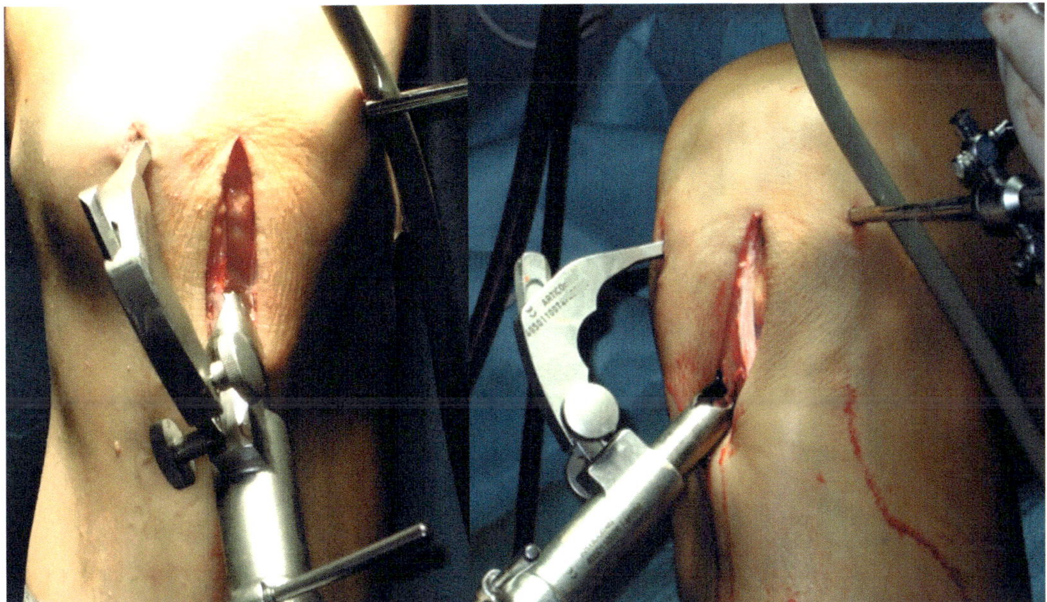

Fig. 6.24 Two options for the tibial tunnel: fix the distal tibial guide in the defect of the tibial tubercle (left) or medial from the tibial tuberosity (anatomically better position) (right)

joint. The correct position can be checked by the length of the tunnel minus the length of the bone cylinder = the depth of the tibial tunnel after implantation (Figs. 6.9 and 6.25).

Femoral Fixation

Take a bone cylinder with a length of 30 mm from the femoral tunnel. Cut it into two pieces.

In case of a **BTB graft**:

- Pull and push the small bone cylinder deep into the femoral tunnel in 120° flexion.
- Push the bone cylinder with the cortical end first into the 9-mm applicator.
- Insert the applicator with pusher through the anteromedial portal to the femoral tunnel.
- Control the bone cylinder through the small slot at the side.
- In maximum knee flexion pull the thread and push the bone cylinder parallel to the graft inside the tunnel.
- A ribbon-like, crescent-shaped graft fixation appears (Fig. 6.20).
- Extend the knee. The graft will be tensioned self-adapted in extension as a "bottom-to-top" fixation (Fig. 6.12).
- Push the cortical bone a little deeper than the surface of the notch (Fig. 6.25).

In case of a **tendon bone graft**:

- Analogous to the hamstring (Figs. 6.12, 6.13, and 6.14).
- Check stability.
- Go back to flexion. Pull strongly on the thread.
- Pull out or cut the thread.

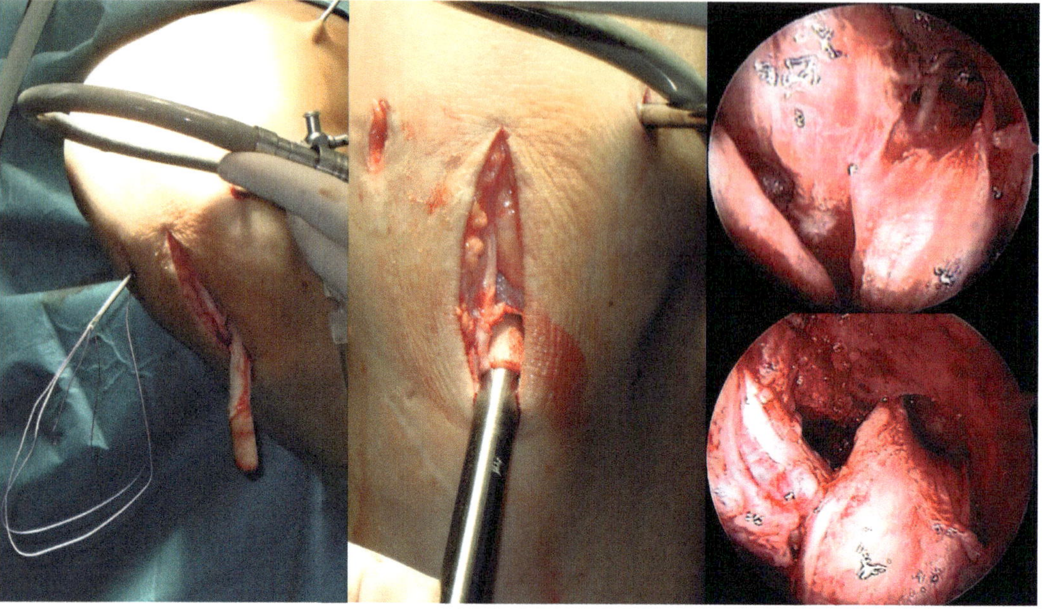

Fig. 6.25 Pull in the graft into the tunnels from distal (left). Simultaneously push in the tibial bone cylinder (middle). Fix it near the original insertion with bone dowels on the femoral side too (analogous to the hamstring) and mimic a ribbon-like anterior cruciate ligament reconstruction

6.3.2.5 Possible Peri-operative Complications

- Femoral/and or tibial fixation is not stable: limit extension in 20° knee flexion in a brace for 4 weeks postoperatively (Table 6.2).
- Femoral posterior blow out: if possible variation to a more high noon position for another femoral tunnel.
- Tibial fixation is unstable: push the cylinder into the tibial tunnel and fix it with a K-wire as a cross-pin for 4–6 weeks, then remove.
- Osteoporotic bone/revision surgery: threads on the femoral and tibial side can each be fixed over a small bone bridge outside the tunnels at the medial tibia and lateral femoral condyle.

6.3.2.6 Closure

- Reinsert the rest of the bone cylinders into the tibial defect and tunnel.
- Close the peritendon over the tendon defect with an absorbable suture.
- Close the subcutaneous and skin layers in a standard fashion
- Intra-articular drainage.
- Simple dressing.
- Apply a flexed knee splint for 1–2 days.
- Plain radiograph control on the same day (Fig. 6.26) or DVT for the correct position of the bone dowels (Figs. 6.27, 6.28 and 6.29).
- MRI in other questions of the graft, e.g. capsule, menisci, cartilage, bone, etc. (Fig. 6.30).

6.3.2.7 Postoperative Course

As for the hamstring.

6.3.2.8 Early-Phase Postoperative Complications

- Swelling
- Stiffness in flexion and/or extension
- Thrombosis
- Atrophy of the quadriceps muscle
- Quadriceps weakness
- Patellar tendinopathy
- Anterior knee pain

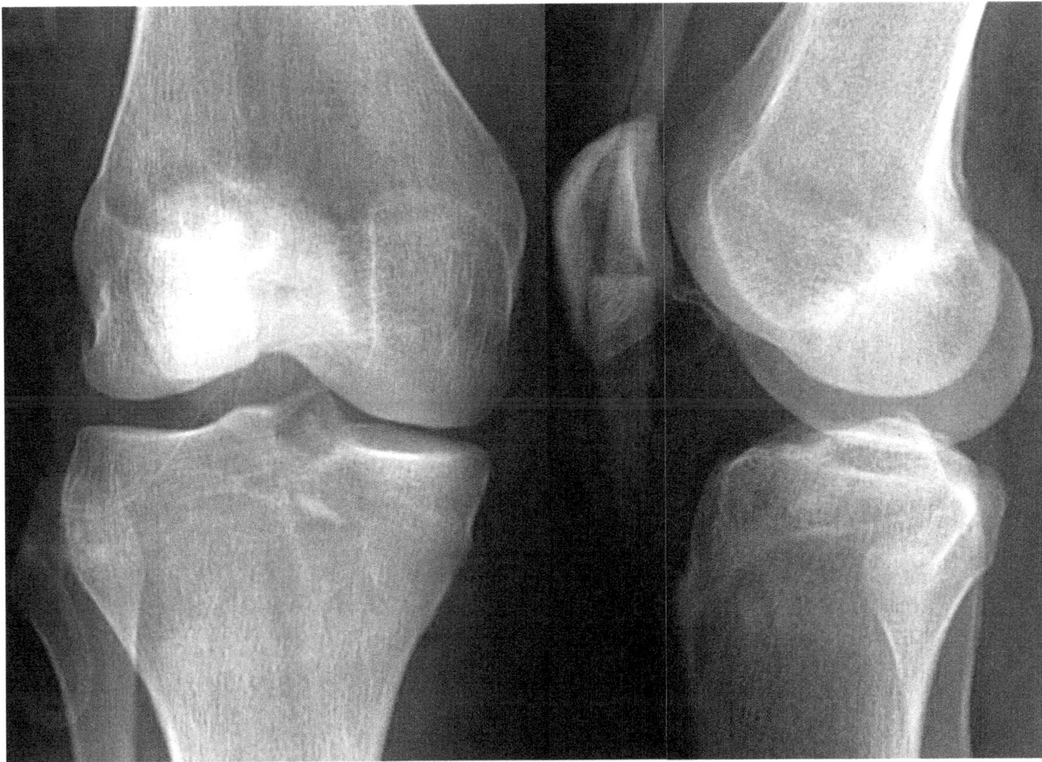

Fig. 6.26 Plain radiograph of a right knee control on the same day shows the position of the tunnels and bone dowels from the front (left) and side (right)

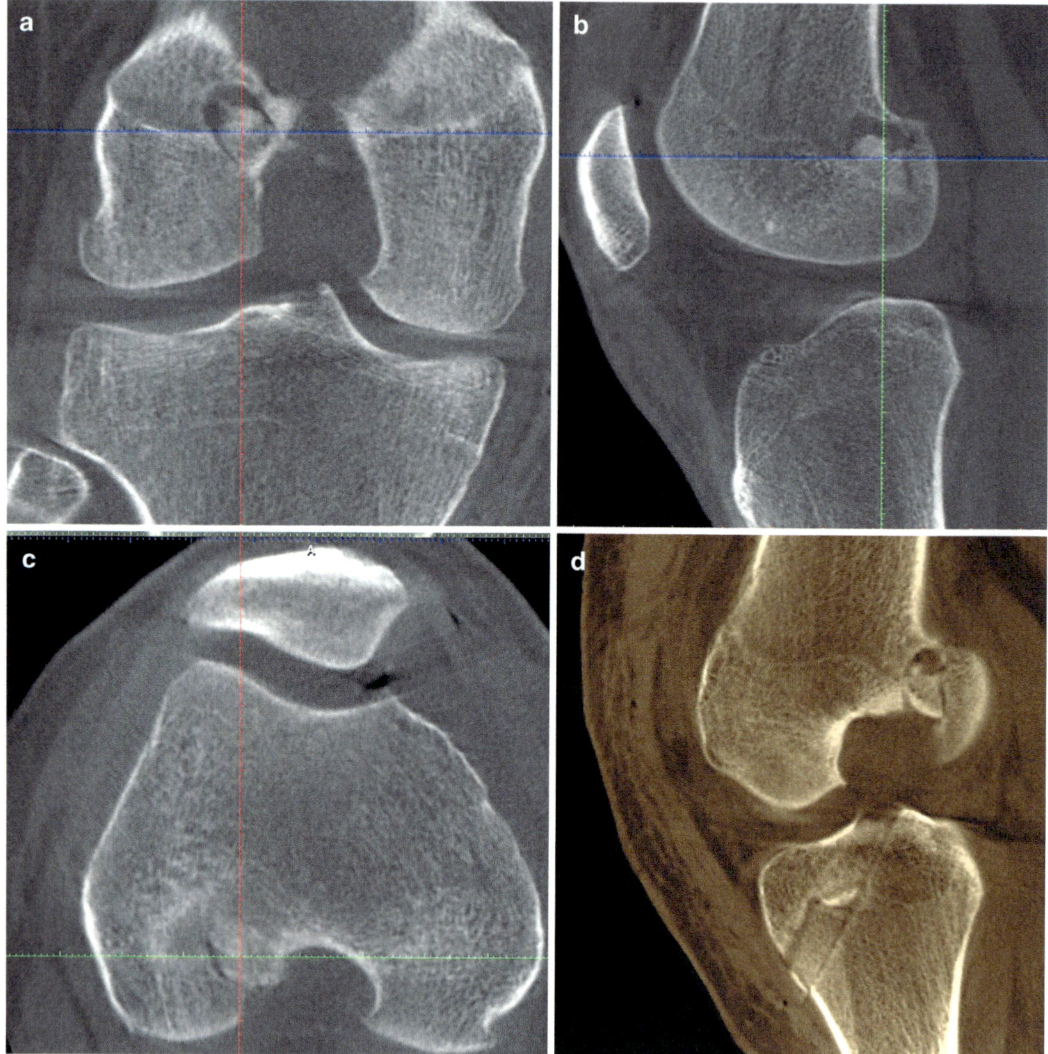

Fig. 6.27 Digital volume tomography (DVT) of a right knee postoperatively with positions of the bone dowels: in the front view, femoral tunnel (**a**); side view femoral tunnel, ribbon-like fixation (**b**); coronal view, femoral tunnel (**c**); angulated 3D tibial and femoral tunnel filled with two bone dowels anchored at the joint line and original insertion; proximal, with femoral fixation at the original insertion (**d**). DVT is a multi-slice computed tomography device, and a two cone-beam CT device [8–11] (Chap. 2)

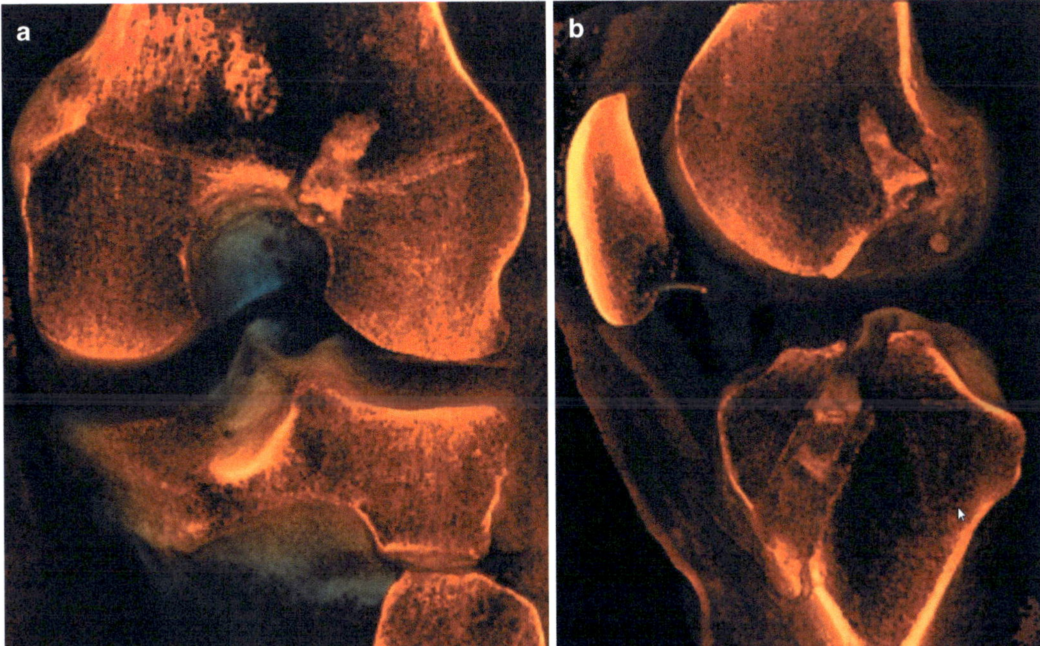

Fig. 6.28 Digital volume tomography of a right knee postoperatively coloured in 3D (three-dimensional rendering with a distance of 0.2 mm each slide) to enhance the contrast with the position of the bone dowels in the femoral tunnel close to the original insertion from posterior (**a**) and the tibial tunnel filled with two bone dowels near the joint line from the side (**b**)

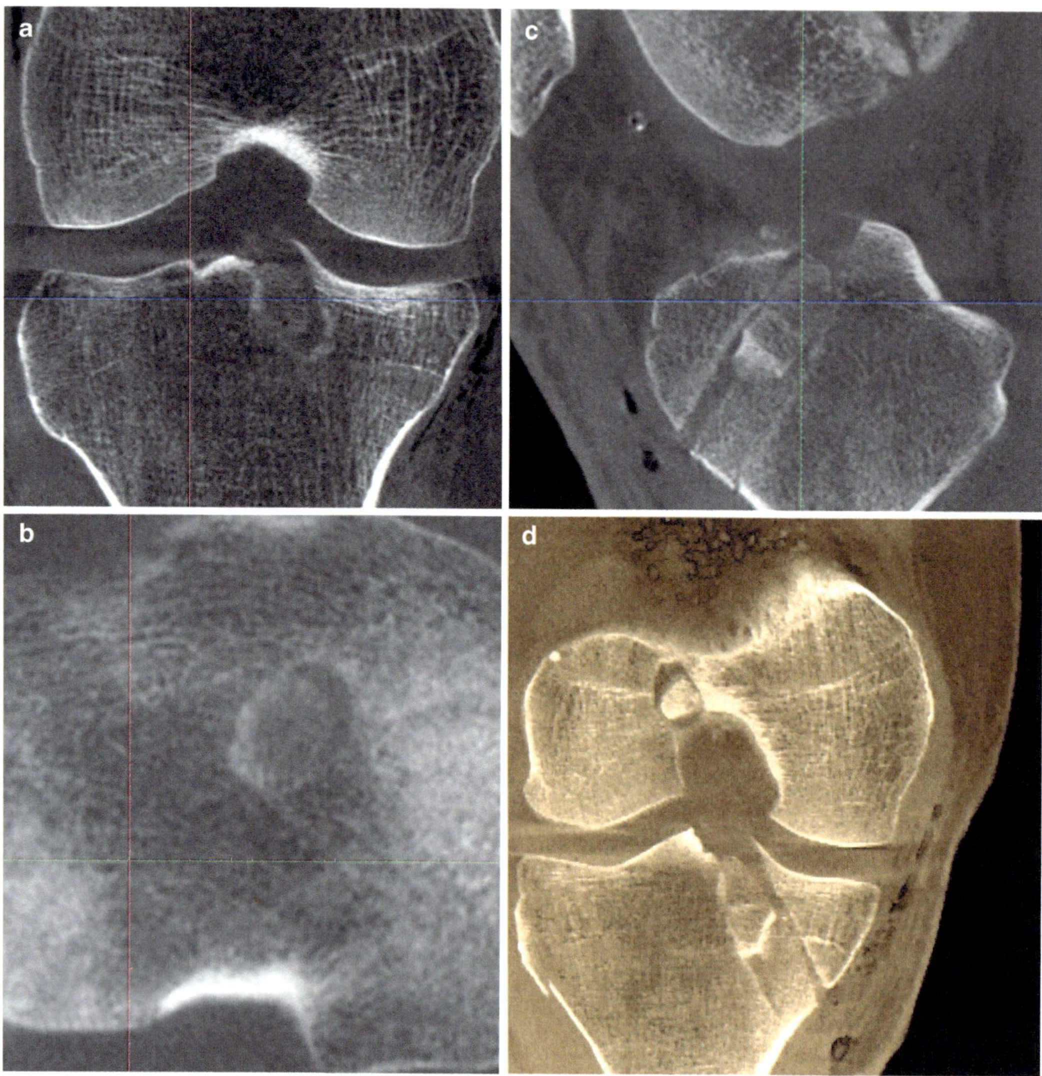

Fig. 6.29 Digital volume tomography of a right knee postoperatively. The tibial tunnel with a C-shaped bone plug laterally (**a**, **b**) and anatomical fixation at the original insertion (**c**, **d**)

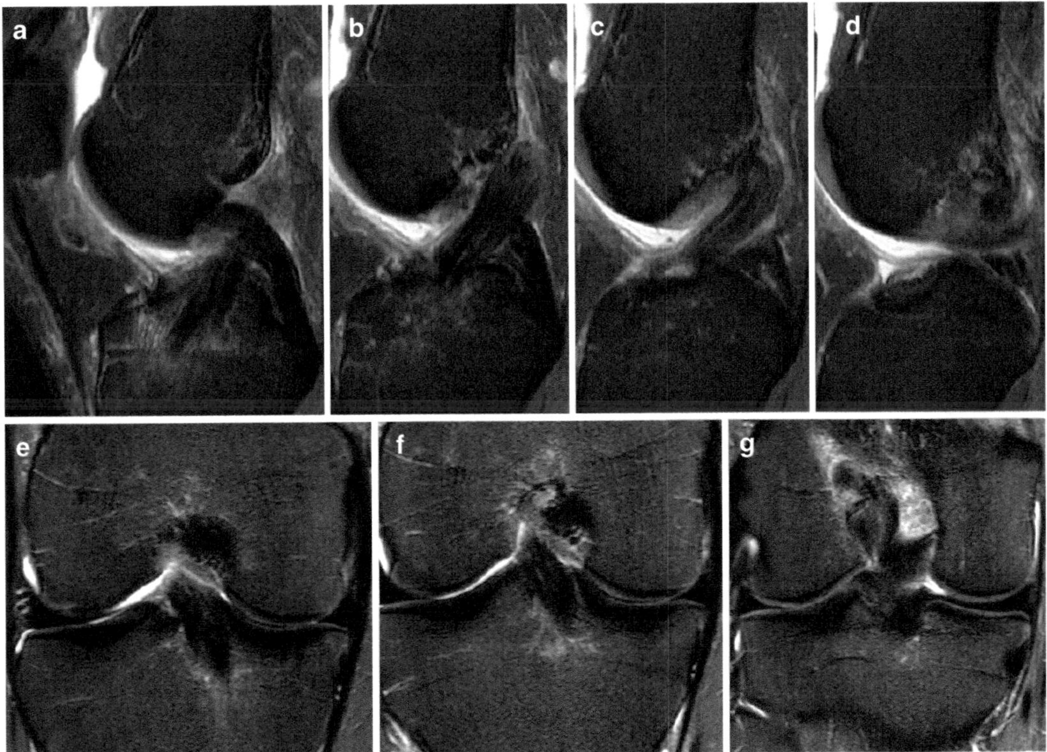

Fig. 6.30 MRI of a left knee after 3 months. Anatomically ribbon-like bony integration of the hamstring graft in the sagittal and frontal cut. Almost no fluid in the tunnels. A flat insertion on the tibia side (**a**, **b**, **c**, **e**, **f**). Femoral insertion is also flat and ribbon like (**d**, **g**)

References

1. Felmet G. [ALL-PRESS-FIT, a new surgical method with femoral and tibial Press Fit fixation]. Arthroskopie. 1999;12:299–304.
2. Felmet G. [ACL Reconstruction with proximal and distal press fit fixation (ALL PRESS FIT) with SDI (Surgical Diamond Instrument) Instruments]. Osteosynth Int. 2000;8(Suppl 1):173–4.
3. Felmet G. [ALL PRESS FIT, a near the origin ACL Reconstruction with Semitendinosus & Gracilis Tendon, a New Surgical Technique] in 21. In: Kongress der deutschsprachigen Arbeitsgemeinschaft für Arthroskopie (AGA), 2004, Luzern, Switzerland; 2004.
4. Felmet G. Implant-free press-fit fixation for bone-patellar tendon-bone ACL reconstruction: 10-year results. Arch Orthop Trauma Surg. 2010;130(8):985–92.
5. Felmet G. Anatomic double bundle single tunnel foreign material free ACL-reconstruction – a technical note. Muscles Ligaments Tendons J. 2011;1(4):148–52.
6. Felmet G. Foreign material-free ACL reconstruction with hollow miller: a biological and anatomic method for every ligament. Tech Orthop. 2013;28(2):166–75.
7. Felmet G. Reconstruction of the anterior cruciate ligament without foreign materials: bone dowel method. In: Jones TVSKH, Kelberine F, McConnell JS, editors. EFOST surgical techniques in sports medicine - knee surgery. Soft tissue, vol. 1. London: JP Medical Ltd; 2015. p. 132.
8. Koivisto J, et al. Effective radiation dose of a MSCT, two CBCT and one conventional radiography device in the ankle region. J Foot Ankle Res. 2015;8:8.
9. Koivisto J, et al. Assessment of effective radiation dose of an extremity CBCT, MSCT and conventional X ray for knee area using MOSFET dosemeters. Radiat Prot Dosim. 2013;157(4):515–24.
10. Koivisto J, et al. Effective radiation dose in the wrist resulting from a radiographic device, two CBCT devices and one MSCT device: a comparative study. Radiat Prot Dosim. 2018;179(1):58–68.
11. Pallaver A, Honigmann P. The role of cone-beam computed tomography (CBCT) scan for detection and follow-up of traumatic wrist pathologies. J Hand Surg [Am]. 2019;44(12):1081–7.

12. Felmet G. "Aquasprint" in the early functional rehabilitation program after ACL reconstruction. In: Frenzel G, Wuschech H, editors. Arthroskopische Gelenkchirurgie, Gestern-Heute-Morgen Standortbestimmung. Berlin: Kongress Compact Verlag; 2002. p. 188–96.
13. Felmet G. [The significance of proprioceptive vibration training in postoperative treatment after ACL reconstruction]. In: DGOOC, 2004, Berlin; 2004.
14. Krautter A, et al. Instrumented arthrometry of the anterior cruciate ligament. A comparison. Biomed Tech. 2012;57:4299.
15. Runer A, et al. The evaluation of Rolimeter, KLT, KiRA and KT-1000 arthrometer in healthy individuals shows acceptable intra-rater but poor inter-rater reliability in the measurement of anterior tibial knee translation. Knee Surg Sports Traumatol Arthrosc. 2021.

7 Healing Response of the ACL with Bone Incision

Conservative treatment of partial anterior cruciate ligament (ACL) ruptures is associated with a high failure rate, and often patients undergo ACL reconstruction. To save the ACL, use the stump and reattach it to the origin is a resource preserving thinking.

Sutures of the ACL remnant are mostly unsuccessful. Newer investigations seem to be more successful [1, 2]. The natural nutrition by only one vessel from the proximal femoral side by the medial genicular artery could be the reason why ruptures in the middle or distal part mostly do not heal.

"Healing response" uses the remnant of the ACL stump in the case of an ultra-femoral rupture. A bone marrow stimulation of the femoral attachment on the ligament side and preparing of the notch can be helpful.

Good results in juvenile competitive athletes have been described by Steadman et al. [3], as well as in older active athletes but also in comparison with the ACL replacement [4]. The rate of re-ruptures after a regular indication of healing response is in the long term of 5 years' follow-up comparable with ACL replacement [5]. Other investigations found in adult patients an association with a high revision rate of secondary ACL reconstruction, comparable with primary conservative treatment.

Healing response did not result in better outcomes than conservative treatment [6].

One biologically anatomical bottleneck seems to be exclusive femoral arterial nutrition by the medial genicular artery. Our experience and investigations underlined the importance of an early time of surgery to use the regular biological potencies combined with a strict indication as well as compliance in the postoperative rehabilitation. The repositioning of the distal ACL remnant pressed into a femoral bone incision seems to be enough for a healing response [7, 8]. Intraligamentary application of concentrated autologous growth factors (platelet-rich plasma [PRP]/autologous-conditioned plasma [ACP]) may support this healing process [9]. ACL stump trephination and concomitant intraligamentary application of ACP revealed promising results at mid-term follow-up to treat partial ACL lesions as partial ruptures [10].

The best indication for healing response treatment is a fresh rupture of the ACL at the femoral origin, or rather "ultra-femorally" located tear. MRI is unable to find a safe indication for the use of healing response. Only arthroscopy supports finding the indication showing the complete lesion with the position and quality of the ACL remnant.

A large volume of the cruciate ligament stump is needed (Fig. 7.1). A partial rupture with similar conditions is suitable for healing response [10]. Planning the surgery and education of the patient should include both options for surgical support. This allows a strict and correct indication for a successful healing response for the patient's benefit.

G. Felmet, *Press-Fit Fixation of the Knee Ligaments*, https://doi.org/10.1007/978-3-031-11906-4_7

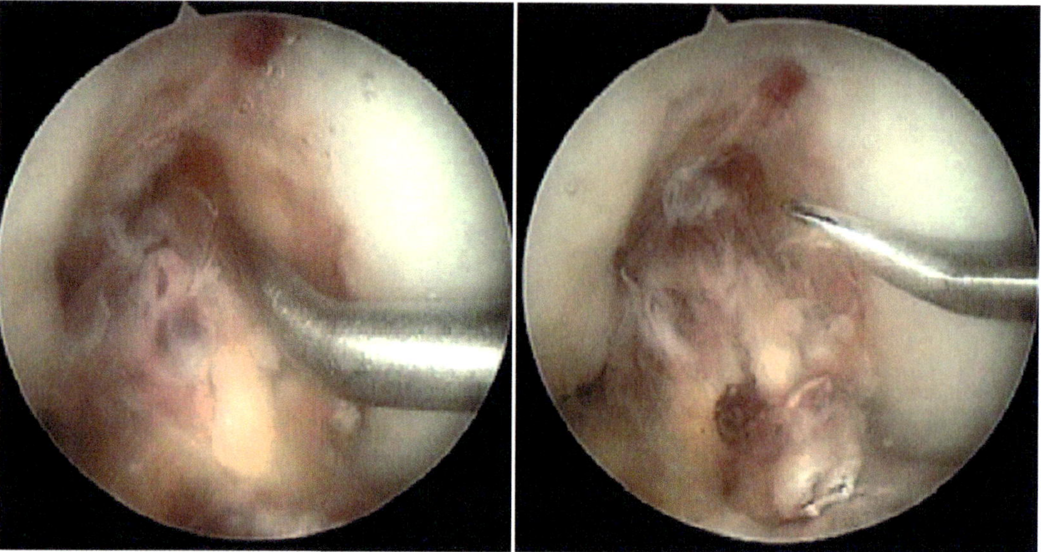

Fig. 7.1 A 5-day-old complete anterior cruciate ligament rupture repositioned with micro-pick combined with bone marrow stimulation at the femoral attachment

7.1 When to Apply Surgery and Healing Response?

The highest biological potential for reattachment and healing is in the first 3–6 weeks after trauma. In a few individual cases a successful supply up to months later was observed. (Never give up and give biology a chance!)

Steadman described after bone marrow stimulation a repositioning of the remnant with all fibres and described good results [3, 4] (Fig. 7.1). Motivated by this and experience of more than 30 years we modified the technique stepwise. Bone marrow stimulation can be performed with a rasp, micro pic, small chisel or a curved chisel. A little unhappy about leaving the stump repositioned incorrectly, we searched for a small area for bone fixation without an implant. The best solution was found to be using a curved chisel to create a small bone cut on the femoral side.

Table 7.1 Graduation of partial to complete ruptures of the anterior cruciate ligament (ACL) in accordance with Angele et al. [10]

	Graduation of partial to complete ACL rupture
Grade 1	Haemorrhage ACL without structural injuries, synovial surface intact
Grade 2	Slight structural injuries with separated fibres out of the synovial tube
Grade 3	Tear of the synovial tube with structural changes in one bundle
Grade 4	Significant structural loss of substance in both bundles
Grade 5	Only minimal residual fibres of the ACL to the femoral insertion

Optimising the indication we classified partial lesions to complete ruptures according to the graduation in 5°, as described by Koch et al. [10].

The ruptures we treated with fixation in a bone scale were grade 4–5: complete ruptures with loss of substance in both bundles (Table 7.1).

7.2 Surgical Technique

A small bone cut is created anterior of the anatomical femoral insertion. This is performed through the anteromedial portal with knee flexion of about 120°. The stump is carefully pulled open longitudinally; the fibres are disentangled to maximum length and stretched with a small chisel or pick to obtain a maximum length. The fibres were reinserted into the gap of the bone cut and pressed inside with the chisel itself. Stabilized then in about 30–40° knee flexion. Waterflow is to be stopped. The stable fluid protects the fibres on the bone scale. This can be explained by the flow behavior of liquids and gases, which was described by the Swiss physicist Daniel Bernoulli in the eighteenth century [7].

Use of arthroscopy is preferred.

- Have a good look inside.
- Check the notch (small or wide)
- If necessary clean the notch (Fig. 7.2)
- Check the quality of the stump
- Be sure that the rupture is on the ultra-femoral side
- Pull the stump open longitudinally with a flat chisel or micro-pic
- Trephination with a micro pick in the posterior area of the femoral insertion at the posteromedial and posterolateral bundle is suggested
- Flex the knee to 120°, set a bone cut and bone scale with a curved chisel at the anterior insertion of the anteromedial bundle (Fig. 7.3)
- Push the fibres of the ACL stump into the bone gap
- Stop water inflow (Fig. 7.3)
- Keep position in 20–30° knee flexion
- Stabilize knee in flexion with a splint or a brace
- Drainage is not recommended

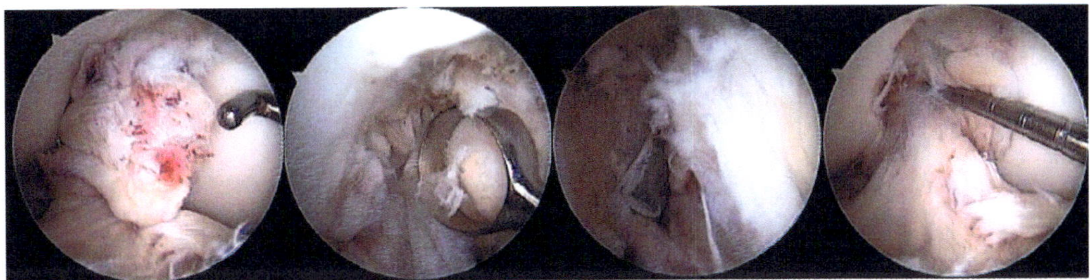

Fig. 7.2 Ultrafemoral anterior cruciate ligament (ACL) rupture, 2 weeks after trauma. Left to right: ACL stump. Cleaning the notch with a curette. Check the femoral side and length of the stump

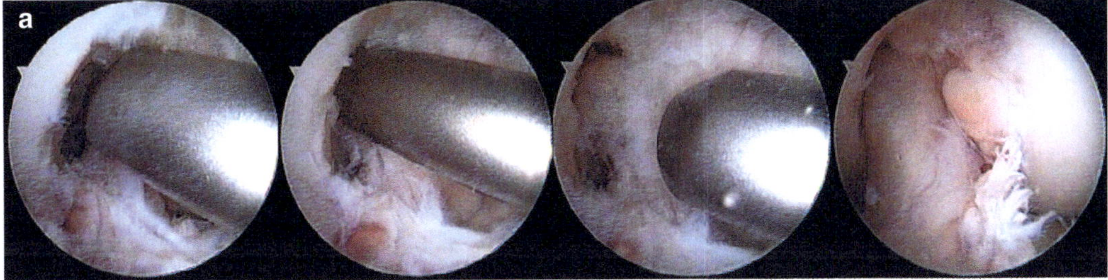

Fig. 7.3 (**a**) Bone cut and bone scale prepared with a curved chisel at the anterior original insertion. The proximal fibres of the stump are squeezed into the open bone scale. (**b**, **c**) ACL rupture with proximal scar tissue and insufficiency (**a**). The stump is disentangled to maximum length and stretched with a small chisel or pic to get a maximum length (**b**). A curved chisel is making the bone cut in 120° knee flexion (**c**). The opened fibres have the length to be squeezed and inserted by chisel into the bone gap at the anterior original insertion

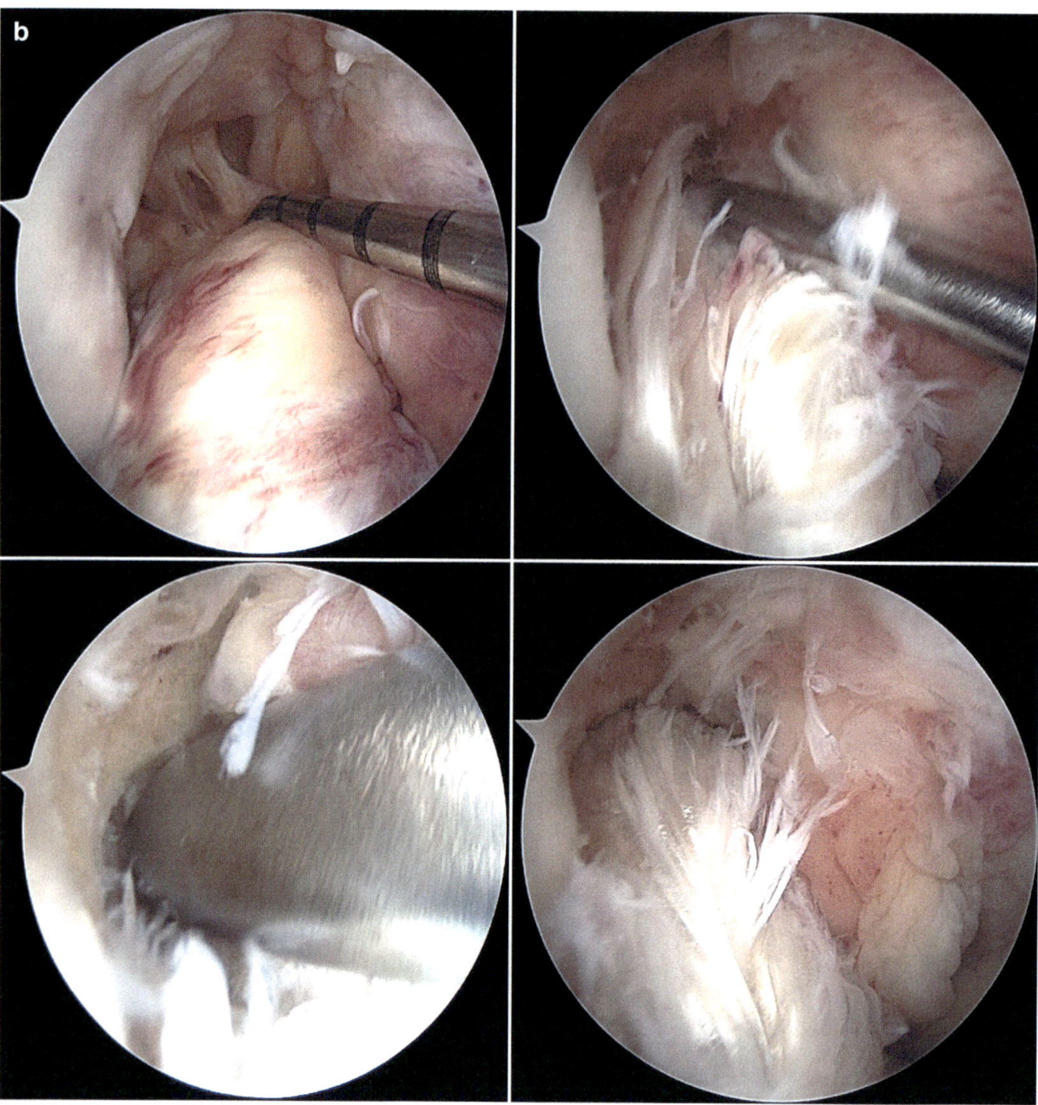

Fig. 7.3 (continued)

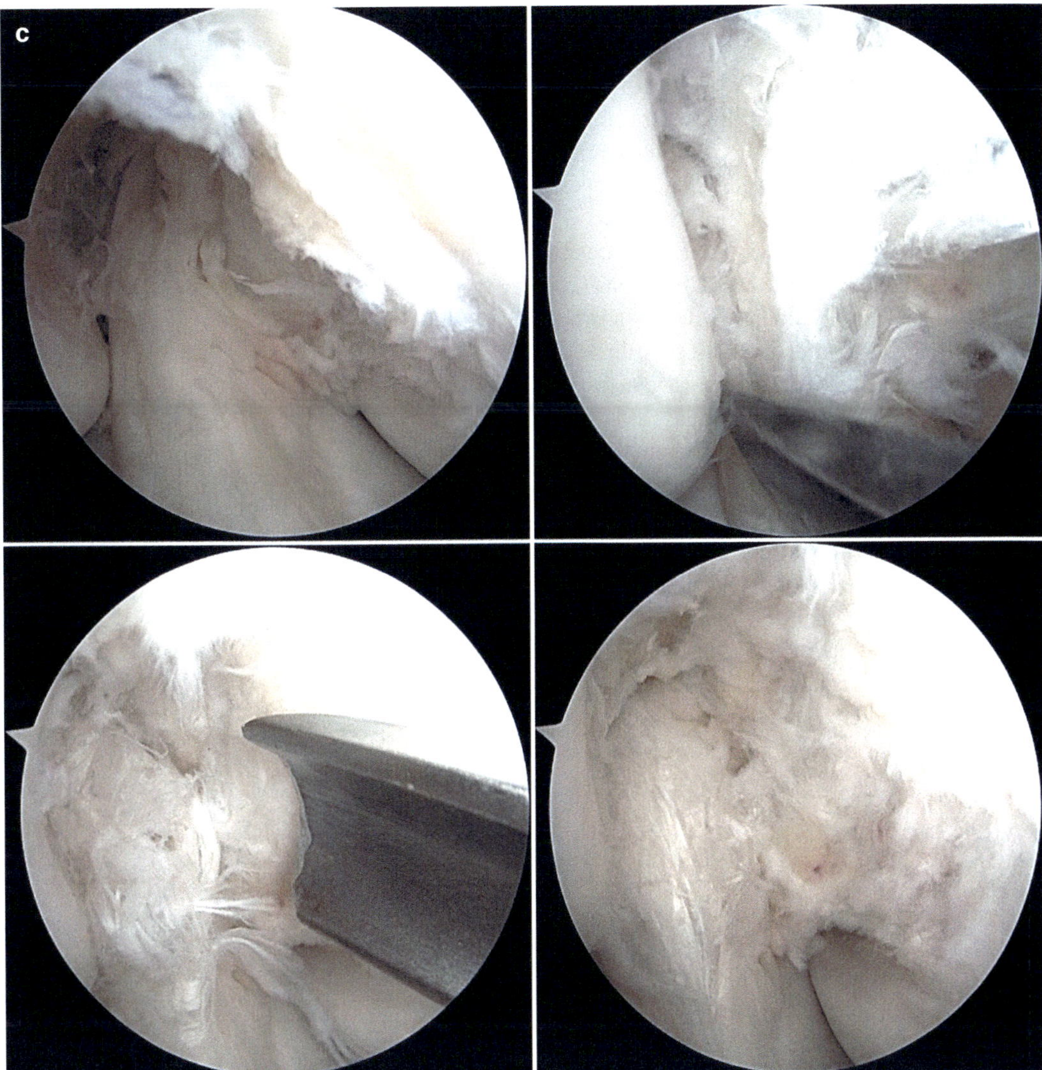

Fig. 7.3 (continued)

7.3 Rehabilitation

- Do not extend the knee after surgery for the next 4 weeks (Table 7.2).
- A brace is to be continuously used with a limited range of motion:
  - Up to the second week 0–30–70
  - third/fourth week 0–30–90
  - fifth/sixth week 0–0–unlimited
- Weightbearing can be started after approximately 8–10 days.
- Training can be performed as co-contraction of quadriceps and ischiocrural muscles (Table 7.2).
- Check-up and measurements with the ArticoMeter (digital Rolimeter) start after 3 months, and continue at 6, 9 and 12 months postoperatively, then annually (Table 7.2).

7.4 Our Own Results

In a prospective study since 2009/10 113 Patients with arthroscopically identified ultra femoral ACL tears were treated with healing response with bone cut and followed over 4.7 years. Excluding criteria: Lost in controles (4). Multidirectional instabilities (2). Focal chondral lesions (2). Incomplete partial ACL lesions (20).

Re-Ruptures in 9 patients with an adequate trauma (10%) 11–25 months post-op. Arthroscopy showed a intermediate ACL rupture and no rupture in the ultra-femoral area of the reinsertion of the healing response. Six of this patient had poor training condition and inadequate reflex behaviour of the vastus medialis of the quadriceps muscle. Another 6 patients could not be completed over all. 76 patients were evaluated (Table 7.2, Fig. 7.4).

An early functional rehabilitation was performed generally. Significantly less muscular atrophy of quadriceps and ischiocrural muscles was recorded postoperatively compared to ACL reconstructions with hamstring or Quadriceps tendon in

Table 7.3 Results after a 3-year follow-up with anterior cruciate ligament-healing response in a bone cut

Healing response with a follow-up of 4.7 years	
Years follow-up	4.7 (3.6–5.8)
N	76 (86%)
Age at injury	29.2 (13–53)
M/F	43/33
Trauma: skiing/soccer/handball	9 (12%)/29 (16%)/38 (50%)
Meniscus lesion: medial/lateral/both	14 (19%)/7 (9%)/5 (7%)
IKDC subjective A/B	73 (96.5%)
IKDC objective A/B	72 (94.7%)
Lachman test with ArticoMeter (digit. Rolimeter)	1.12 (±0.88 mm)
Lachman A 0–2.9 mm	72 (94.7%)
Lachman B 3–5.9 mm	4 (5.3%)
Pivot shift negative	69 (90.8%)
Pivot shift positive	4 (5.3%)
Pivot glide	7 (5.3%)
Tegner activity:	
Pretrauma	7.1
Follow-up	5.5

IKDC International Knee Documentation Committee

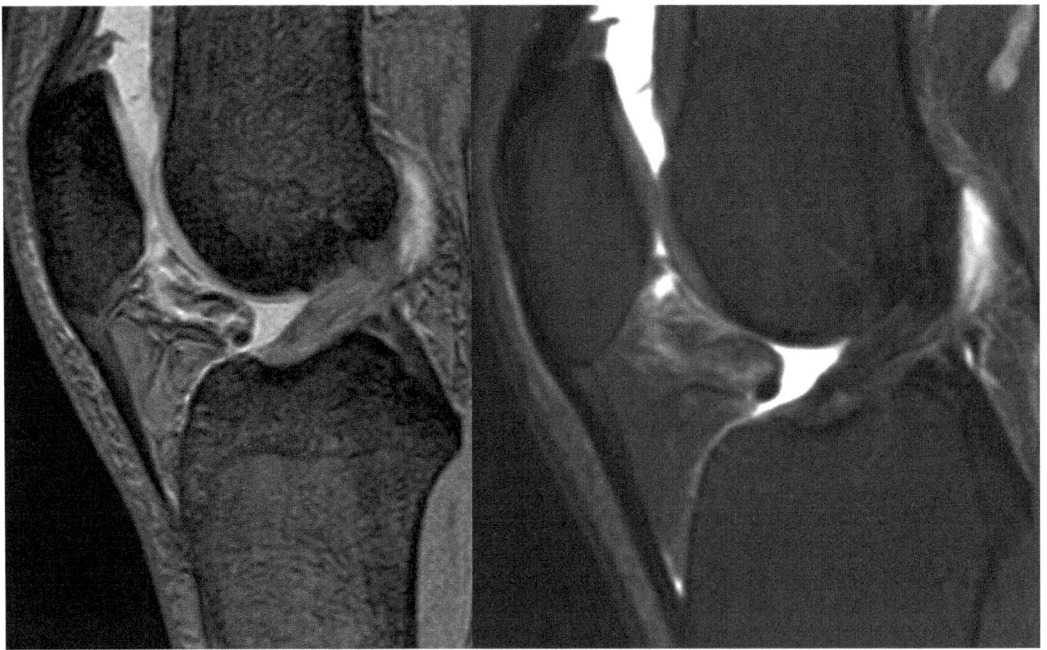

Fig. 7.4 Female skier, 32 years old, MRI 9 months after healing response in stable function

Table 7.2 Rehabilitation plan B is suggested to distress the anterior cruciate ligament in unstable fixation (without further damage, which requires a different programme). Complete extension is not allowed in healing response for 4 weeks. Co-contraction of quadriceps and ischiocrural muscles start immediately. An adapted systematic step-by-step program is to set. Some suggestions of exercises and equipment are made. (Aquasprint can be performed as adult in 50- to 70-cm-deep water. The water stabilizes like a brace.)

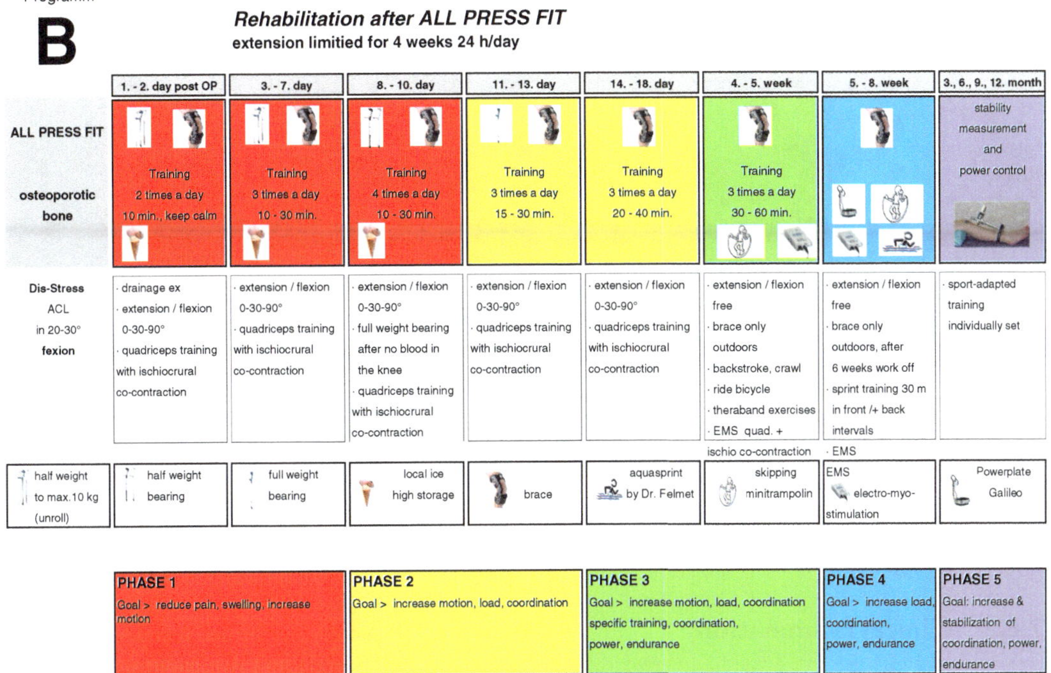

the same time. Laxity investigations with digital Rolimeter (Articometer) [11, 12], stability and coordination tests were performed after 3, 6 , 9, 12 months, then year by year with good results.

After 12–18 months 63% of the patients returned to their previous sport, mostly german soccer. Similarly good results were obtained after 3 years of FU [8]. Nevertheless the activity score over all was not recovered in the Tegner score [7, 8, 13].

7.5 Healing Response in the Posterior Cruciate Ligament

Diagnostic of a posterior cruciate ligament (PCL) lesion needs a careful and attentive examination.

Spontaneous posterior drawer easily can be overlooked.

After a second look, some primary PCL lesions with a diagnosis of an “ACL instability” turn out to be a PCL insufficiency.

Conservative treatment of a fresh PCL lesion is benign and successful when it is detected shortly after the trauma during the first 3–6 weeks. It is more a question of using a straight splint or a PCL Jack brace.

To our knowledge, there are no reports in literature on the PCL healing response in humans. Only a few reports exist about a healing response of the PCL in animals. Bone marrow stimulation in animal models on the PCL were more cellular and a more organized extracellular matrix was required than the repair tissue in the non-stimulated group [14]. Also, the healing process was faster in the bone marrow injection group [15]. Positive effects on ACL healing response with ACP have been reported [10].

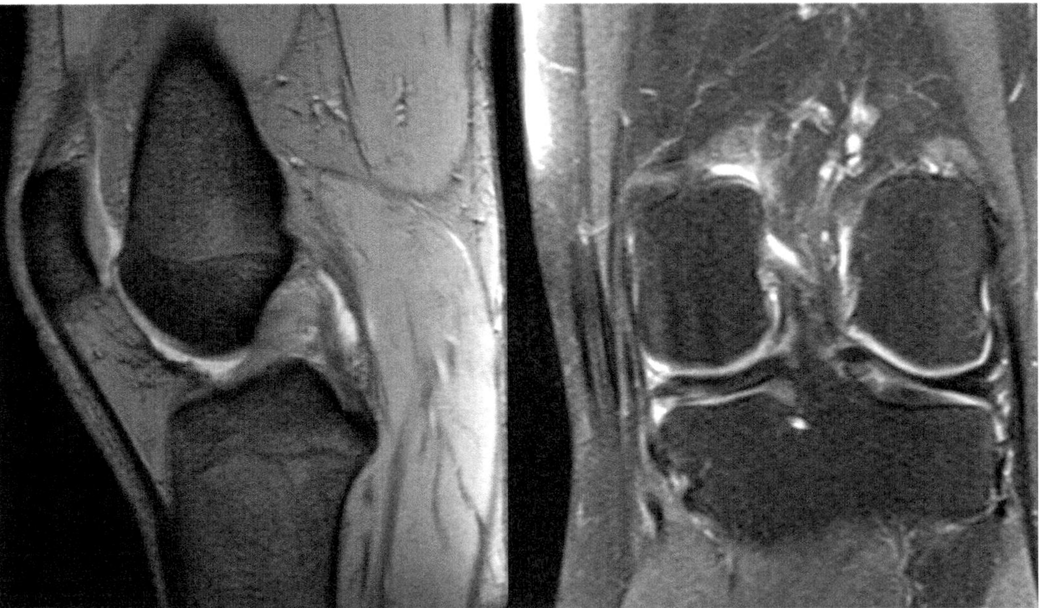

Fig. 7.5 MRI diagnostic of a posterolateral rupture

7.6 Diagnostics

7.6.1 Clinical Examination

- Instability with a posterior drawer
- ArticoMeter (digital Rolimeter)
- X-ray if possible under posterior tibial stress (check fractures, possibly CT/ Digital Volume Tomography (DVT) CBCT: Cone beam (CT)
- MRI with incomplete signal and avulsion of the PCL (Fig. 7.5)
- In the case of co-morbidity of the ACL, address the PCL first.

7.7 Indication

Healing response in a PCL lesion in the

- First 6 weeks with an objective instability of
- A posterior drawer of more than 8 mm
- Conservative treatment is not wanted by the patient or not possible because of co-morbidity

7.8 Technique and surgery

Surgery is typically performed using arthroscopy. Two anterior portals and two high posterior portals are necessary (Fig. 7.6). After addressing menisci, cartilage and collateral damage the posterior knee joint is prepared carefully. After resection of synovial structures inspect the PCL remnant.

- A good volume and remainder of the PCL stump is needed (Fig. 7.7).
- Check instability and reposition the stump ends (Fig. 7.7).
- Pulled open longitudinally and stretched the ends with a small chisel or pick to get a maximum length (Fig. 7.8).
- Check the distance and contact of the ends to each other under the anterior drawer (Fig. 7.8).
- Stop water flow.
- Drainage inside from the anterior portals is suggested.

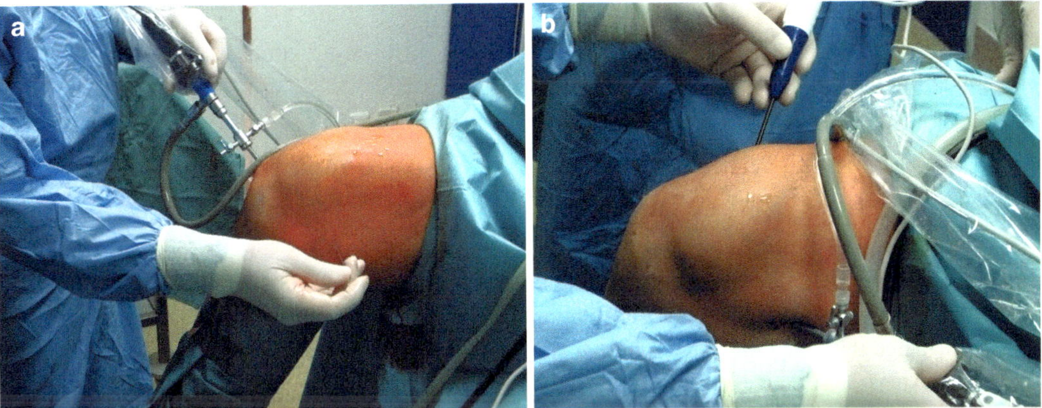

Fig. 7.6 (**a**, **b**) Posterior arthroscopic portals medially and laterally

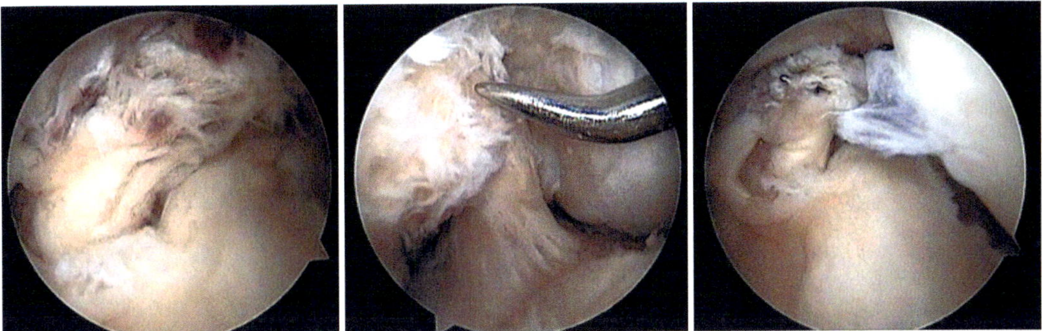

Fig. 7.7 Five-week-old posterior cruciate ligament rupture with posterior instability

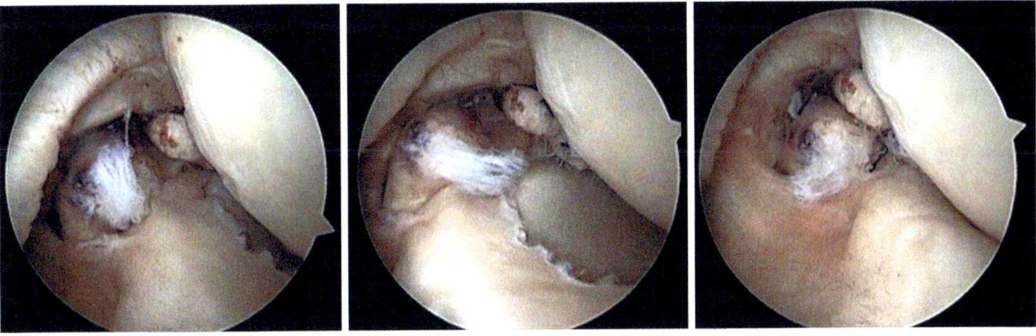

Fig. 7.8 Posterior cruciate ligament stump with femoral and tibial stump pulled open longitudinally and the stretched ends positioned each end to end

7.9 Rehabilitation

Straight splint and pillow to push the tibial head anterior or the PCL Jack brace (Fig. 7.9) (without any break, 24 h a day) for 12 weeks. Flexion is allowed in the PCL Jack brace (Fig. 7.9) after 6 weeks.

All exercises address the extensor muscles (quadriceps). Active exercises are also possible with the support of electro myostimulation (EMS). Change the brace only under active and complete extension. Passive mobilisation under active protection with the anterior drawer carefully after week 4.

Check-up and measurements with the ArticoMeter (digital Rolimeter) start after 3 months, and continue 6, 9, and 12 months postoperatively, then annually (Fig. 7.10).

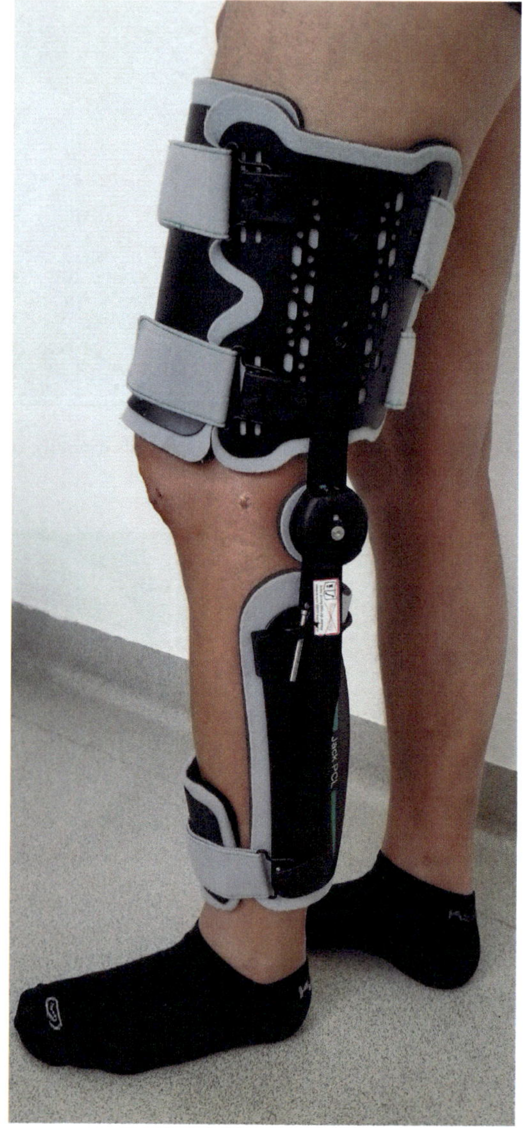

Fig. 7.9 Posterior cruciate ligament Jack Albrecht brace postoperatively for 12 weeks or more

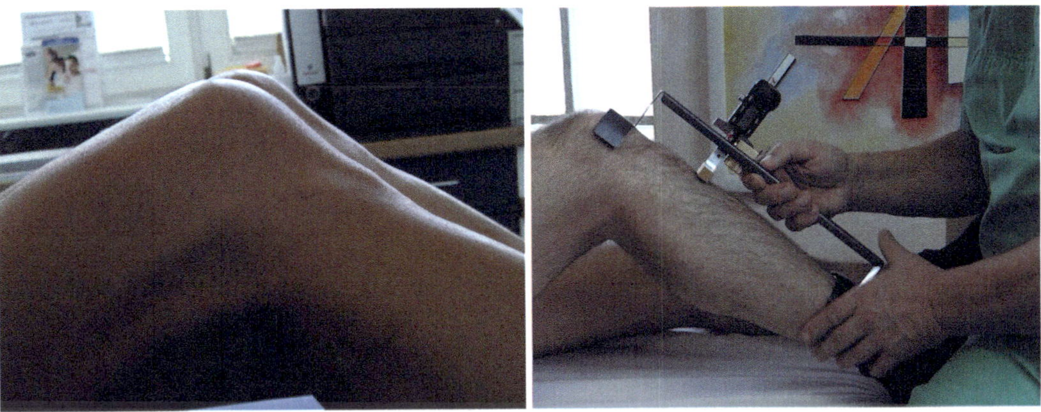

Fig. 7.10 A small posterior drawer in the right knee spontaneously 7 months after healing response *(left)*. Active measurement with ArticoMeter (digital Rolimeter) in 70° knee flexion *(right)* [11, 12]

7.10 Results

From 2009 to 2013 we treated seven patients using this technique as outpatients with no ligament co-morbidities and followed them for up to 4 years. The PCL Jack brace was used in every patient during the first 12 weeks after surgery; rehabilitation management is described above.

Healing response in the PCL is demanding for the surgeon as well as for the rehabilitation. Results have been subjectively and objectively successful for all seven patients (Fig. 7.11). The patients were satisfied; four returned to their original sport but not at the same level. Treatment was performed without any support for the bone marrow, or PRP-analogous substances (Table 7.4). An important key to success seems close contact with the physiotherapist and systematic controls with the patient.

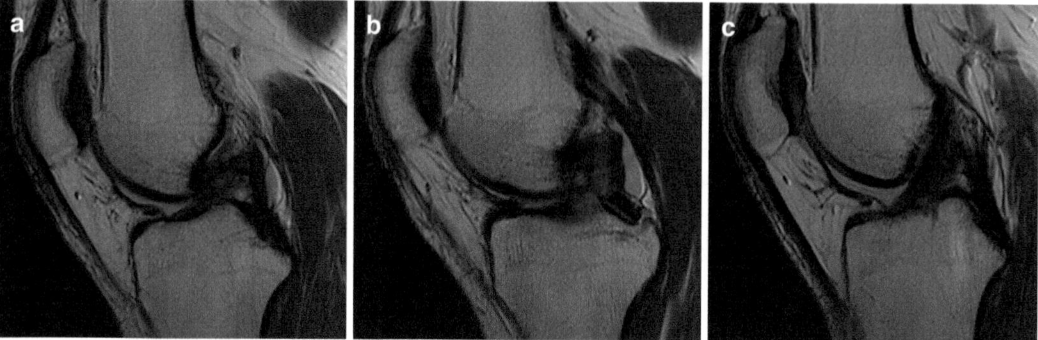

Fig. 7.11 MRI 7-month postoperative healing response: (**a**, **b**) posterior cruciate ligament reintegrated and angulated with obvious scar tissue. Correct signals of the anterior cruciate ligament of this patient (c)

Table 7.4 Results of healing response treatment at the posterior cruciate ligament in seven patients with 3-year follow-up

PCL healing response at 3-year follow up	
Years follow-up	2.9 (2.2–4.1)
N (%)	7 (100%)
Age at injury	26, 4 (21–52)
M/F	M5/F2
Trauma: Skiing/Soccer/Handball	1 (14%)/3 (43%)/3 (43%)
Meniscus lesion: medial/lateral/ both	1 (14%)/0/3 (43%)
IKDC subjective A/B	74 (96.9%)
IKDC objective A/B	71 (93.1%)
Preoperative posterior drawer in 70° with ArticoMeter	8.9 ± 1.3 mm
Postoperative posterior drawer in 70° with ArticoMeter	1.9 (± 1.5 mm)
Spontaneous posterior drawer 1–3 mm	2 (29%)
Tegner activity:	
Pretrauma	7.4
Follow-up	5.3

IKDC International Knee Damage Committee

7.11 Conclusion

Healing response works as well in ACL ruptures as in PCL ruptures.

Good to very good clinical results in patients after healing response treatment could be achieved in the medium- to long-term follow-up with stability. In comparison with a reconstruction, the healing response procedure is an alternative treatment option for acute, proximal ACL ruptures ultra-proximal ACL ruptures.

References

1. DiFelice GS, van der List JP. Clinical outcomes of arthroscopic primary repair of proximal anterior cru¬ciate ligament tears are maintained at mid-term fol¬low-up. Arthroscopy. 2018;34(4):1085–93.
2. Achtnich A, et al. [Arthroscopic refixation of acute proximal anterior cruciate ligament rupture using suture anchors]. Oper Orthop Traumatol. 2017;29(2):173–9.
3. Steadman JR, et al. A minimally invasive technique ("healing response") to treat proximal ACL inju¬ries in skeletally immature athletes. J Knee Surg. 2006;19(1):8–13.
4. Steadman JR, et al. Outcomes following healing response in older, active patients: a primary ante¬rior cruciate ligament repair technique. J Knee Surg. 2012;25(3):255–60.
5. Jorjani J, et al. [Medium- to long-term follow-up after anterior cruciate ligament rupture and repair in healing response technique]. Z Orthop Unfall. 2013;151(6):570–9.
6. Wasmaier J, et al. Proximal anterior cruciate ligament tears: the healing response technique versus conserva¬tive treatment. J Knee Surg. 2013;26(4):263–71.
7. Felmet G. Healing response – indications and results. In: World Sports Trauma Congress & 7th EFOST Congress, 2012, London; 2012.
8. Felmet G. ACL & PCL healing response – indica¬tion and results. In: SICOT International Orthopedics, 2016, Wuerzburg, Germany; 2016.

9. Di Matteo B, et al. Biologic agents for anterior cruciate ligament healing: a systematic review. World J Orthop. 2016;7(9):592–603.
10. Koch M, et al. Intra-ligamentary autologous conditioned plasma and healing response to treat par-tial ACL ruptures. Arch Orthop Trauma Surg. 2018;138(5):675–83.
11. Krautter A, et al. Instrumented Arthrometry of the anterior cruciate ligament. A comparison. Biomed Tech (Berl), 2012(issue-s1-R/bmt-2012-4299/bmt-2012-4299).
12. Runer A, et al. The evaluation of Rolimeter, KLT, KiRA and KT-1000 arthrometer in healthy individuals shows acceptable intra-rater but poor inter-rater reliability in the measurement of anterior tibial knee translation. Knee Surg Sports Traumatol Arthrosc. 2021.
13. Felmet, G., Healing response in complete proximal ACL tears 4,7 y FU, in 19th ESSKA Congress 11-15 May 2021. 2021: virtual.
14. Rodkey WG, Arnoczky SP, Steadman JR. Healing of a surgically created partial detachment of the posterior cruciate ligament using marrow stimulation: an experimental study in dogs. J Knee Surg. 2006;19(1):14–8.
15. Kim E, et al. The effect of intra-articular autogenous bone marrow injection on healing of an acute posterior cruciate ligament injury in rabbits. Arthroscopy. 2011;27(7):965–77.

8 ACL Revision After Re-Rupture

The ACL failure rate is reported to be between 3.2% and 27% (mean 11.8%) [1].

The most common reasons for failure of an anterior cruciate ligament (ACL) graft are incorrect positioning of the drill channels and insufficient fixation. In many cases, one-stage revision and the appropriate corrections are possible.

Autografts had better outcomes than allografts in revision ACL reconstruction, with lower postoperative laxity and rates of complications and reoperations. However, after excluding irradiated allografts, outcomes were similar between autografts and allografts. Overall, the choice of graft at revision ACL reconstruction should be on an individual basis considering, for instance, the preferred technique of the surgeon, whether a combined reconstruction is required, the type of graft that was previously used, whether the tunnels are enlarged, and the availability of allograft [2].

This study compared the results of revision surgery of autologous versus allogenous patellar tendon grafts for revision surgery of the ACL in a 5-year follow-up and found similar stability in both patellar tendon grafts [3].

A meta-analysis compared clinical outcomes of primary ACL reconstruction with hamstring tendon autografts versus soft-tissue allografts and showed that soft-tissue allografts are inferior to hamstring tendon autografts [4].

Latest reviews report a range of clinical failures in several series and objective clinical failures (range, 0–82%) was >5% in 15 of the 16 series and >10% in 12 of them. Most frequent complications were knee stiffness and anterior knee pain, whereas reoperations were primarily debridement and meniscectomies. The proportion of re-ruptures after revision ACL reconstruction was <5% in the majority of the studies in this review and 0% in 8 of the 16 series [5].

With an increase in ACL revisions graft options are also challenging. Concomitant injuries to the affected knee, such as chondral and meniscal lesions, are more common in the ACL revision than in primary ACL reconstruction. Patients undergoing ACL revision have lower rates of return to sport when compared with primary ACL surgery [6].

8.1 Diagnostics

As described in "clinical investigations" check the history of trauma and surgery, documents and images and instability and co-morbidity. Tunnels are analyzed and measured for exact planning.

1. Plain X-rays (Fig. 8.1)
2. MRI scans (Fig. 8.2)
3. CT scans (Fig. 8.3)
4. Digital volume tomography (DVT (CBCT)) (Figs. 8.4 and 8.5)

G. Felmet, *Press-Fit Fixation of the Knee Ligaments*, https://doi.org/10.1007/978-3-031-11906-4_8

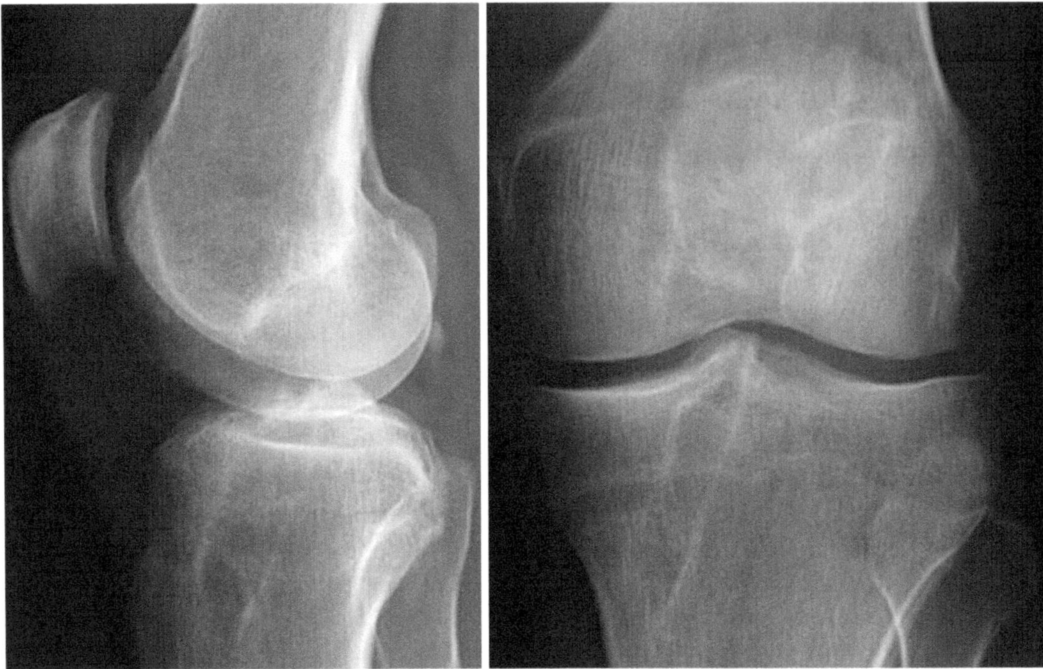

Fig. 8.1 Plain X-ray (weight-bearing if possible) as an overview for tunnels, bone stock, degenerative reaction, and morphology

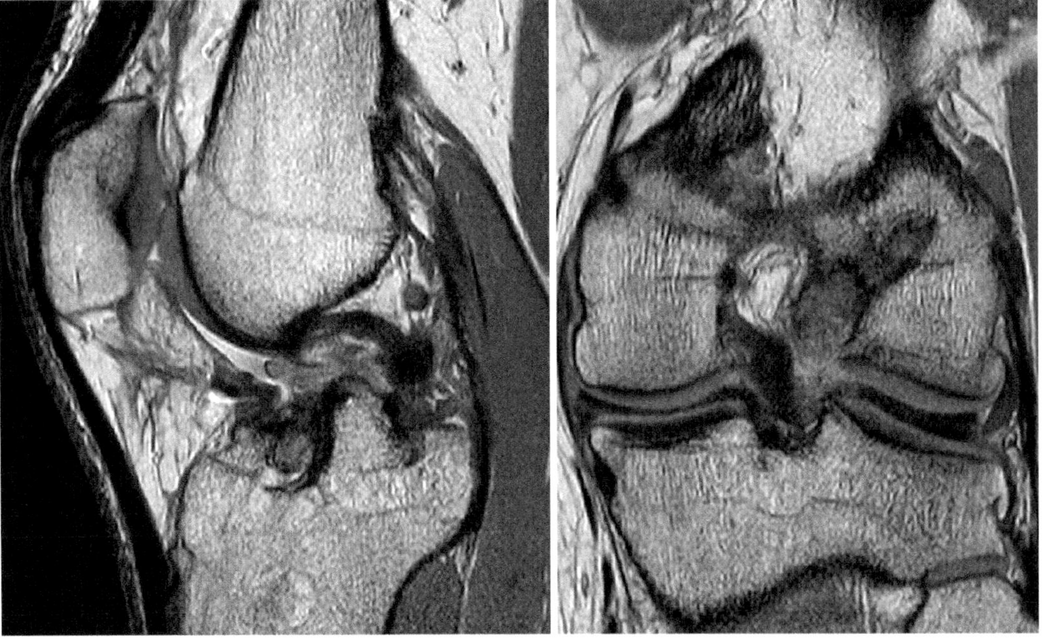

Fig. 8.2 The MRI shows ligaments, cartilage, menisci, soft tissue, inflammation, and bone bruising in T1 and T2 weighting in different morphologies. Algorithm and strategy in cases of correct or incorrect tunnels, enlargement, with /without screws for single-stage surgery with any graft

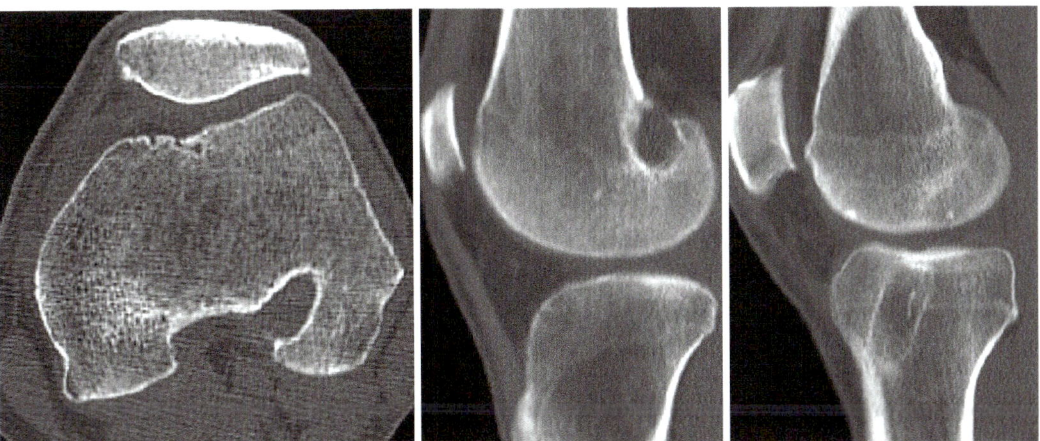

Fig. 8.3 Computed tomography of tunnel enlargement, osteolysis, and bone morphology. Usually 3 mm each slide, 3D reconstruction possible

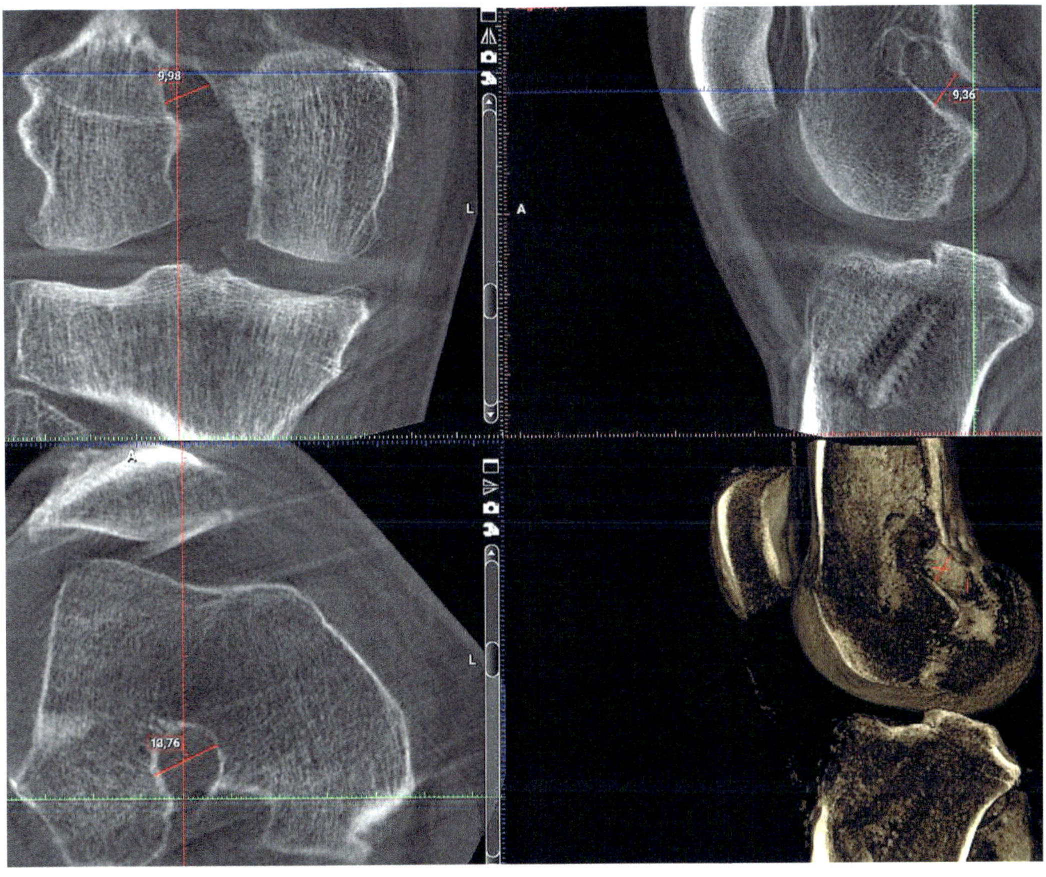

Fig. 8.4 Digital volume tomography DVT (CBCT) for tunnel enlargement, osteolysis, and bone morphology. DVT (CBCT) has a high resolution with 0.2-mm steps each slide, low radiation, and 3D reconstruction in less than 30 s (here femoral tunnel measurement). DVT (CBCT) is a multislice computed tomography device or two cone-beam CT device [7–10]

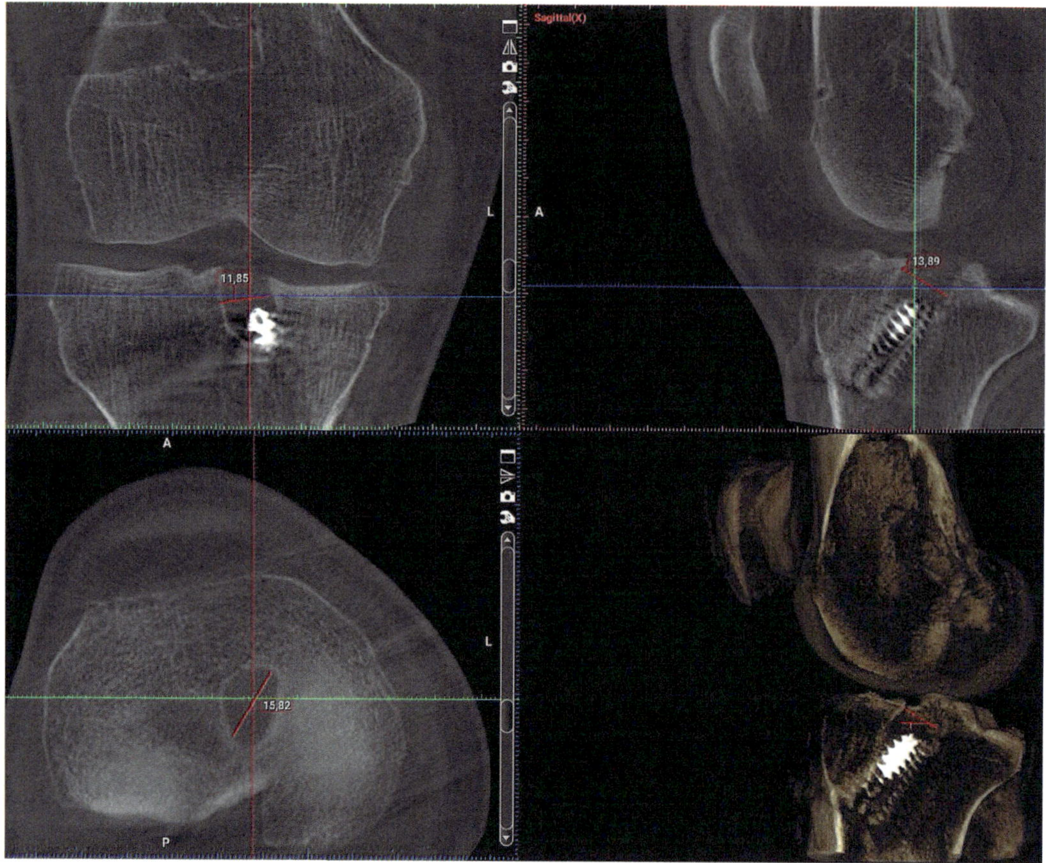

Fig. 8.5 Digital volume tomography (DVT (CBCT)) for tunnel enlargement, osteolysis, and bone morphology. DVT (CBCT) has a high resolution by 0.2-mm steps each slide, low radiation, and 3D reconstruction in less than 30 s (here tibial tunnel measurement and metal screw)

The bone stock is to be checked for osteoporosis, defects, implant tunnel position, and enlargement.

8.2 Surgical Management and Planning

Revision after ACL re-rupture is mostly accompanied by tunnel widening.

Foreign material interference screws made of metal can be positioned deep inside the tunnels or outside (Fig. 8.5). Screws from absorbable material mostly still exist or are incompletely absorbed. Sutures or threads can usually be taken out. Endobutton at the femoral side should be left. Suture disks are mostly be found on the tibial side.

This foreign material should usually be removed. Metal screws can cause large defects in the bone stock that make a single-stage procedure impossible. Bio-screws (not absorbable) with an intact substance can be over-drilled and left to help fixation. Absorbable screws have to be removed.

The set-up with a hollow reamer, guiding devices, measuring instruments, diamond and crown cutter, harvester, and applicator in different diameters, mostly 9–11 mm, are helpful (Figs. 8.6, 8.7, and 8.8).

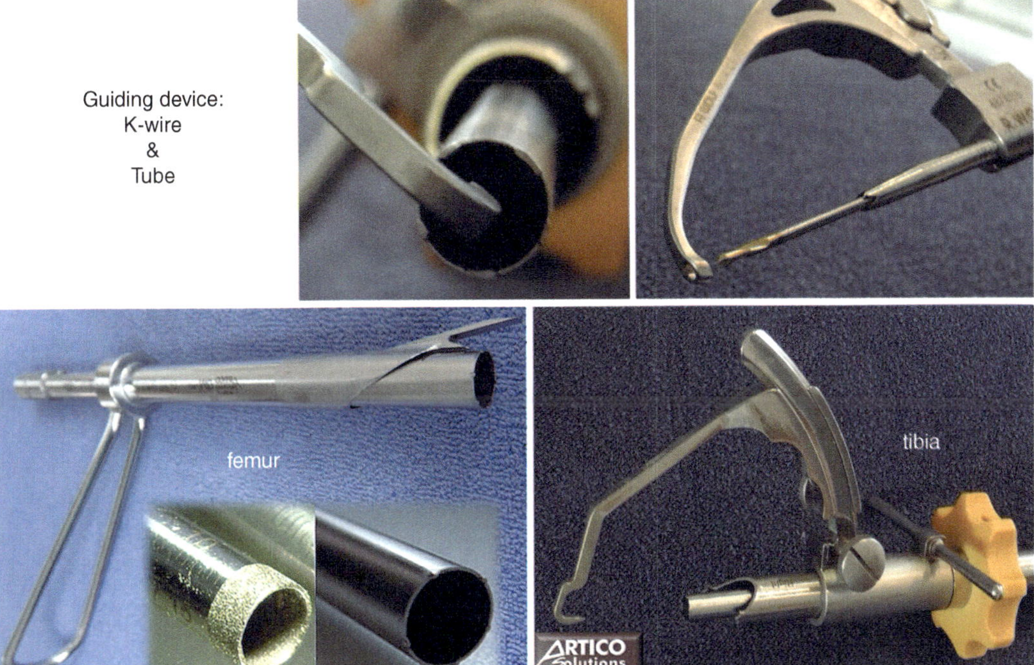

Fig. 8.6 Guiding devices are also helpful in revision. K-wire guiding devices can be used for hollow reamers with an extra internal guide. Tubed guiding devices are for hollow reamers

Tunnels con be positioned (a) correctly, (b) incompletely incorrectly, or (c) totally incorrectly.

Totally incorrect tunnels often allow direct reconstruction and correct positioning of the new tunnels. Anatomical tunnels with no enlargement can be filled with an oversized bone dowel in both sides to fix the graft press-fit (Fig. 8.9).

As described in Chaps. 5 and 6 we developed a surgical technique to close the defect and fix the graft in an anatomical position with bone dowels in a single step based on "all press-fit" fixation on the femoral and tibial side [11–14] (Figs. 8.6, 8.7, and 8.8). Good results have also been reported with oversized homologous bone cylinder and press-fit fixation in the former tunnel in a single-stage revision [15].

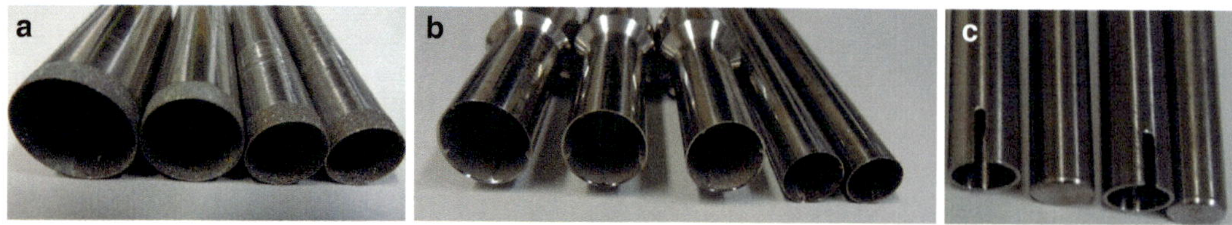

Fig. 8.7 (**a**) Diamond hollow reamer, (**b**) extractors harvest the cylinder out of the bone, (**c**) different applicators are filled with bone cylinders or cancellous bone chips for the tunnel. Different sizes are available, 9–11 mm are mostly used for revision

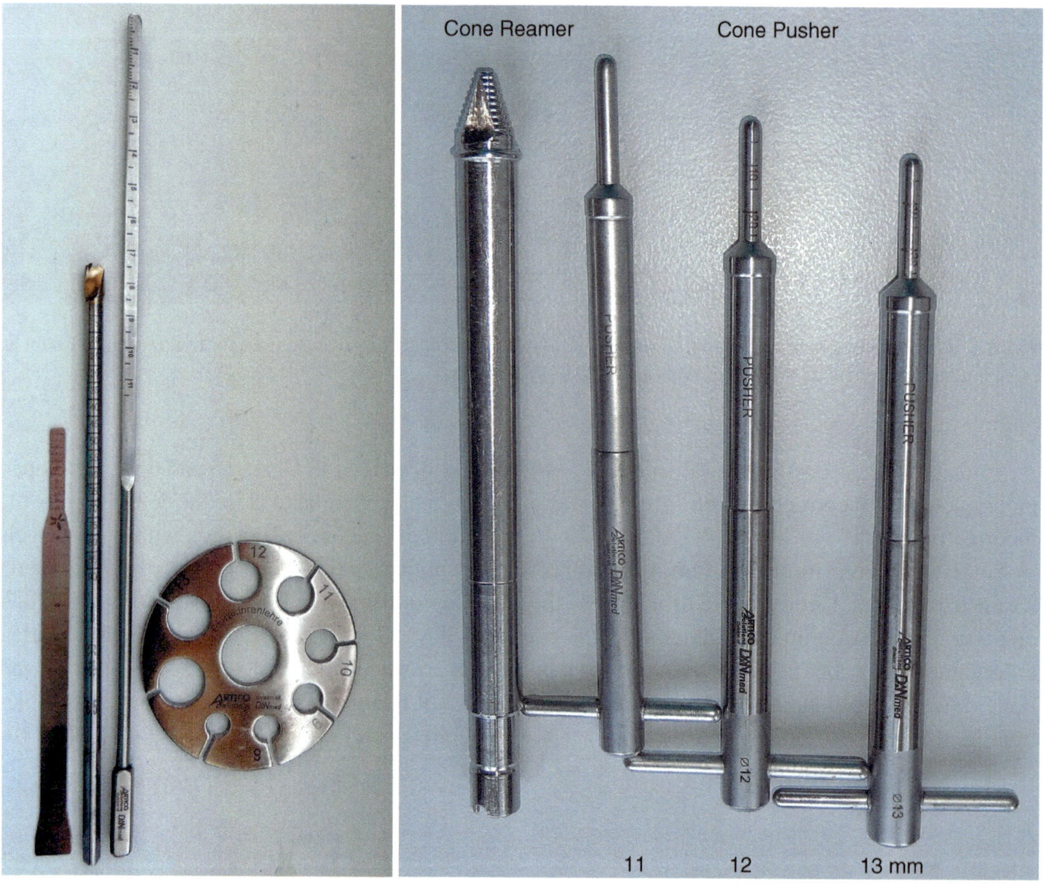

Fig. 8.8 Different rulers are used to measure defects intraoperatively. Cone reamer and cone pusher ease the "tibial" approach and compact the tunnel

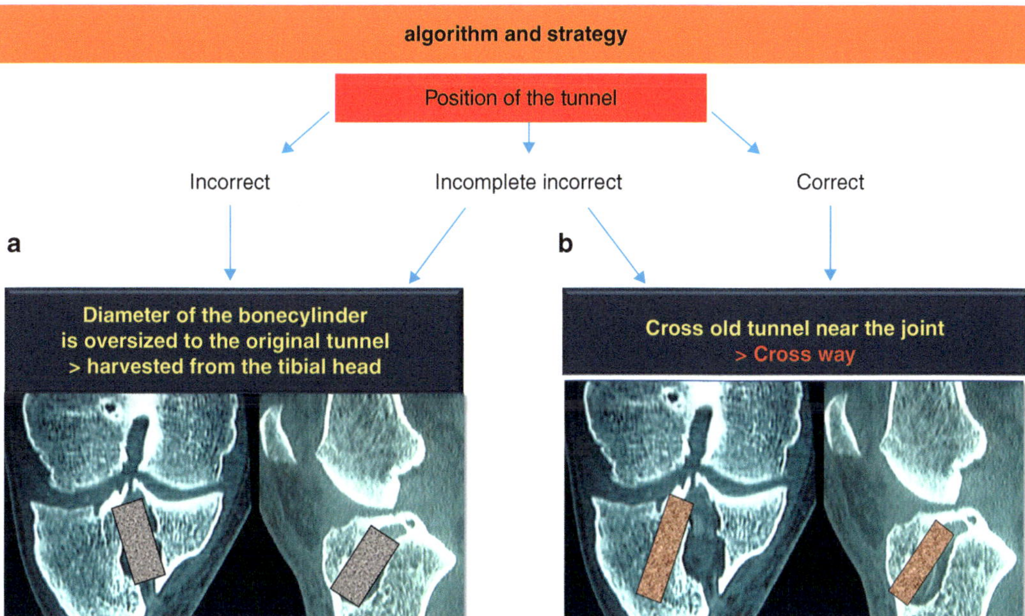

Fig. 8.9 Single-stage algorithm and strategy in cases of (1) correct, (2) incompletely incorrect, (3) incorrect tunnels. Fixation with oversized bone cylinder (autologous from the tibial head or homologous bone cylinder (a) in the same tunnel (b) with "cross way" as a bypass to the old tunnels

8.3 How to Make Decision

ACL revision is demanding. Depending on variable individualities a single-stage or two-stage revision is to be discussed. Individual facts and check-lists may guide toward a sophisticated algorithm (Fig. 8.9).

1. Check if:
   (a) The position of the tunnels is correct
   (b) The position of the tunnels is incompletely incorrect
   (c) The position of the tunnels is totally incorrect
   (d) The tunnels are enlarged 9 mm or more
   (e) Bone stock is stable
   (f) There is no osteopenic bone
   (g) There is no blow out of the tunnels

A. If the tunnels are correct (a), not enlarged (no d) with good bone quality (with e, f, g) a one-stage ACL reconstruction might be possible (Fig. 8.10)
   – Check the remaining graft and decide on a method from Chap. 6.

B. If the tunnels are only half incorrect (no c, d) but acceptable for a biomechanically correct new reconstruction, with good bone quality (no e, f, g)
   – Check for a one-stage ACL reconstruction if a "crossway" Plan B could work (Figs. 8.11, 8.12, and 8.13).

C. If (A) and (B) are not possible with a strong indication
   – Decide on a two-stage procedure and restore the bone stock first.

8.3.1 Single-Stage Revision

Bio-absorbable, mechanically stable implants can be left. Metal and implants should be removed. Tunnels can be checked by CT or DVT (CBCT). During surgery the width and bone quality can be proven by different-sized pushers (Fig. 8.7).

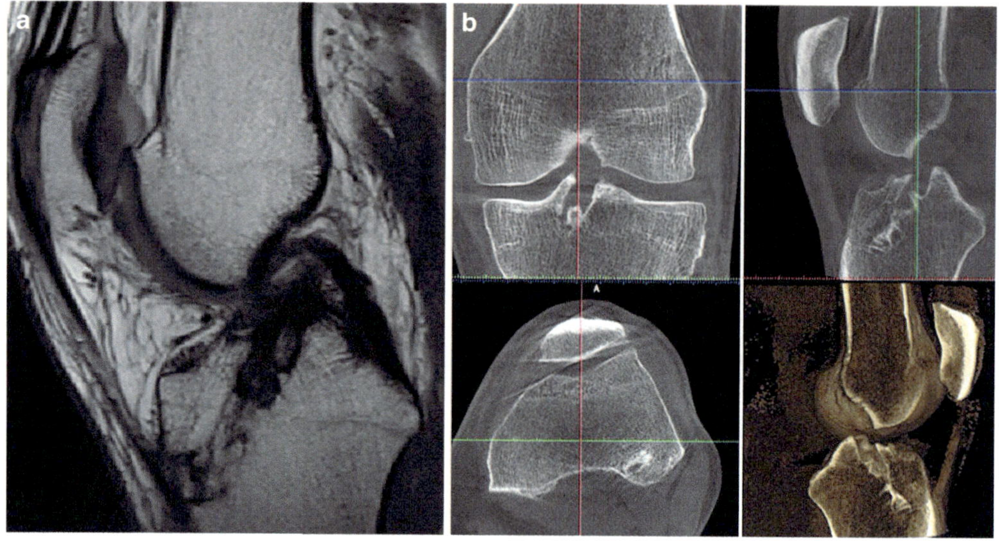

Fig. 8.10 (**a**) MRI and (**b**) digital volume tomography show correct tunnel placement and bone-stock without tunnel enlargement after "all press-fit" material-free anterior cruciate ligament reconstruction

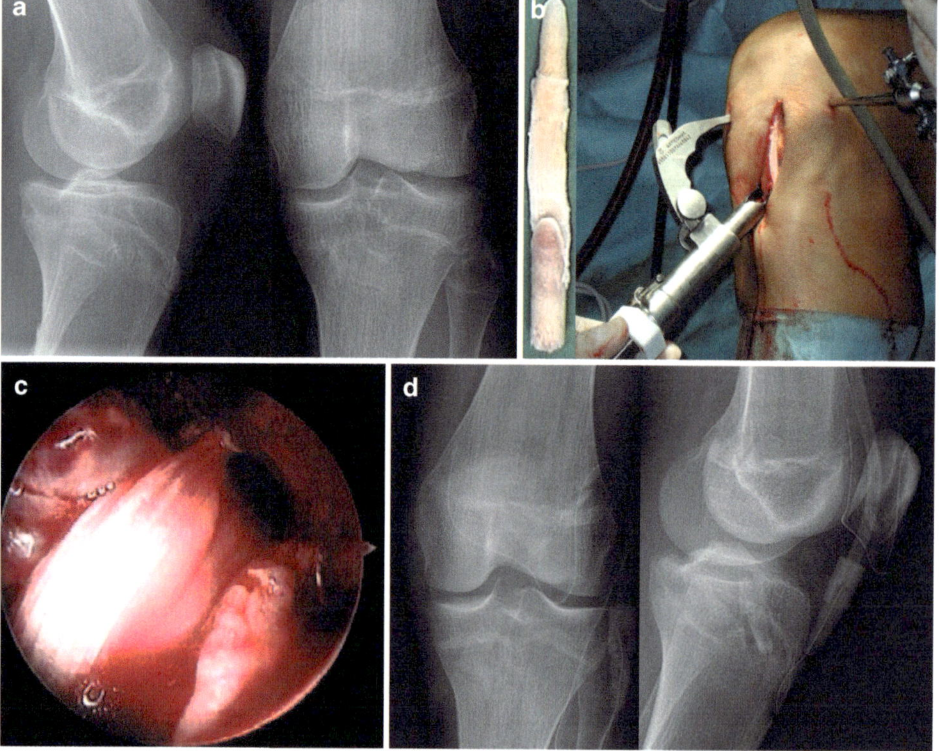

Fig. 8.11 One-stage reconstruction (same tunnel) after re-rupture in a 19-year-old man after material-free hamstring reconstruction. (**a**) X-rays show correct tunnels, no enlargement. (**b**) Middle third of patellar bone–tendon–bone is harvested, the original tunnel is used. (**c**) Ribbon-like all press-fit anterior cruciate ligament reconstruction. (**d**) Correct position of the bone cylinder

Depending on your choice and graft:

1. Patellar tendon–bone or
2. Quadriceps tendon–bone is harvested with a bone cylinder with a hollow reamer with an adequate diameter (Fig. 8.12).
3. Quadruple hamstring is armed with a bone cylinder on one side from the tibial tunnel or tibia head. In the case of a wrongly positioned tunnel, the new graft is inserted in the correct position (Fig. 8.13).

   Harvest the bone cylinder with "all press-fit" instruments larger than the tunnel for press-fit fixation.

   Check the bypass and "crossway" (Figs. 8.12 and 8.13).

   Plan B: for the "crossway" the tibial tunnel is positioned beside or through the tibial tuberosity (the latter is good to use with the patellar BTB graft). The new tunnel crosses the old and hits at the correct anatomical insertion. Correctly positioned tibial tunnels are used again and filled with an oversized bone cylinder from the tibia head (harvested with a hollow reamer) to fix the graft press-fit in one step. The graft is inserted from distal and fixed press-fit in the tibial tunnel near the plateau. The bone cylinder overlaps the prior tunnel. The graft is now fixed on the femoral side press-fit with a bone dowel "bottom to top" in 120° knee flexion.

Fix the graft on the femoral side with a bone cylinder from this tunnel or from the tibial head and follow the procedure from Chap. 6. The use of an homologous bone cylinder should be considered.

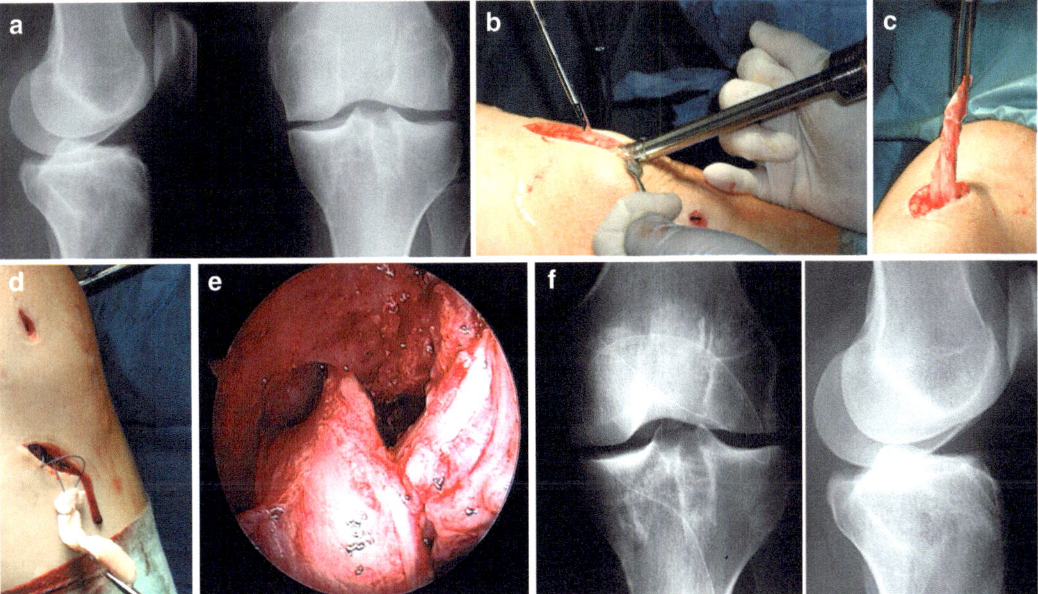

Fig. 8.12 One-stage reconstruction ("cross way") after re-rupture in a 28-year-old man after material-free patellar bone–tendon–bone reconstruction, primarily fixed over a central tunnel through the tibial tuberosity. (**a**) X-rays show correct tunnels. (**b**, **c**) Middle third of the quadriceps tendon is harvested as a tendon–bone graft. (**d**) The tibial antero-medial tunnel position is used and crosses the old tunnel inside the joint. (**e**) Ribbon-like all press-fit anterior cruciate ligament reconstruction. (**f**) Correct position of the bone cylinder and graft

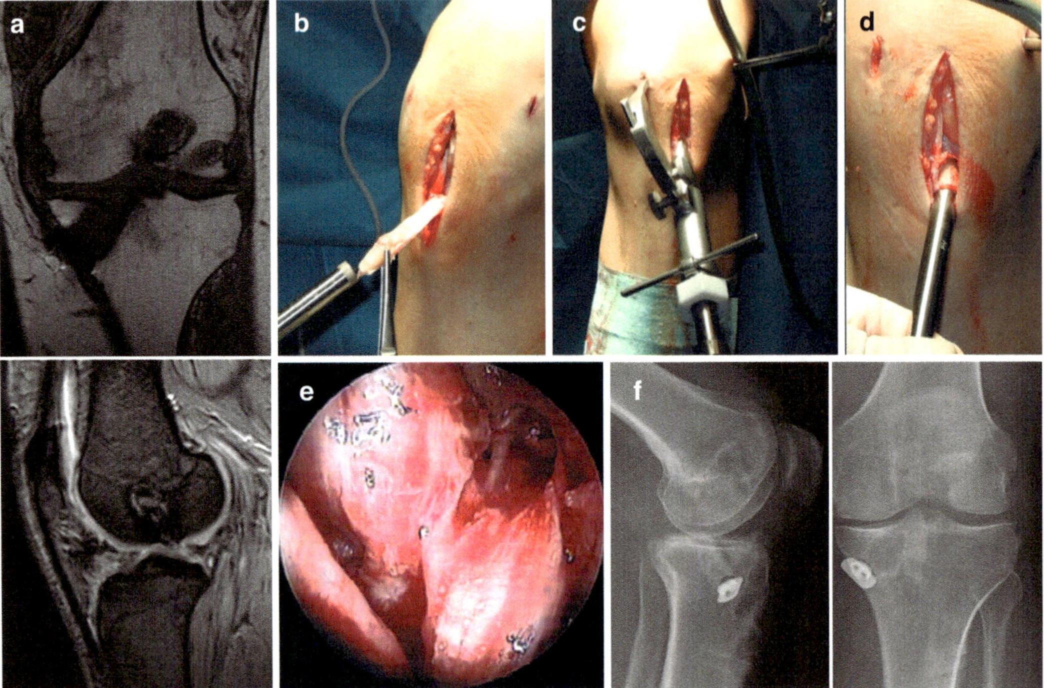

Fig. 8.13 One-stage reconstruction ("cross way") after malreplacement with hamstring in a 48-year-old woman. (**a**) MRI malpositioned tunnels and enlargement on both sides. (**b**) Middle third of a patellar bone–tendon–bone (BTB) is harvested. (**c**) The central tunnel through the tibial tuberosity (defect from the harvested BTB graft) is created (**d**) and the graft is fixed press-fit. (**e**) The stabile ACL reconstruction is ribbon like. (**f**) Correct position of the tibial bone cylinder (leave the suture disk in place to protect the soft tissue)

8.4 Rehabilitation

- In stable fixation extension is allowed: rehabilitation program plan A is suggested (Table 8.1)
- In osteopenic or unstable fixation extension should be limited to 20–30° for 2–4 weeks postoperatively: rehabilitation program plan B is suggested (Table 8.2)

8.4.1 Two-Stage Revision

The bone stock is to be restored and the defects have to be closed with either autologous bone or homologous bone.

Bone stock can be restored by autologous bone, e.g., from the iliac crest. The "all press-fit" instruments the hollow reamer and the harvester are helpful.

Homologous cancellous bone chips complete and ease the surgery for the patient and doctor (Fig. 8.14). If there is no contraindication, the use of gentamycin with 80 mg/15 cm^3 is recommended in a mix with autologous blood and cancellous bone chips. The use of autologous bone is possible. The tunnels are revised and cleaned completely from the rest of graft, screws, threads, etc. (Fig. 8.15). Both tunnels are filled with compacted cancellous bone chips by an applicator (Figs. 8.14, 8.16, and 8.17). Graft implantation in a second stage press-fit fixation as shown is usually possible after 3–4 months (Fig. 8.18).

The principles shown can also be used for all kinds of revision and bone defects, such as the PCL.

The results of single-stage and two-stage revision after 4 years show better anterior stability in the group of two-stage revisions (Table 8.3). Single-stage revision seems to save time and allows the patient to make a little earlier return to

Table 8.1 Rehabilitation plan A is suggested in stable fixation (without further damage, which requires a different program). Complete extension is allowed and a systematic step-by-step program is possible. Some suggestions of exercises and equipment are made. Aquasprint can be performed as an adult in water 50–70 cm deep

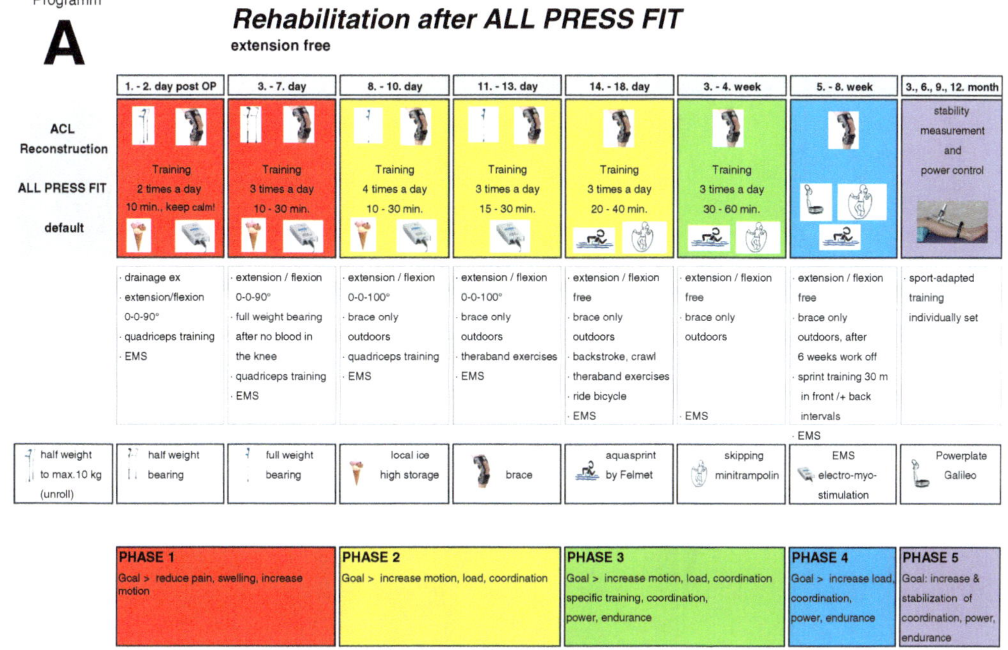

Table 8.2 Rehabilitation plan B is suggested in osteoporotic or unstable fixation (without further damage, which requires a different program). Complete extension is not allowed for 2–4 weeks to dis-stress the ACL. An adapted systematic step-by-step program is to be set. Some suggestions of exercises and equipment are made. Aquasprint can be performed as an adult in water 50–70 cm deep

Anterior cruciate ligament single-stage versus two-stage revision 4-year follow-up		
Only first re-rupture	Single stage	Two stage
Years of surgery	2008–2016	2015–2019
Years of follow up	4 (2.8–6.1)	3.5 (2.6–4.2)
N=	32	39
Age at injury	31.2 (19–43)	36.4 (19–57)
Male/female	14/18	18/21
Graft: P-BTB/Hamstring/Quadriceps tendon (from the ipsilateral side)	(5)-(11)-(16)	(1)-(9)-(29)
IKDC subjective A/B	91%	96%
IKDC objective A/B	95%	97%
IKDC total A/B	87%	91%
KT 1000/digital Rolimeter, mm	1.89 mm (±0.88)	1.11 mm (±0.66)
Lachman A 0–2.9 mm	92%	97%
B 3–5.9 mm	7%	2%
Pivot shift negative	63%	88%
Glide	21%	18%
Tegner activity		
Pretrauma	6.9	7.1
Follow-up	4.4	5.7
Complications	Tibial loosening 3, femoral loosening 1, infection 0, fracture 0	Tibial loosening 0, femoral loosening 0, infection 0, fracture 0
Osteoarthritis, femoral–patellar	23%	21%
Osteoarthritis gap increasing	4%	3%

P-BTB patellar bone–tendon–bone, *IKDC* International Knee Documentation Committee

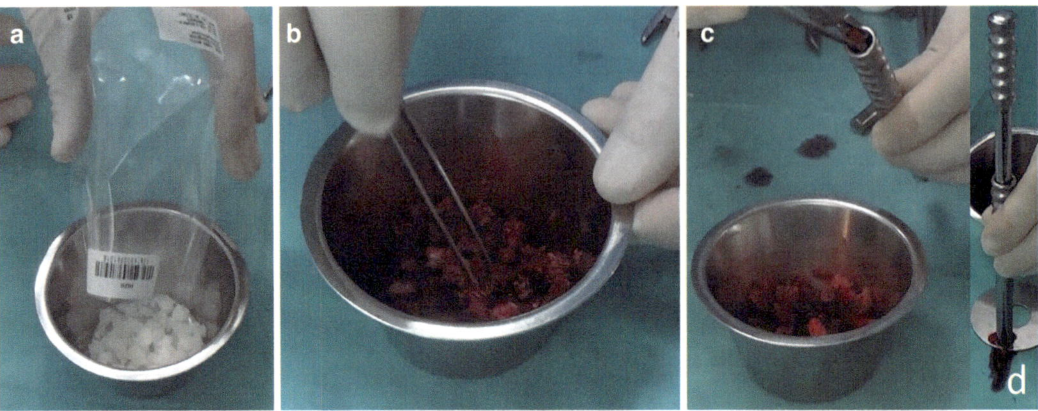

Fig. 8.14 Homologous (**a**) cancellous bone chips, (**b**) mixed in gentamycin 80 mg/15 cm^3 and autologous blood, (**c**) bone chips are placed into the applicator, and are (**d**) compacted by the pusher before application into the defect

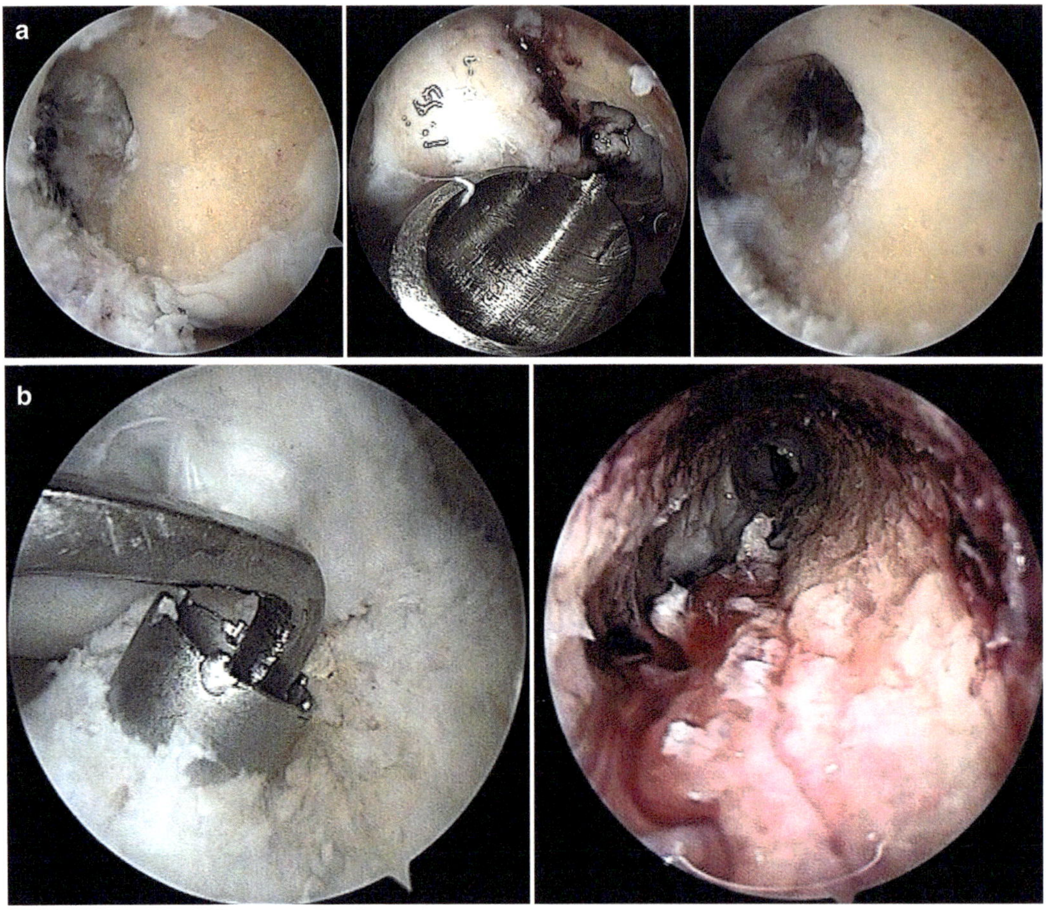

Fig. 8.15 Cleaning the tunnels. (**a**) Femoral tunnel after notch plastic, femoral tubed guide, and harvested femoral tunnel (from left). (**b**) Tibial guide with crown cutter, tunnel with the rest of the old graft (from left)

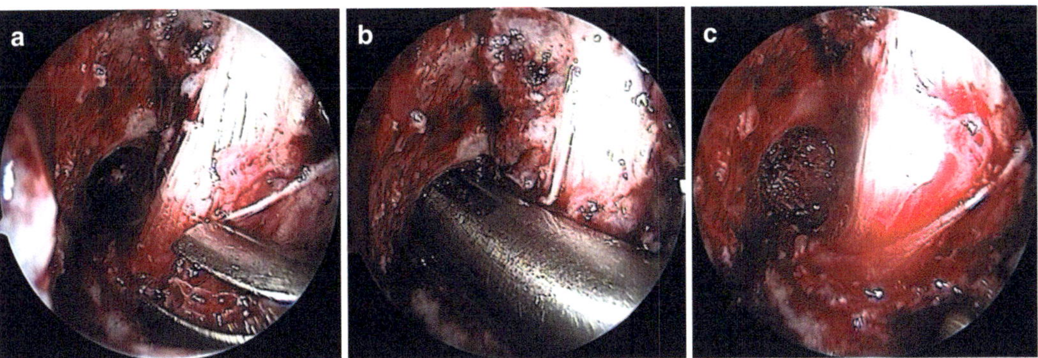

Fig. 8.16 Filling the femoral tunnel of a right knee from the antero-medial portal (**a**) applicator loaded with compacted cancellous bone chips, (**b**) filling the tunnel using a pusher, and (**c**) closing the defect

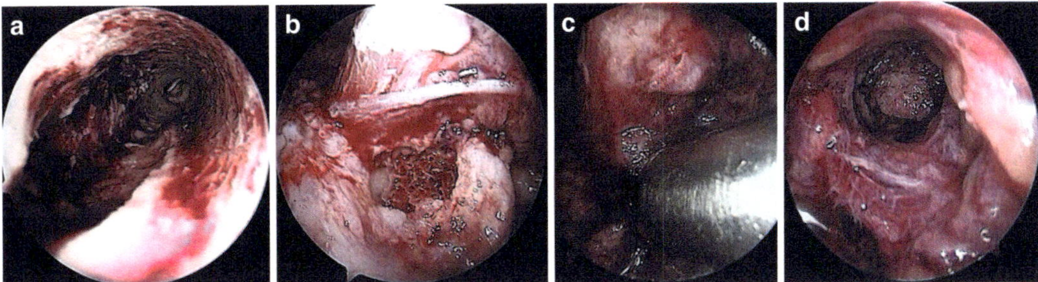

Fig. 8.17 (**a**) Tibial tunnel of a right knee from distally; (**b**) compacted bone chips pushed up from distally; (**c**) bone chips are blocked by a pusher through the antero-medial portal; (**d**) closed tibial tunnel

sport. Comorbidities in the meniscus and cartilage play a role in both groups. Also, the competence of muscles and psychological readiness are important factors in a return to sport in the long term. Single-stage procedures showed a little less anterior stability but no disadvantages with regard to a return to sport. Those who had complete or incomplete wrongly positioned tunnels had the most individual benefit from anterior stability. Advantages of time of 3–4 months in a single-stage procedure and return to sport are individual but are not significant in the long term. The indication for a single-stage procedure must fulfill strong criteria in the correct positioning of the tunnels and bone-stock quality. Comorbidities and intrinsic factors such as anatomical and biomechanical axis in varus/valgus, bone morphology, and posterior tibial slope should be considered [16–23] (Fig. 8.19) (Chaps. 1 and 2).

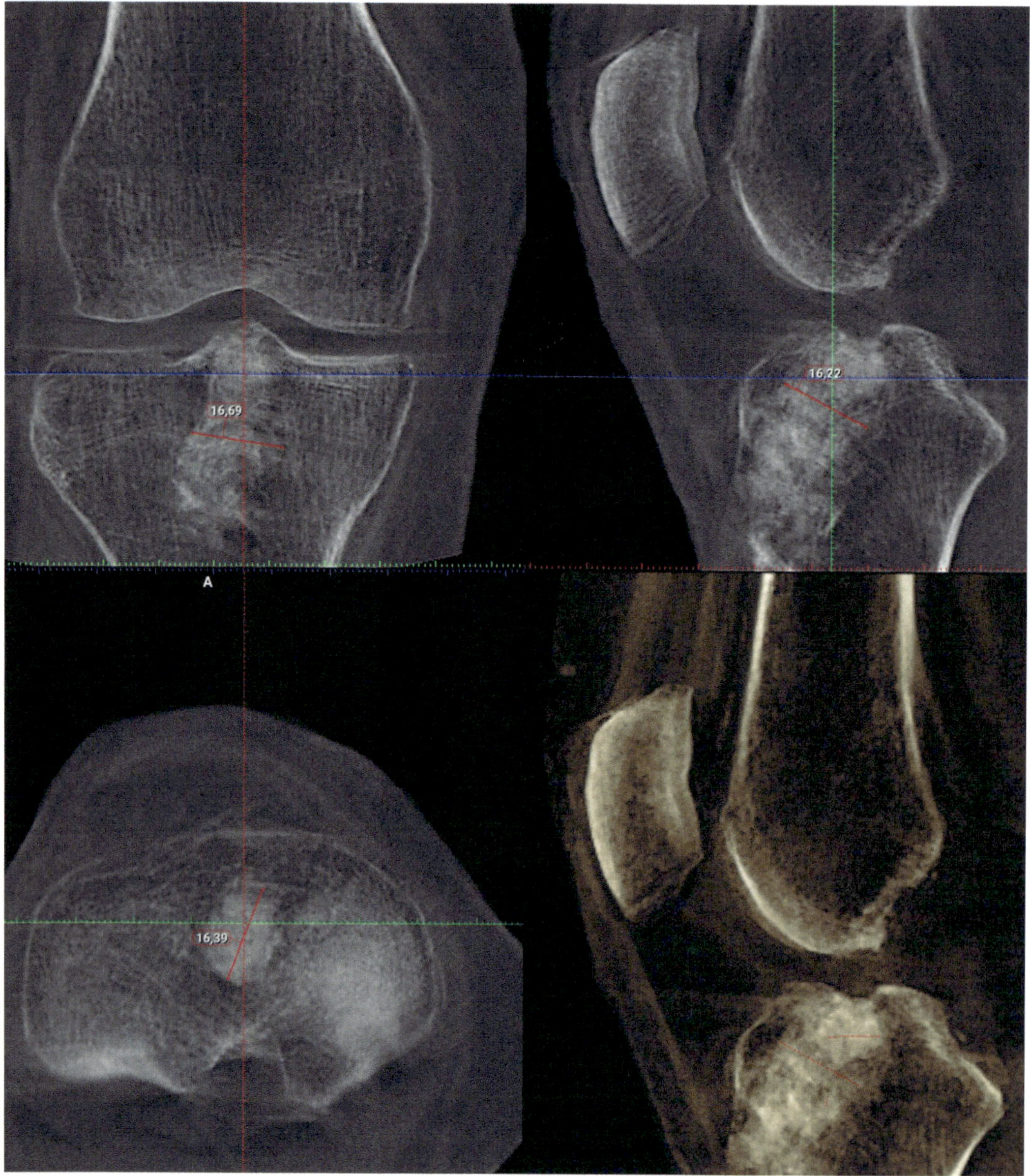

Fig. 8.18 Large defect in osteopenic bone 4 months after bone-stock revision with homologous cancellous bone chips

Table 8.3 The results of single-stage and two-stage revision after 4 years: better anterior stability in the group with a two-stage revision. Those with complete or incompletely wrongly positioned tunnels had the most benefit from anterior stability. Advantages of time with 3–4 months in a single stage and return to sport are individual but are not significant in long term

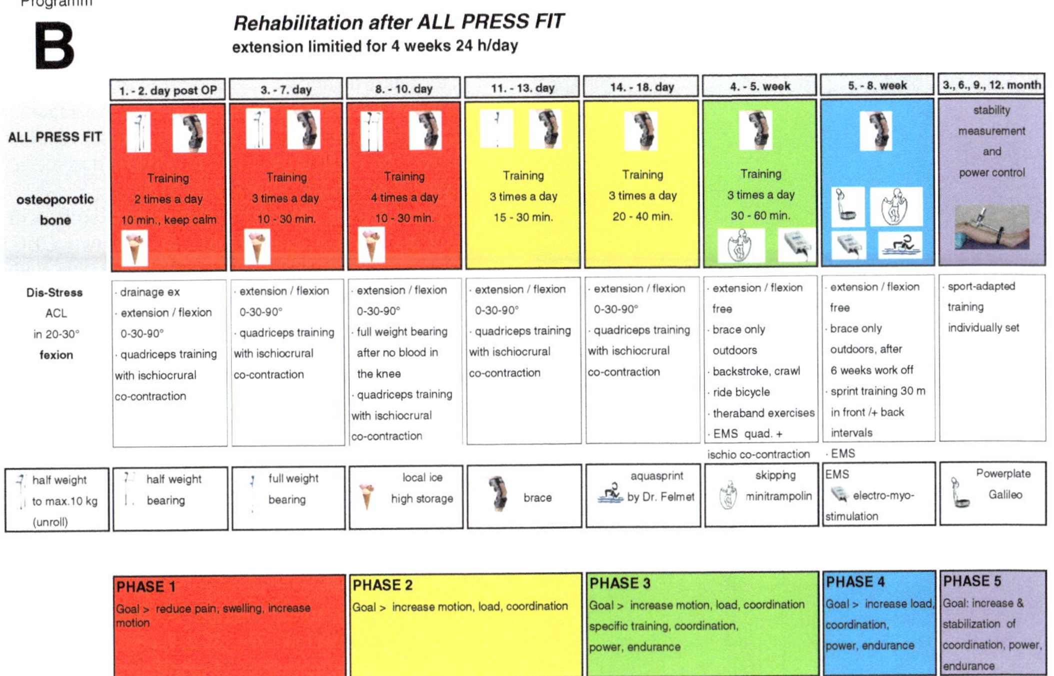

Advantages of the ACL all press-fit and bottom-to-top method

- Autologous replacement
- Biologically simple, reproducible, self-adapted tensioning of the graft
- For every graft
- Ease of revision
- Ease of osteotomy to correct the tibial slope and axis

Hollow reamer—crown cutter

- Press-fit standard
- Tubed or K-wire guiding devices
- Minimized bone loss "bone recycling"
- Osteochondral autologous transfer surgery with the same instruments

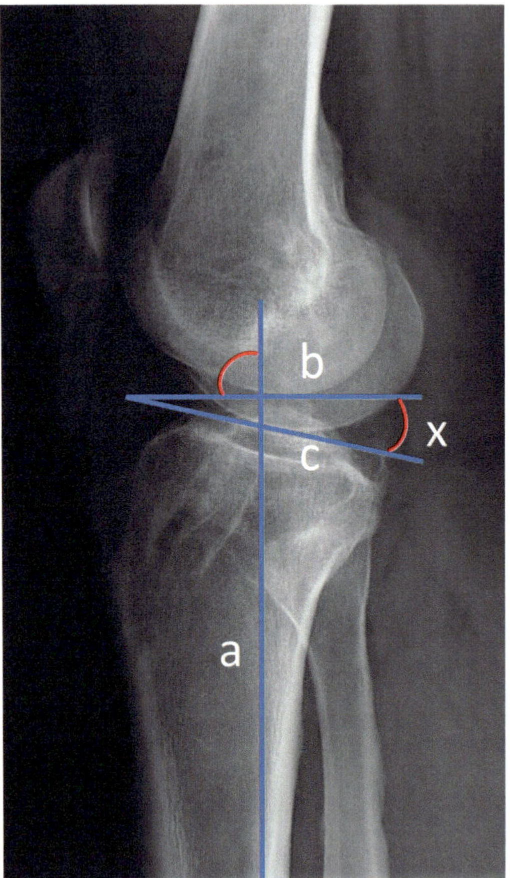

Fig. 8.19 Biomechanical intrinsic risk factors for overload and re-ruptures such as an increased tibial posterior slope should be considered [16, 18, 20, 21] (Chaps. 1–3)

References

1. Crawford SN, Waterman BR, Lubowitz JH. Long-term failure of anterior cruciate ligament reconstruction. Arthroscopy. 2013;29(9):1566–71.
2. Grassi A, et al. Does the type of graft affect the outcome of revision anterior cruciate ligament reconstruction? a meta-analysis of 32 studies. Bone Joint J. 2017;99-b(6):714–23.
3. Mayr HO, et al. Revision of anterior cruciate ligament reconstruction with patellar tendon allograft and autograft: 2- and 5-year results. Arch Orthop Trauma Surg. 2012;132(6):867–74.
4. Wang HD, et al. Comparison of clinical outcomes after anterior cruciate ligament reconstruction with hamstring tendon autograft versus soft-tissue allograft: a meta-analysis of randomised controlled trials. Int J Surg. 2018;56:174–83.
5. Grassi A, et al. What is the mid-term failure rate of revision ACL reconstruction? A systematic review. Clin Orthop Relat Res. 2017;475(10):2484–99.
6. Horvath A, et al. Outcome after anterior cruciate ligament revision. Curr Rev Musculoskelet Med. 2019;12:397–405.
7. Koivisto J, et al. Effective radiation dose of a MSCT, two CBCT and one conventional radiography device in the ankle region. J Foot Ankle Res. 2015;8:8.
8. Koivisto J, et al. Assessment of effective radiation dose of an extremity CBCT, MSCT and conventional X ray for knee area using MOSFET dosemeters. Radiat Prot Dosim. 2013;157(4):515–24.
9. Koivisto J, et al. Effective radiation dose in the wrist resulting from a radiographic device, two CBCT devices and one MSCT device: a comparative study. Radiat Prot Dosim. 2018;179(1):58–68.
10. Pallaver A, Honigmann P. The role of cone-beam computed tomography (CBCT) scan for detection and follow-up of traumatic wrist pathologies. J Hand Surg [Am]. 2019;44(12):1081–7.
11. Felmet G. [ALL-PRESS-FIT, a new surgical method with femoral and tibial Press Fit fixation]. Arthroskopie. 1999;12:299–304.
12. Felmet G. Implant-free press-fit fixation for bone-patellar tendon-bone ACL reconstruction: 10-year results. Arch Orthop Trauma Surg. 2010;130(8):985–92.
13. Felmet G. Anatomic double bundle single tunnel foreign material free ACL-reconstruction – a technical note. Muscles Ligaments Tendons J. 2011;1(4):148–52.
14. Felmet G. Foreign material-free ACL reconstruction with hollow miller: a biological and anatomic method for every ligament. Tech Orthop. 2013;28(2):166–75.
15. Demyttenaere J, Claes S, Bellemans J. One-stage revision anterior cruciate ligament reconstruction in cases with excessive tunnel osteolysis. Results of a new technique using impaction bone grafting. Knee. 2018;25(6):1308–17.
16. Feucht MJ, et al. The role of the tibial slope in sustaining and treating anterior cruciate ligament injuries. Knee Surg Sports Traumatol Arthrosc. 2013;21(1):134–45.
17. Feucht MJ, Tischer T. [Osteotomies around the knee for ligament insufficiency]. Orthopade. 2017;46(7):601–9.
18. Napier RJ, et al. Increased radiographic posterior tibial slope is associated with subsequent injury following revision anterior cruciate ligament reconstruction. Orthop J Sports Med. 2019;7(11):2325967119879373.
19. Rahnemai-Azar AA, et al. Increased lateral tibial plateau slope predisposes male college football players to anterior cruciate ligament injury. J Bone Joint Surg Am. 2016;98(12):1001–6.
20. Tischer T, et al. The impact of osseous malalignment and realignment procedures in knee ligament surgery: a systematic review of the clinical evidence. Orthop J Sports Med. 2017;5(3):2325967117697287.

21. Wordeman SC, et al. In vivo evidence for tibial plateau slope as a risk factor for anterior cruciate ligament injury: a systematic review and meta-analysis. Am J Sports Med. 2012;40(7):1673–81.
22. Bayer S, et al. Knee morphological risk factors for anterior cruciate ligament injury: a systematic review. J Bone Joint Surg Am. 2020;102:703–18.
23. Schillhammer CK, et al. Arthroscopy up to date: anterior cruciate ligament anatomy. Arthroscopy. 2016;32(1):209–12.

9 Repair of Cartilage Defects with Mosaicplasty: Osteochondral Autograft Transfer

Osteochondral defects are detected as isolated or as comorbidities in all joints. Repair of cartilage defects is difficult up to impossible. Autologous chondrocyte transplantation (ACT) using various techniques and autologous repair using bone-marrow stimulation have been established. Growth factors (PRP) or analogous therapies suggest activation in stem cells.

This chapter shows the transplantation of osteochondral cylinders from non-weight-bearing areas of the joint to the area of damage and focal lesion. The principle here is shown by working with different sizes of diamond wet grinding hollow reamers. A micro-cutter can also be used, and with restrictions the crown cutter as well. It shown in this chapter because of this additional benefit from press-fit fixation and the use of hollow reamers.

Autologous osteochondral transplantation by Hangody et al., Hungary, uses small autologous bone cylinders harvested with sharp hollow tubes punched out of a non-weight-bearing area such as the medial or lateral patellar grove. Then, they are implanted in place of the damaged cartilage in a weight-bearing zone [1, 2]. With good to excellent results in 92%, it was seen as an alternative for small and medium-sized focal chondral and osteochondral defects of weight-bearing surfaces of the knee and other weight-bearing synovial joints [2]. Good to excellent results were obtained for the ankle without adverse effects on the (donor) knee [3]. Authors also saw that the method is limited by the defect size and the number of plugs to be taken at the donor site [4, 5].

Osteochondral transplantation is seen to achieve long-term coverage of the defect with hyaline cartilage. Donor site morbidity at the patellofemoral joint after the harvest of several cylinders and pain syndromes were observed. Therefore, the technique was suggested to be limited to two cylinders with a maximum diameter of 12 mm and one further cylinder with a smaller diameter [6, 7]. Also, good results for defects measuring 2–10.5 cm^2 were reported [8, 9]. Mega OATS procedures are also reported with a 15-mm osteochondral bone cylinder overlapping the defect at the medial femoral weight-bearing area [10].

Alterations of cartilage following OATS repair were reported after 6 and 12 months. Use of quantitative polarised light microscopy and other histopathological methods revealed a number of unique localised alterations of the collagen network in both adjacent host and implanted cartilage in OATS-repaired defects, associated with abnormal chondrocyte organisation. These alterations are consistent with mechanobiological processes and the direction and magnitude of cartilage strain [11].

G. Felmet, *Press-Fit Fixation of the Knee Ligaments*, https://doi.org/10.1007/978-3-031-11906-4_9

9.1 Indications

- Osteochondral focal defects within the weight-bearing zone of the femoral condyle after traumatic, post-traumatic, osteochondrosis dissecans, and focal osteochondronecrosis lesions.
- Osteochondral autograft transfer (OAT) is typically used for younger patients (under 50) with isolated cartilage damage, with healthy cartilage available for transfer.
- Defect size should not be more than 2–4 cm^2.
- Comorbidities such as ligament instabilities and malalignment should be addressed before or simultaneously with the OAT intervention.

9.2 Pre-operative Assessment

9.2.1 Clinical Assessment

Basic signs of cartilage tear:

- Patients describe swelling, sometimes a crepitus or locking or a giving way. Pain is variable.
- A patient may also feel pain when climbing stairs or when the knee bears weight as it straightens.
- Examination assesses the amount of swelling and the location of pain. Both can limit the range of motion. The examiner also investigates through gentle manipulation ligament instability for anterior/posterior cruciate ligaments, collateral ligaments, and menisci.

  Further physical assessment:

- Investigate frontal laxity in extension. If present, this could indicate an additional peripheral ligamentous lesion.
- Investigate the presence of pain at the joint line, which could indicate a meniscal tear.

9.2.2 Imaging Assessment

9.2.2.1 Radiographs

- Anteroposterior and lateral views detect possible osteochondral defects.

9.2.2.2 Magnetic Resonance Imaging (MRI)

- MRI is useful for detecting focal chondral defects and bone bruise as a marker and extent of the lesion. Donator sites can be checked.
- Anterior/posterior cruciate ligaments, collateral ligament tears are visible as disorganization of the ligament fibres and also lesions at the menisci.

9.2.2.3 Timing of Surgery

- Surgery takes place once inflammation around the knee has mostly resolved.
- The patient must display good quadriceps strength.
- The knee joint must be pain free and be able to flex actively to at least 120°.

9.3 Surgical Preparation

9.3.1 Surgical Equipment

- The osteochondral autograft transfer system (OATS) includes a wet grinding hollow reamer system with micro crown cutter or diamond hollow reamer of different diameters (8–18 mm)
- Harvester, applicator, and pusher in diameters of 8 to 18 mm
- Universal hollow reamer adapter (Figs. 9.1 and 9.2)

9.3.1.1 Drill with Jacobs Connector

- Wet grinding hollow reamer harvest osteochondral bone cylinder with water cooling in high precision and an intact cancellous bone

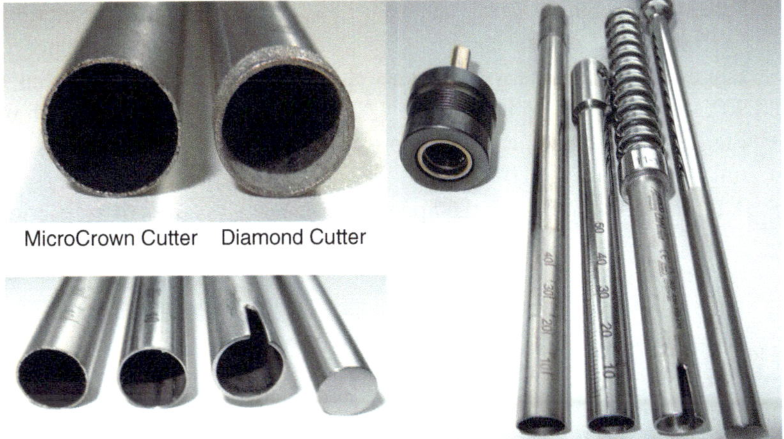

Fig. 9.1 Basic instrument set for wet grinding hollow reamers: micro-crown cutter or diamond cutter, harvester, applicator, pusher, and a universal adapter

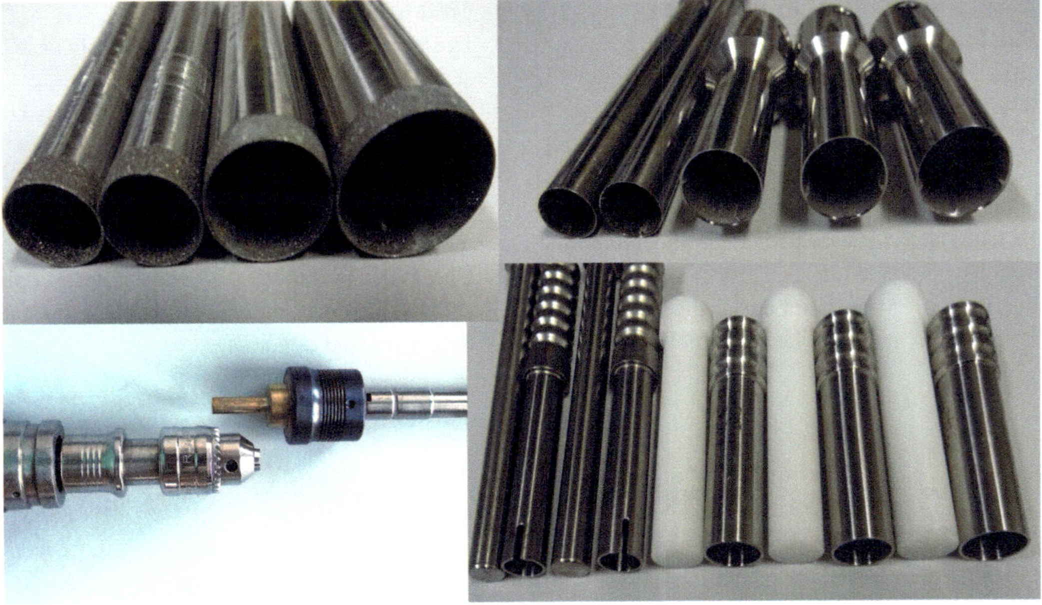

Fig. 9.2 Mega OATS wet grinding, hollow reamer. Diameter 12–16 mm is mostly used. Each size needs an extractor, applicator, and pusher

cylinder for press-fit fixation in complementary sizes

- For small diameters from 6 to 10 mm single-use OATS facilities are available (without wet grinding hollow reamer) and only a sharp harvester
- Complete arthroscopic set with a shaver
- An arthroscopy pump is not used routinely

Equipment positioning:

- The arthroscopic tower faces the surgeon on the opposite side of the table at the level of patient's shoulder

Patient positioning:

- Lay the patient supine with the knee flexed at 90°, stabilised in a leg holder.
- Ensure that the knee can be mobilised from full extension up to 120° flexion
- A tourniquet is applied to the upper thigh

Further preparation:

- Transplantation of material justifies antibiotic prophylaxis

9.4 Surgical Technique

9.4.1 Arthroscopy

9.4.1.1 Portals

- Inflate the tourniquet to 350 mmHg. Exsanguinate the limb before making the first incision
- Place anterolateral and anteromedial portals for scope insertion
- The high anterolateral portal should be placed 1.5–2 cm above the lateral joint line and 1 cm lateral to the margin of the patellar tendon at a palpable soft spot
- The anteromedial portal should be placed opposite, 1 cm above the lateral joint line and 1 cm lateral to the margin of the patellar tendon
- Assess by inspection and probing the menisci, cartilage, and ligaments

Preparation and Planning:

- Start having a good overview.
- Resect the villous synovia and hypertrophic plica.
- Treat meniscal tears and synovial impingement.
- Treat ligament instability first.
- Decide to perform OAT simultaneously or in a second surgery.
- Check the focal defect and measure the size (Fig. 9.3).
- Check the donator site superior medially and laterally to the notch or above the sulcus terminalis.
- Check the portal with a needle arthroscopically for a perpendicular approach on the defect site and donor site.

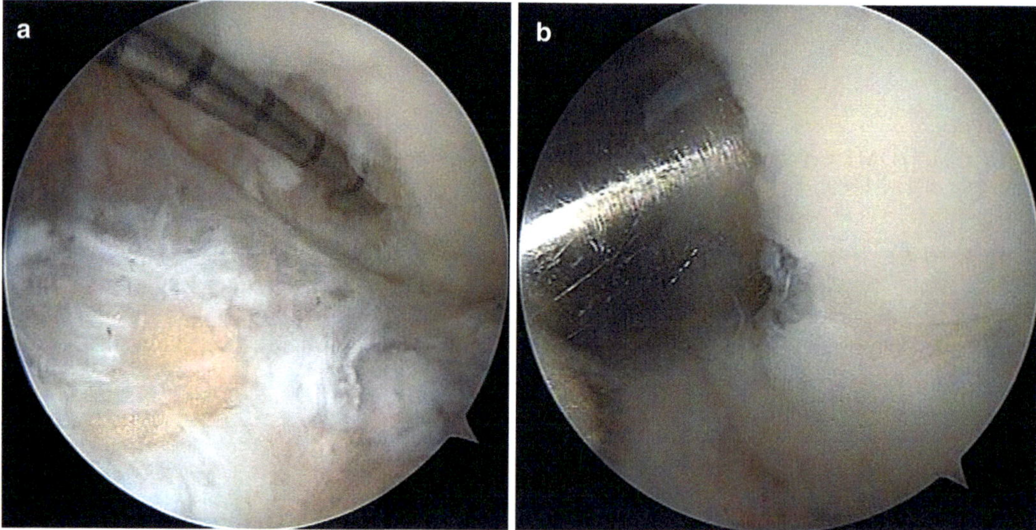

Fig. 9.3 Measure the size of the defect (**a**). Probe with a size analogue extractor (**b**) and push the extractor to make bone contact

Harvesting an osteochondral bone cylinder at the defect site:

- Make a vertical skin incision and open the perpendicular approach at the femoral condyle.
- Hollow reamer and harvester of small diameter can be managed arthroscopically.
- Diameters of more than 12 mm for mega OATS could need a mini open portal.
- Insert the harvester and check the size.
- Try to overlap the defect with one large sized of harvester (mega OAT; Fig. 9.3) or use smaller sizes and add cylinders to mosaicplasty.
- The recipient harvester is impacted to the bone and cuts the cartilage.
- The hollow reamer of the same size is inserted perpendicularly, drilled to a depth of 15 to 20 mm and removed (Fig. 9.4).
- The harvester is then impacted to the same depth.
- Insert the small rod into the end of the connector for a T-handle.
- Rotate the harvester 90° clockwise twice with its T-handle. The harvester is removed. A bone socket is created. (Fig. 9.5).
- Use a pusher and harvest the osteochondral bone cylinder out of the harvester.
- Place the bone cylinder into a saline bath.

Harvesting osteochondral bone cylinder at the donator site:

- Make a vertical skin incision and open the perpendicular approach at the donor site.
- Donor sites are medial or lateral above the sulcus terminalis (Fig. 9.6) or in maximum flexion (minimum of 120°) from the posterior femoral condyle typically for mega OATS

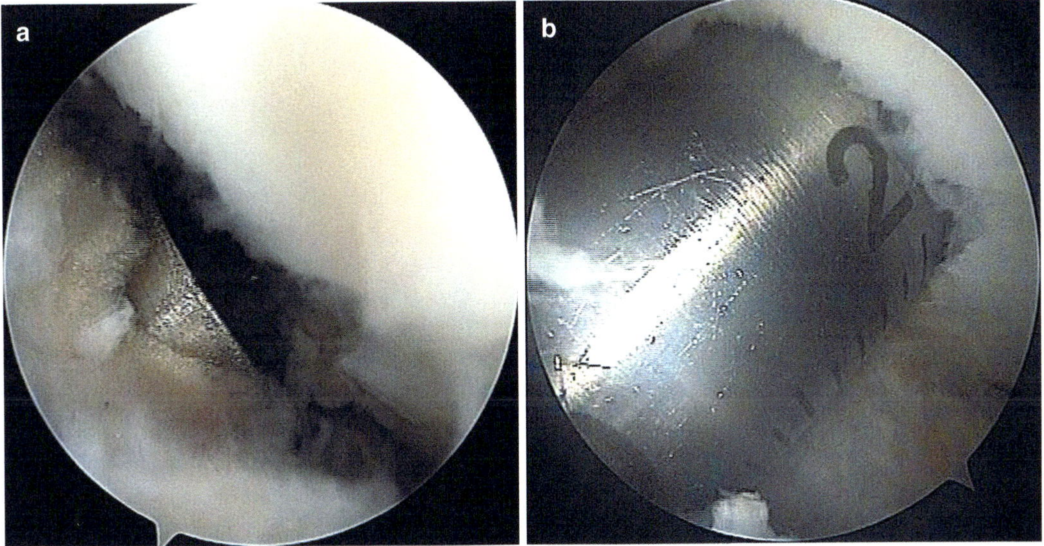

Fig. 9.4 Insert the hollow reamer (**a**). Mill (wet grinding) to the 20-mm marking (**b**)

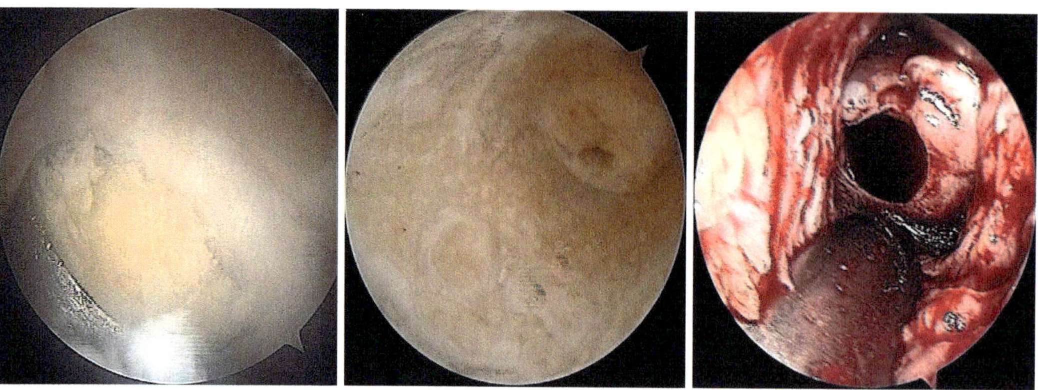

Fig. 9.5 Insert the extractor, rotate 90° clockwise, and harvest the bone cylinder

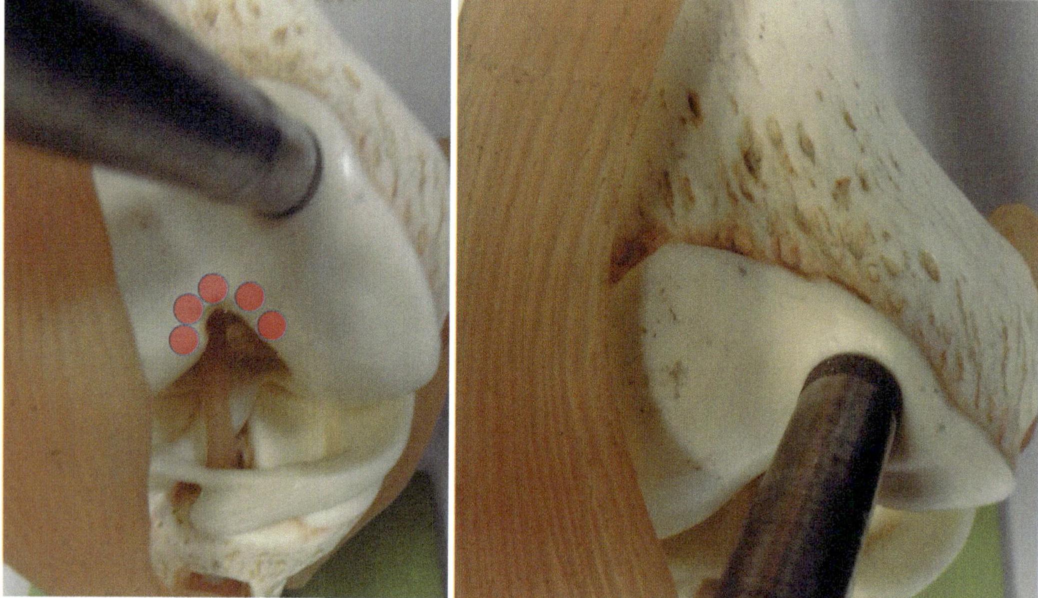

Fig. 9.6 Donor site for mega-OATS: medial trochlea. Red circles mark the donor site also for mosaicplasty superior to the notch

(Fig. 9.7) or superior to the notch for mosaicplasty (Fig. 9.6).

- Hollow reamer and harvester of small diameter can be managed arthroscopically.
- Diameters of more than 12 mm for mega OATS need a mini open portal.
- Check the alignment to the surface you harvested from the defect site.
- Insert the harvester and check the size, one step higher than the defect size.
- The recipient harvester is impacted to the bone and cuts the cartilage.
- The hollow reamer of the same size is inserted perpendicularly and drilled to a depth of 15 to 20 mm as at the defect site and removed.
- The harvester is then impacted to the same depth (Fig. 9.3).
- Insert the small rod into the end of the connector for a T-handle.
- Rotate the harvester 90° clockwise twice with its T-handle. The harvester is removed and creates a bone socket.
- Use a pusher and harvest the osteochondral bone cylinder out of the harvester (Fig. 9.5).
- Do not place the bone cylinder into a saline bath to prevent swelling.

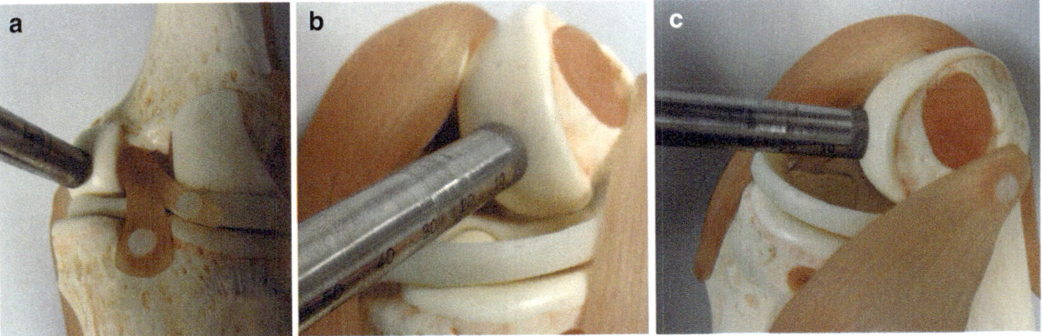

Fig. 9.7 Posterior approach (**a**), anterior approach in 120° knee flexion (**b**, **c**)

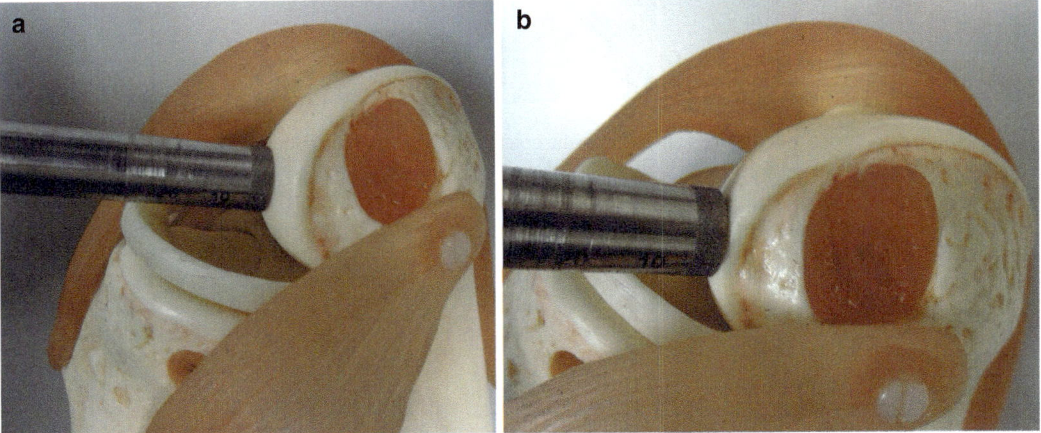

Fig. 9.8 Donor site of the dorsal femoral condyle with different convexity, central (**a**) and lateral (**b**) to align the defect site. Caveat: thinner cartilage at the edge

9.4.2 Transfer of Osteochondral Bone

9.4.2.1 Resurface the Lesion

- Check the length of both cylinders and adjust the donor cylinder to the length of the defect cylinder with respect to the depth of the socket.
- Check the alignment of the surface and adjust the position to prevent steps (Fig. 9.8).
- Insert the osteochondral bone cylinder from the donor site into the applicator.
- Position the applicator perpendicular to the socket of the defect site.
- Insert the osteochondral bone cylinder perpendicularly into the recipient socket.
- Final seating is performed using the pusher. Fixation is performed press-fit (Fig. 9.9).

9.4.2.2 Fill the Donor Site

- Take the bone cylinder from the defect site and clean the cortical bone.
- Insert the bone cylinder with the cortical bone up into an applicator of this size.
- Position the applicator perpendicular to the socket of the donor site.
- Insert the bone cylinder perpendicularly into the recipient socket.
- The size of the bone cylinder is one size smaller than the socket of the donor site.
- Tilt the bone cylinder to one side and seat it with a pusher (Fig. 9.9).

9.4.2.3 Individual Variations

- Larger defects can be treated with an overlapping of transferred bone cylinders step by step with mega OATS [10] (Fig. 9.10).

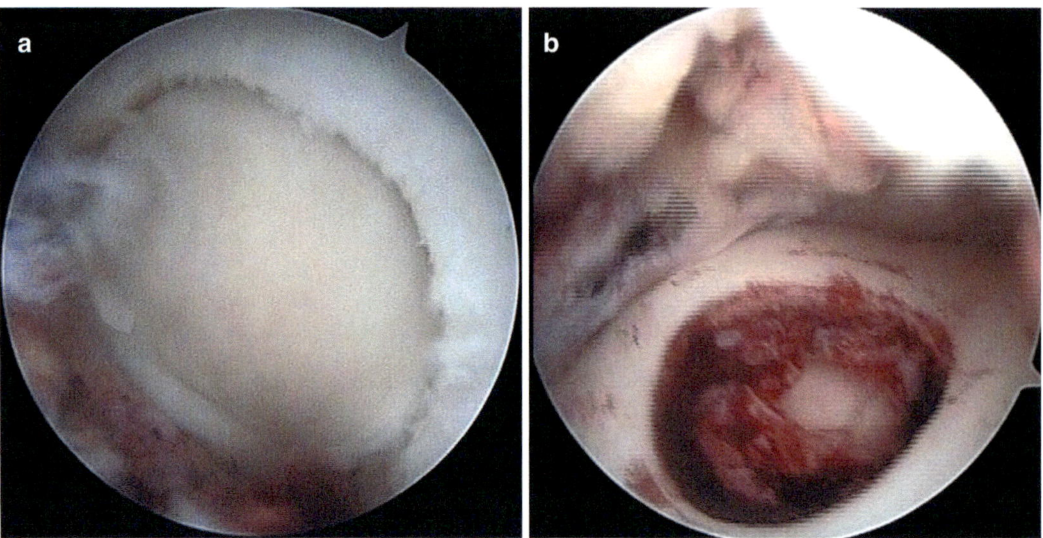

Fig. 9.9 Take the osteochondral bone cylinder from the donator site and insert it at the defect site (**a**). Implant the bone cylinder from the defect site into the socket of the donator site (**b**)

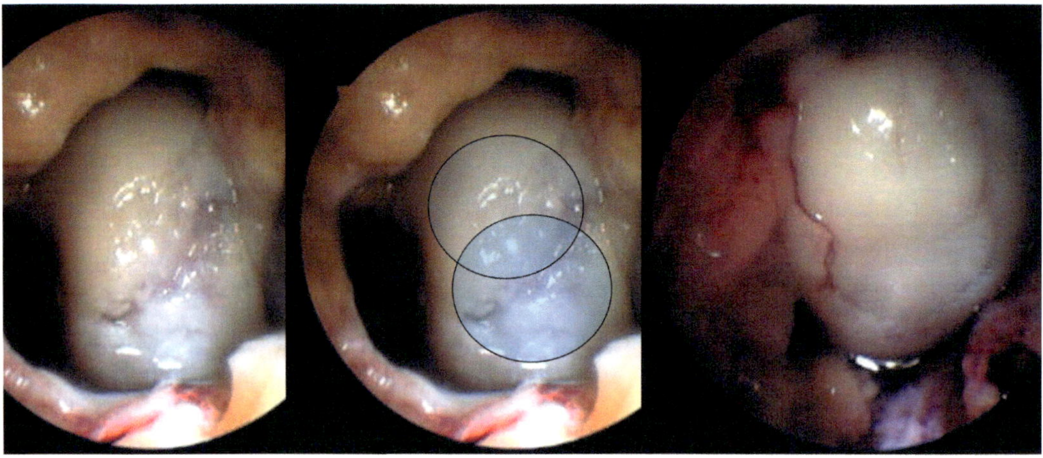

Fig. 9.10 Mega OATS: 15-mm osteochondral bone cylinder overlap. Donor site: medial trochlea and posterior medial femoral condyle [10]

- Typically mosaicplasty consists in adding several small osteochondral bone cylinders side by side with smaller gaps between the cylinders in the resurfaced defect site [1, 2].

9.4.2.4 Possible Peri-operative Complications

- Short bone cylinder from donor site > carefully insert final seating.
- Donator site bone cylinder too long > cut it to the size of the recipient socket.
- The bone cylinder from the defect site is not fixed in the socket of the donor site > rotate the bone.
- The cylinder is positioned 90° crosswise and pushed into the socket press-fit.
- Different chondral thickness but congruent articular surface > wait and see (Fig. 9.11).

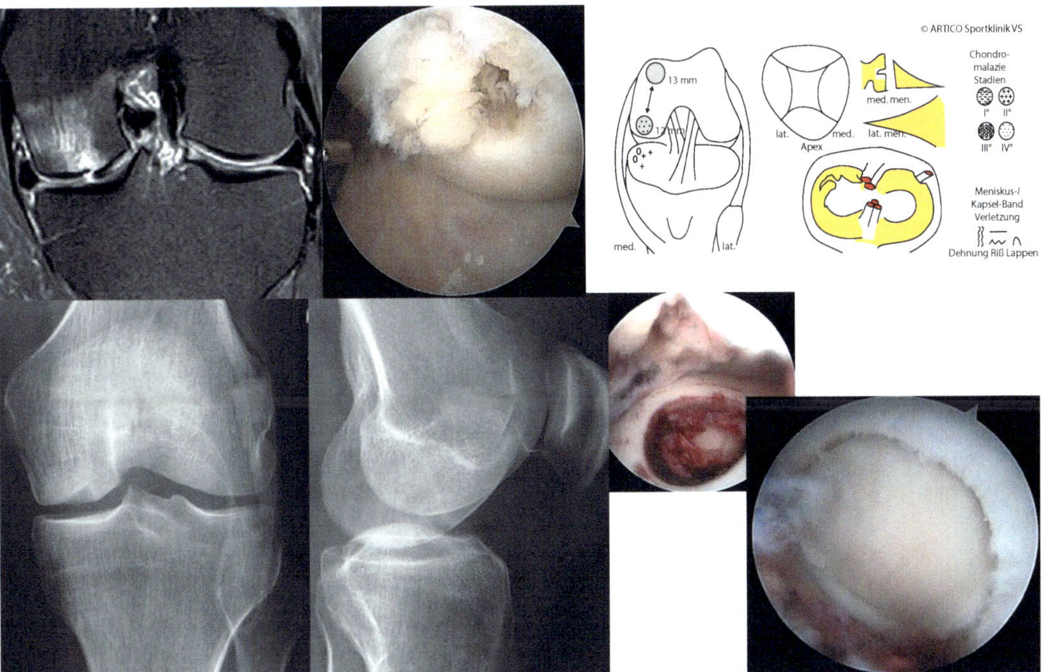

Fig. 9.11 Osteochondral necrosis with a 12-mm defect at the medial femoral weight-bearing zone, 47-year-old male, left knee

9.4.3 Closure

- Close the capsule with an absorbable suture.
- Use drainage.
- Close subcutaneous and skin layers in a standard fashion.
- Simple dressing.
- Apply a rigid straight knee splint.

Post-operative course:

- Postoperative regimen
- Medications: pain killer, nonsteroidal anti-inflammatory drugs (NSAIDs)
- Passive continuous motion treatment for 4–6 weeks
- Weight-bearing: 25 kg after 3 weeks
- Full weight-bearing after 6 weeks
- Immediate mobilization without limitation
- Isometric quadriceps contractions and ischio-crural contractions
- Plain radiographs postoperatively and after 6 weeks to check healing of the bone transfer

Early-phase postoperative complications:

- Swelling
- Stiffness in flexion and/or extension

References

1. Hangody L, et al. Mosaicplasty for the treatment of articular defects of the knee and ankle. Clin Orthop Relat Res. 2001;391 Suppl:S328–36.
2. Hangody L, et al. Autologous osteochondral grafting – technique and long-term results. Injury. 2008;39(Suppl 1):S32–9.
3. Gautier E, Kolker D, Jakob RP. Treatment of cartilage defects of the talus by autologous osteochondral grafts. J Bone Joint Surg Br. 2002;84(2):237–44.
4. Jakob RP, et al. Autologous osteochondral grafting in the knee: indication, results, and reflections. Clin Orthop Relat Res. 2002;401:170–84.
5. Marcacci M, et al. Arthroscopic autologous osteochondral grafting for cartilage defects of the knee: prospective study results at a minimum 7-year follow-up. Am J Sports Med. 2007;35(12):2014–21.
6. Schnettler R, Horas U, Meyer C. Autologous osteochondral transplants. Orthopade. 2008;37(8):734–42.
7. Agneskirchner JD, et al. Large osteochondral defects of the femoral condyle: press-fit transplantation of

the posterior femoral condyle (MEGA-OATS). Knee Surg Sports Traumatol Arthrosc. 2002;10(3):160–8.
8. Braun S, et al. The 5.5-year results of MegaOATS – autologous transfer of the posterior femoral condyle: a case-series study. Arthritis Res Ther. 2008;10(3):R68.
9. Brucker PU, Braun S, Imhoff AB. [Mega-OATS technique – autologous osteochondral transplantation as a salvage procedure for large osteochondral defects of the femoral condyle]. Oper Orthop Traumatol. 2008;20(3):188–98.
10. Felmet G. Repair of cartilage defects with mosaicplasty – osteochondral autograft transfer. In: Tiburtius HJ, Klos VS, Kelberine F, Khan W, editors. EFOST surgical techniques in sports medicine – knee surgery vol. 2: bone and cartilage; 2016. p. 29–35. p. 128.
11. Raub CB, et al. Microstructural remodeling of articular cartilage following defect repair by osteochondral autograft transfer. Osteoarthr Cartil. 2013;21(6):860–8.

10 Management of Quality and Complications

Anterior cruciate ligament (ACL) reconstruction today is a safe and standardized surgical procedure. Beside technical and individual requirements, as in any other surgical technique, a learning curve is necessary. The impact of surgical factors for postoperative failure is reported to be 22–79% [1–3]. Particularly the learning curve for tunnel positioning anatomically and correctly is between 30 and 50 cases. This is one of the important factors for failure [2, 4].

This chapter is shows different workflows, strategies for possible complication management, as well characteristics of quality control.

10.1 Preoperative Planning

Before the operation starts patients' correct identity and labeling of the limb have to be performed according to the "WHO Surgical Safety Checklist" to ensure and increase patients' safety [5] (Fig. 10.1).

A preoperative examination, with the patient relaxed under anesthesia, is indispensable. Translational stability (anterior versus posterior), collateral ligaments, and instabilities in rotation are identified and documented. In the case of a tourniquet and an electric leg holder good padding of the extremity is necessary. To avoid irritation of the skin the padding can be covered by adhesive film.

To avoid tourniquet-associated complications such as sensitivity disorders, early infection, or disorders in wound healing the tourniquet period should not exceed 120 min [6]. The level of pneumatic tourniquet is adapted to the patient with values between 250 and a maximum of 350 mmHg.

G. Felmet, *Press-Fit Fixation of the Knee Ligaments*, https://doi.org/10.1007/978-3-031-11906-4_10

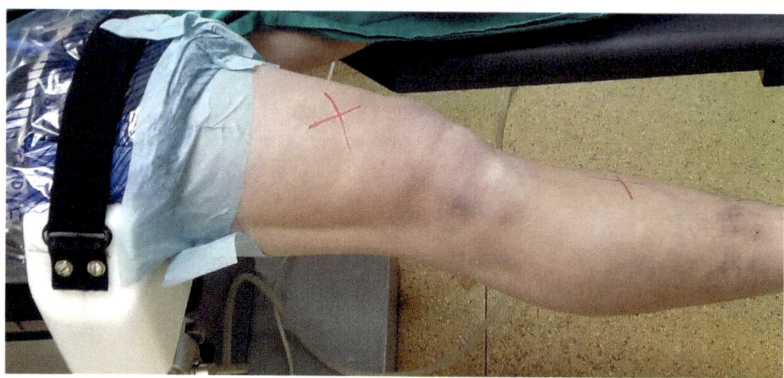

Fig. 10.1 Patient's correct identity and labeling of the limb has to be performed according to the "WHO Surgical Safety Checklist" to ensure and increase patients' safety

10.2 Tendon Removal

The graft is to be harvested sufficiently long and thick. Because of the individual preferences of the patient and the surgeon, advantages and disadvantages of different grafts suggest a plan A and B for alternative procedures. This must also be taken into account in the preliminary discussion and legal clarification. This is especially helpful in unforeseeable complications of graft removal or even loss of the graft.

10.3 Tunnel Position

Incorrect tunnel position is the greatest cause of graft insufficiency in about 70–80% [1]. Drilling the femoral tunnel in particular has the greatest potential for failure. A femoral tunnel that is positioned too far ventrally is the most common technical error [7].

The trans-tibial drilling with an extra-anatomical tunnel location is associated with poor visualization of the posterior femoral condylar wall, confusion with the "resident's ridge," and a high rate of error. The tubed femoral guiding device allows checking after a marking drill to control the position. Alternatively, the tunnel position can be evaluated radiologically on fluorescence radiography. The tibial tunnel should be placed anatomically correct neither too ventral nor dorsal avoiding a notch impingement or hyperlaxity Stäubli and Rausching [8].

10.4 Graft Insertion and Fixation

After creating the tunnels the graft is typically pulled over the tibial tunnel into the femoral tunnel (bottom to top) [9]. The threads should be strong enough. The tunnel should be clean and soft tissue eliminated preventing a stop. The tibial stump should not be resected completely to seal the gap to the tunnel.

1. Check the diameter of the tibial graft with the bone cylinder. Enlarge the tunnel to this diameter with the cone-pusher. Stop at 1 cm under the tibia plateau.
2. Now the graft is pulled inside the tunnel. Step-by-step the tibial bone cylinder is pushed deeper. In the case of hard bone it can be impossible to deepen the graft. Pull out the complete graft with a Kocher clamp or Kantrowitz clamp. Enlarge the tunnel again as needed. Start implantation again.
3. In the case of loss or destruction of the tibial bone cylinder, harvest a new one from the tibial head and insert it again into the graft (Fig. 10.2).
4. In the case of an unstable fixation or blow out of the tibial tunnel use a K-wire for a temporary fixation for 6 weeks. Alternatively, use a thread and fix it at the tibial bone-cylinder. Fix the graft over a bone bridge at the tibial tunnel side (Fig. 10.3).
5. Femoral fixation can be fixed by an additional or oversized bone cylinder from the tibial head (Fig. 10.2).

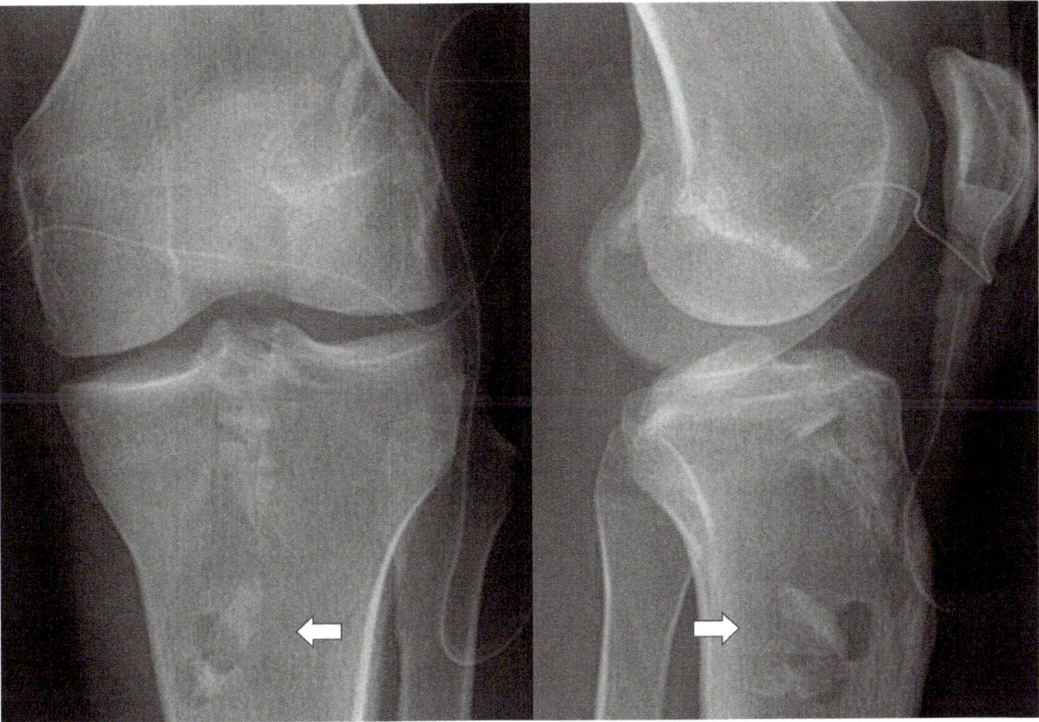

Fig. 10.2 In the case of loss or destruction of the tibial bone cylinder, harvest a new one from the tibial head (arrows) and insert it again into the graft

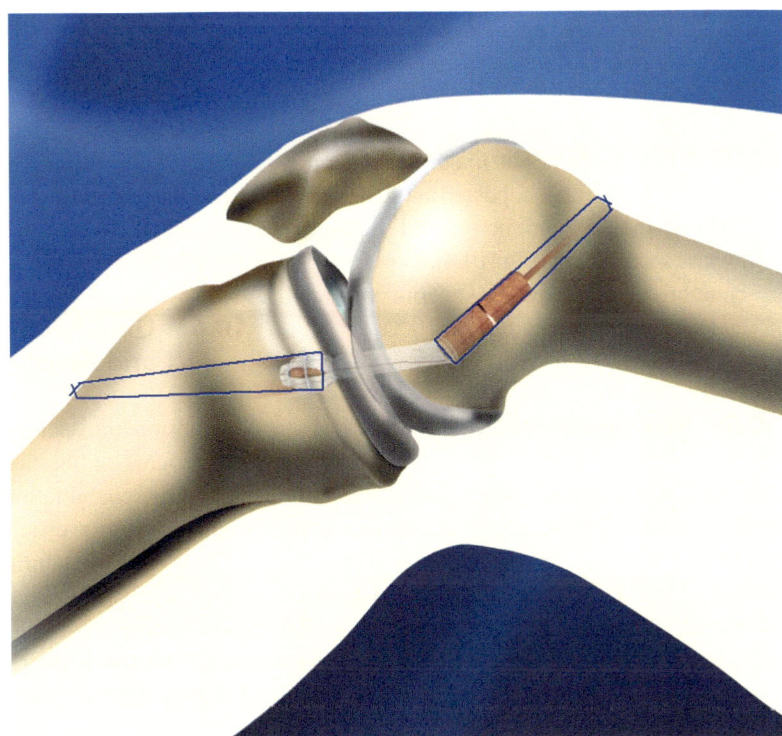

Fig. 10.3 Femoral side is not fixed: in revision or osteoporotic soft bone, posterior blow out, the "pull-in thread" can be guided through a bypass second drill. Fix it over the bone bridge thus created, superior to the lateral condyle with a knot. The tibial side is unstable: pull the tibial bone cylinder with an extra thread down and fix it with a knot over a bone-bridge

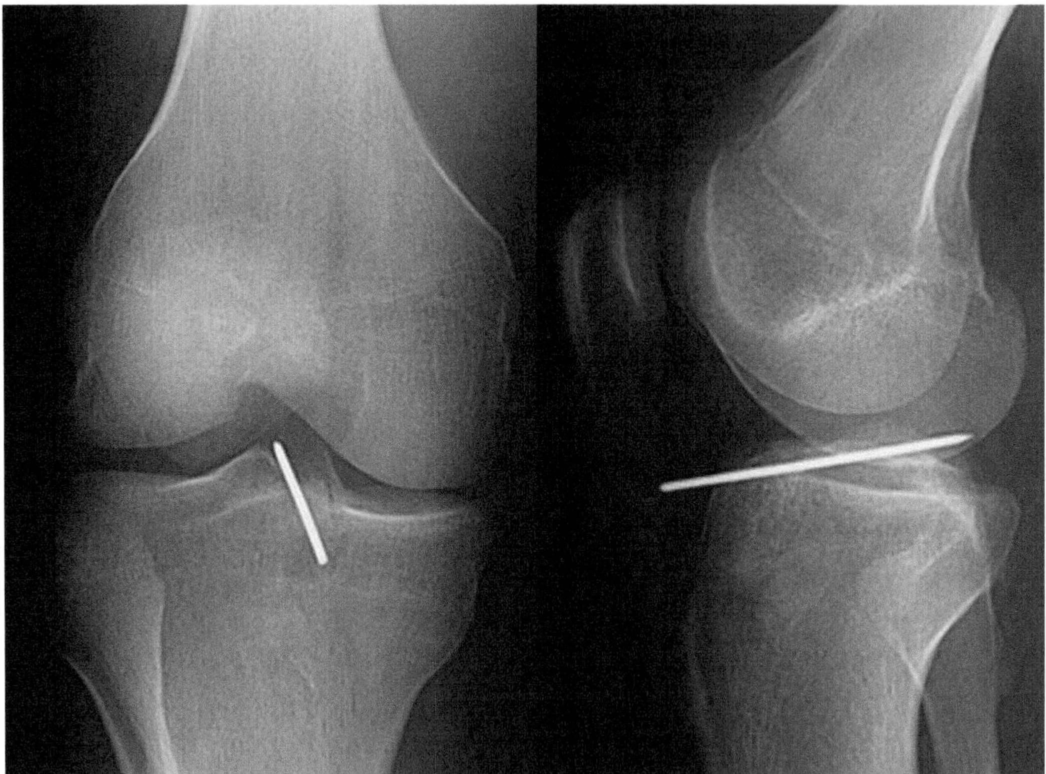

Fig. 10.4 In the case of an unstable fixation or blow out of the tibial tunnel, use a K-wire for a temporary fixation for 6 weeks. Alternatively, use a thread and fix at the tibial bone cylinder. Fix the graft over a bone bridge on the tibial tunnel side

6. The femoral side is not fixed: in revision or osteoporotic soft bone, posterior blow out, the "pull-in thread" can be guided through a bypass second drill (Fig. 10.4). Fix it over the bone bridge thus created, superior to the lateral condyle with a knot (Fig. 10.3).

10.5 Postoperative Infection

Although postoperative knee infections after ACL reconstruction are rare, it is a serious complication with a potential indication for arthroscopic lavage, synovectomy, and revision of the ACL. Realize and act immediately. The effusion is punctured and the blood examined [10, 11]. The incidence of corresponding infections could be reduced by incubation of the tendon grafts in vancomycin (5 mg/ml), with success from the previous average 1.4% to almost 0% [12, 13].

10.6 Quality Control and Benchmarks

The postoperative check-ups of stability and clinical progress in the first weeks are the surgeon's duty. The rehabilitation program is defined with physiotherapists, coaches, and team physicians.

Transversal stability and pivot shift after 3/6/9/12 months are recommended. Instrumented stability tests such as the ArticoMeter, Rolimeter, or KT 1000 are favored and recommended [14, 15] (Fig. 10.5.). Side-to-side stability should be better than 3 mm. Typical quotes of a Lachman

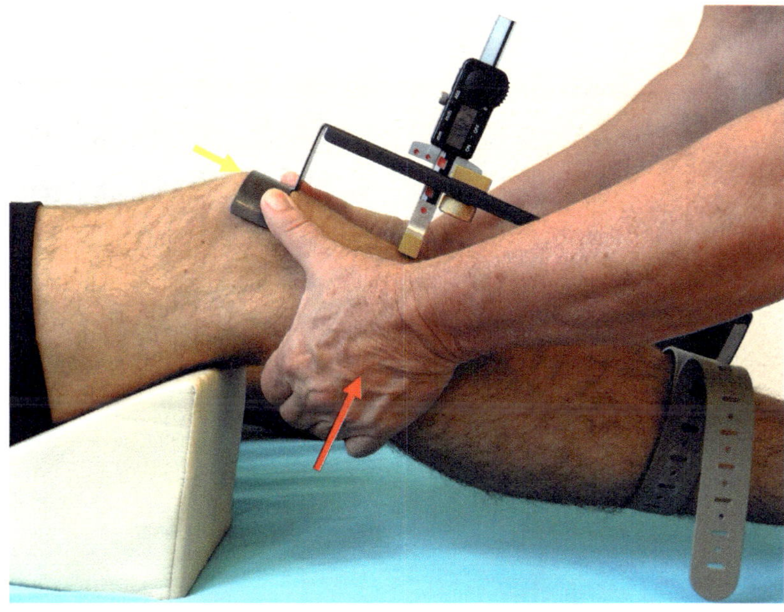

Fig. 10.5 Instrumented stability tests such as the ArticoMeter, Rolimeter, or KT 1000 are favored and recommended [14–16]. Side-to-side stability should be better than 3 mm

rate of approximately 70% and a negative pivot shift rate of around 78%, each with a anteromedial drilling technique have been reported [17]. Regular tests for coordination, muscle strength, and agility are important during rehabilitation and for decision making regarding a return to sport and competition (see Chap. 11).

References

1. Kamath GV, et al. Revision anterior cruciate ligament reconstruction. Am J Sports Med. 2011;39(1):199–217.
2. Ma Y, et al. Failed anterior cruciate ligament reconstruction: analysis of factors leading to instability after primary surgery. Chin Med J. 2013;126(2):280–5.
3. MARS Group (Collaborators: Wright RW, Huston L, Haas AK, Spindler KP, Nwosu SK, Allen CR, Anderson AF, Cooper DE, DeBerardino TM, Dunn WR, Lantz BB, Stuart MJ, Garofoli EA, Albright JP, Amendola AN, Andrish JT, Annunziata CC, Arciero RA, Bach BR Jr, Baker CL 3rd, Bartolozzi AR, Baumgarten KM, Bechler JR, Berg JH, Bernas GA, Brockmeier SF, Brophy RH, Bush-Joseph CA, Butler JB 5th, Campbell JD, Carey JL, Carpenter JE, Cole BJ, Cooper JM, Cox CL, Creighton RA, Dahm DL, David TS, Flanigan DC, Frederick RW, Ganley TJ, Gatt CJ Jr, Gecha SR, Giffin JR, Hame SL, Hannafin JA, Harner CD, Harris NL Jr, Hechtman KS, Hershman EB, Hoellrich RG, Hosea TM, Johnson DC, Johnson TS, Jones MH, Kaeding CC, Kamath GV, Klootwyk TE, Levy BA, Ma CB, Maiers GP 2nd, Marx RG, Matava MJ, Mathien GM, McAllister DR, McCarty EC, McCormack RG, Miller BS, Nissen CW, O'Neill DF, Owens BD, Parker RD, Purnell ML, Ramappa AJ, Rauh MA, Rettig AC, Sekiya JK, Shea KG, Sherman OH, Slauterbeck JR, Smith MV, Spang JT, Svoboda SJ, Taft TN, Tenuta JJ, Tingstad EM, Vidal AF, Viskontas DG, White RA, Williams JS Jr, Wolcott ML, Wolf BR, York JJ.) Effect of graft choice on the outcome of revision anterior cruciate ligament reconstruction in the Multicenter ACL Revision Study (MARS) Cohort. Am J Sports Med. 2014;42(10):2301–2310.
4. Luthringer TA, et al. The learning curve associated with anteromedial portal drilling in ACL reconstruction. Phys Sportsmed. 2016;44(2):141–7.
5. van Klei WA, et al. Effects of the introduction of the WHO "Surgical Safety Checklist" on in-hospital mortality: a cohort study. Ann Surg. 2012;255(1):44–9.
6. Reda W, et al. Anterior cruciate ligament reconstruction; is a tourniquet necessary? A randomized controlled trial. Knee Surg Sports Traumatol Arthrosc. 2016;24(9):2948–52.
7. Trojani C, et al. Causes for failure of ACL reconstruction and influence of meniscectomies after revision. Knee Surg Sports Traumatol Arthrosc. 2011;19(2):196–201.
8. Stäubli HU, Rauschning W. Tibial attachment area of the anterior cruciate ligament in the extended knee position. Anatomy and cryosections in vitro complemented by magnetic resonance arthrography in vivo. Knee Surg Sports Traumatol Arthrosc. 1994;2(3):138–46.
9. Felmet G. Foreign material-free ACL reconstruction with hollow miller: a biological and anatomic method for every ligament. Techn Orthop. 2013;28(2):166–75.

10. Ascione T, et al. Post-arthroscopic septic arthritis of the knee. Analysis of the outcome after treatment in a case series and systematic literature review. Eur Rev Med Pharmacol Sci. 2019;23(2 Suppl):76–85.
11. Renz N, et al. Enterococcal periprosthetic joint infection: clinical and microbiological findings from an 8-year retrospective cohort study. BMC Infect Dis. 2019;19(1):1083.
12. Phegan M, Grayson JE, Vertullo CJ. No infections in 1300 anterior cruciate ligament reconstructions with vancomycin pre-soaking of hamstring grafts. Knee Surg Sports Traumatol Arthrosc. 2016;24(9):2729–35.
13. Vertullo CJ, et al. A surgical technique using presoaked vancomycin hamstring grafts to decrease the risk of infection after anterior cruciate ligament reconstruction. Arthroscopy. 2012;28(3):337–42.
14. Felmet G, et al. Press-fit ACL reconstruction. In: Norimasa Nakamura SZ, Marx RG, Musahl V, editors. Controversies in the technical aspects of ACL reconstruction: an evidence-based medicine approach. ISAKOS: Springer; 2017. p. 247–61.
15. Krautter A, et al. Instrumented arthrometry of the anterior cruciate ligament. A comparison. Biomed Tech (Berl). (issue-s1-R/bmt-2012-4299/bmt-2012-4299). 2012.
16. Runer A, et al. The evaluation of Rolimeter, KLT, KiRA and KT-1000 arthrometer in healthy individuals shows acceptable intra-rater but poor inter-rater reliability in the measurement of anterior tibial knee translation. Knee Surg Sports Traumatol Arthrosc. 2021.
17. Chen Y, et al. Outcome of single-bundle hamstring anterior cruciate ligament reconstruction using the anteromedial versus the transtibial technique: a systematic review and meta-analysis. Arthroscopy. 2015;31(9):1784–94.

11 Rehabilitation After ACL Reconstruction, Return to Sport and Prevention

This chapter describes rehabilitation after ACL reconstruction, taking into account the all press-fit fixation: standard, after revision, osteoporotic bone fixation, and healing response reinsertion. Biomechanical knowledge is fundamental in early postoperative and subsequent follow-up treatment.

Individual features have to be calculated. Proven and scientific backgrounds are made accessible. Exercises to be implemented without extensive technology are illustrated with examples. Coupled with the experience in athletes and occasional athletes, test options and special technical items are presented and discussed for qualification to return to sport or competition. Rehabilitation begins with exercises of basic sports and part of the prevention program. Prevention is a key issue today from many points of view such as the national economy, individual quality of life, and the cost unit or insurance. This once again underlines the demand for "prevention first."

11.1 Biomechanics of the Anterior Cruciate Ligament and Conclusion for Rehabilitation Exercises

The main principle of the movement of the knee is a roll-slide movement between the femur and the tibia. In detail, however, it becomes more difficult, the extent of the mixing of rolling and sliding in the individual movement phases exactly because the movements of flexion and extension in the main sagittal plane by the automatic initial and final rotation and the arbitrary rotation are superimposed. The crucial ligaments are important stabilizers of the knee and determine the roll-gliding mechanism in knee flexion [1]. The femur and tibia form a connecting rods system, in which the bones resemble plates and the ligaments strings. The strings do not change their lengths with limited elasticity, when the plates are moved around each other. This is important for the first postoperative weeks, because it shows that ACL strain does not necessarily increase in knee flexion exercises, even though the tibia translates forward. The anterior shift of the tibia is compensated for by moving the attachment of the ACL at the femur downward. This model can be backed up by biomechanical data, which show that elongation of the ACL decreases from 2.5% in hyperextension to −0.5% in 40° and then rises up to 1% in 90° knee flexion. The higher tension of the ACL in full extension is a result of limiting tibial forward translation and inducing terminal outward rotation of 14° in the last 20° of extension. Increased tension of the ACL in knee flexion beyond 40° is a result of limiting femoral regression on the tibial slope. If knee flexion goes beyond 90° elongation is greater than 1% [2]. Range of motion (ROM) after an ACL reconstruction is often limited to 0–0-90°.

G. Felmet, *Press-Fit Fixation of the Knee Ligaments*, https://doi.org/10.1007/978-3-031-11906-4_11

Anterior cruciate ligament strain is highly dependent on muscle activation. Maximal pure quadriceps activation between 20 and 40° of knee flexion causes an anterior drawer with an elongation of about 2.5%, for example, 4500 N can cause ACL injury at 20° knee flexion [3]. High moments can be generated through the long lever arm of the patella in this position. To reduce the lever and risk of lengthening the ACL the ROM can be set to 60–90° knee flexion and the pad can be placed at the proximal part of the tibia [4–6]. In a hip-dominant squatting exercise, however, ACL stress is low even though the quadriceps is working, because the hamstrings, especially between 15° and 80° knee flexion, pull the tibia backward, reducing the anterior drawer [7–9]. Some research indicates that strain on the ACL in squatting with maximal load (28 N) is only a tenth of the strain caused by knee extension without resistance (396 N) [10].

Secondly, ACL strain can be influenced by in- and outward rotation. Whereas outward rotation disentangles both ACLs, inward rotation with an anterior drawer generates higher loads on the ACL than each mechanism alone [11]. Inward rotation in low knee flexion angles results in exceptionally high ACL stress, as is common in ACL tears in skiing accidents [12]. In soccer, cleated shoes are responsible for high internal rotation moments, causing the ACL to tear [13, 14]. Malalignment in the foot such as hyperpronation is thought to increase ACL injury risk by inducing internal rotation of the tibia [15–17].

The third factor responsible for ACL stress is the dynamic valgus. Commonly in this movement, hip adduction, femoral internal rotation, knee abduction, tibial internal rotation, and hyperpronation occur [18]. But some studies indicate that valgus collapse can go along with external rotation [19]. Individuals, who demonstrate an 8° greater knee abduction angle, which resembles 2.5-fold knee abduction moment, than the normal population, are at risk for ACL injury [20]. In another study, Myer et al. showed that the risk of subsequent ACL injury increases 17-fold, from 0.4% to 6.8%, if the knee abduction moment goes beyond 25.3 Nm [21]. Simulation indicates that the increase is shallow between 0 and 10 Nm and above 40 Nm, but really steep between 10 and 40 Nm [22]. This could explain why small changes in the leg axis can determine if an ACL tears or not. Moreover, a valgus collapse is often combined with an anterior drawer, which results from quadriceps activity and tibiofemoral compression, or is induced by inward rotation, which can result from a twisted ski [13].

11.2 Biology and Physiology

Understanding of biological and physiological processes are important to understanding of healing, repair, and regeneration of muscle and tendon. The selection of exercises and treatment is adapted on this cascade [23–25] (Table 11.1).

Table 11.1 Overview of the physiological processes after trauma and surgery. Remodeling and maturation take longer in tendon than in muscle

Inflammation phase	
Injury/ incident	Immediate vasoconstriction of the blood flow. Immobilization to reduce pain and swelling
24–48 h post	Vasodilatation and proliferation of tissue. Inflammation. Icing is not recommended as it slows down healing by decreasing lymphatic flow, proliferation, and cell–cell-interactions. Same rules apply for anti-inflammatory drugs. Ice has numbing effects and should only be used for a few minutes for pain relief
Proliferation phase	
5 days	Type III collagen is produced and will be transferred to type I over time. Reconstruction and orientation of the type III fibers depend on stress of movement and weight bearing. That is why exercises in full ROM allowed and weight bearing are so important to guarantee good healing of tissue and scars
Remodeling/maturation	
~3 weeks	Type III collagen is transferred into type I. regaining ROM, proprioceptive and contractile information to allow good healing. Regaining biomechanical qualities of the tissue. Formation of cross-links for greater stiffness. This process is supported by load and mobilization into the end of ROM in exercises. 300–500 days until tissue regains its former function

ROM range of motion

11.3 Rehabilitation

Up to 60% of patients with an ACL reconstruction regain their old level of activity [26, 27] and only up to 44% return to competitive sport [28, 29]. Re-injury rates for ACL vary from 0 to 19% or worse for the ipsilateral side and 7–24% for the contralateral side [30]. Six months postoperatively, when many patients are allowed to return to sports, athletes still have a limb-symmetry index of less than 90% for different athletic tasks. However, not just the performance but also the movement quality is poor [31]. For most patients it takes 2 years until differences are below 5% [32].

Considering the lower functional performance of the involved leg and the higher tendency toward risky movement patterns even before the injury, it is obvious why so many athletes reinjure [18]. This demonstrates the importance of proper rehabilitation after reconstruction. Load and tendon tension stimulate "Remodeling and Maturation" in synthesis of collagen [33], change of structure [34]. Integration and tendon adaption need well dosed stimulus for tendon and muscle [35, 36].

11.3.1 Guidelines for ACL-Reconstruction After All Press-Fit Programs A and B

To simplify rehabilitation and ease an overview of the rehabilitation for all press-fit ACL only we distinguish between program A and program B. Program A allows complete extension from the first day after surgery. Patient and physiotherapist start rapidly with active exercises. After trauma and surgery the vastus medialis is usually difficult to activate. The Jendrassik maneuver is a method of reinforcement and can help in priming vastus medialis activity [37–39] (Fig. 11.1). Therefore, external support such as neuromuscular electrical stimulation is helpful against loss of the quadriceps [40] (Fig. 11.2) (Table 11.2A). Program B is limited in extension for 2–4 weeks in a brace (24 h/day) depending on the indication of unstable graft fixation (osteoporosis) or co-morbidities of other ligaments or capsule or osteochondral lesions. Co-contraction exercises of the quadriceps muscle with the ischiocrural muscles (hamstrings) are suggested (Fig. 11.1) (Table 11.2B). After this early period of limitation program B changes to the issues of program A. Post-traumatic bone density measurements with peripheral quantitative computed tomography) after ACL rupture detected a bone loss of 12% (in individual cases up to 25%) in the tibial head in the first 3 months [41]. Proprioceptive vibration training can be included to support reinforcement of the quadriceps muscle and vastus medialis and may prevent further bone loss [42]. Early initiation of skipping and several short interval sprints of 20–30 m (5-sprint interval) and aquasprint (in knee- to hip-deep water) against water resistance can be started after finishing the early healing period [43] (Fig. 11.3). Freestyle swimming with the leg stroke is also recommended.

11.3.2 First Postoperative Days

11.3.2.1 Heal Slides

In the first few days after ACL reconstruction rest and movement of the full ROM allowed in the pain-free zone is recommended. Rest is important to decrease swelling and reduce further inflammation in the knee. Motion influences tissue growth, induces bio-electrical processes, increases growth of cells, and has a positive effect on scar tissue [44]. Thus, heel slides are one of the most important exercises in the first postoperative weeks until the prescribed range of motion is regained. Immobilization phases that are too long lead to functional and physiological adaptations, which, for example, lead to failure of knee extension [44]. This complication is one of the most common issues after ACL reconstruction [45]. The exercise should be done 6–8 times per day, 10–15 repetitions in three sets (Fig. 11.4).

A variation is to target knee extension in particular with knee extension exercises in standing with low weight bearing on the involved limb (Fig. 11.5).

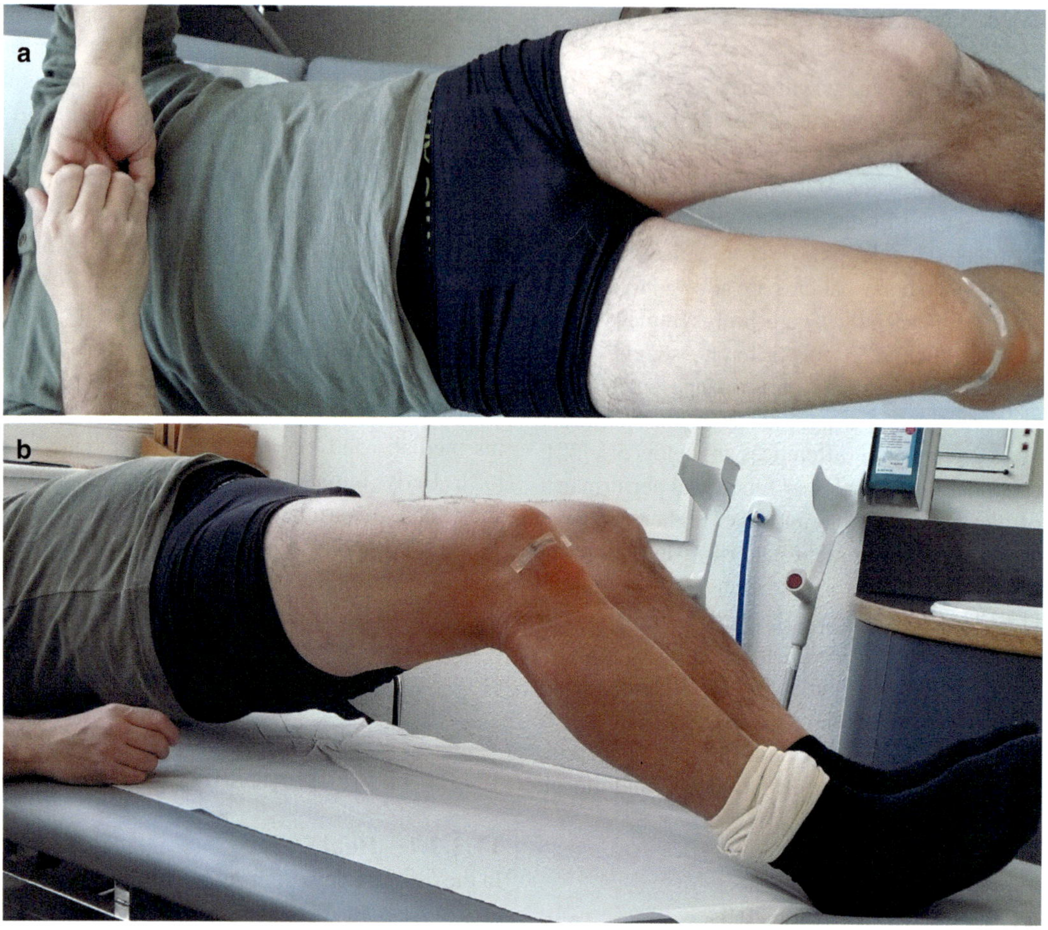

Fig. 11.1 The Jendrasik maneuver is a method of reinforcement and can help in priming vastus medialis activity [37, 38] (**a**). Isometric quadriceps contraction and co-contraction exercises of the quadriceps muscle with the ischiocrural muscles (hamstrings) are suggested with lifting of the hips (**b**)

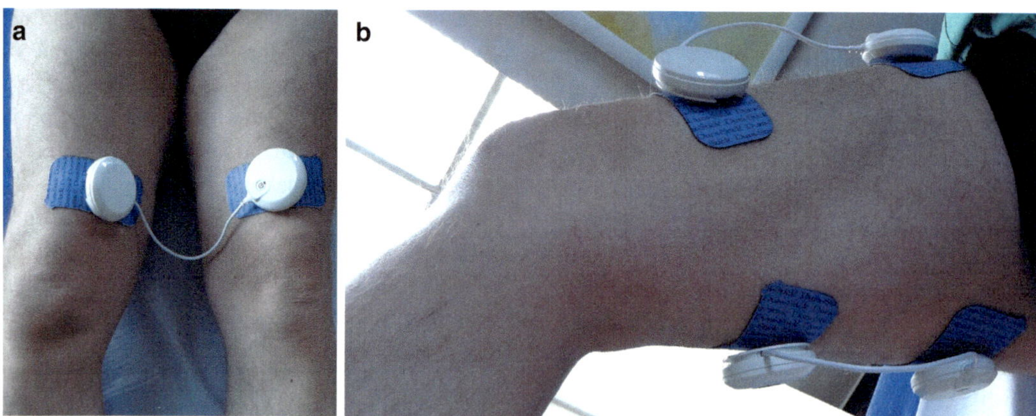

Fig. 11.2 Neuromuscular electrical stimulation combats the loss of the quadriceps [40]. Anode and cathode can be used side to side, stimulating the injured side with the healthy side in the later period (**a**). Quadriceps and ischiocrural muscle stimulation can work in parallel (**b**)

Table 11.2 (**A**) Rehabilitation program is reduced to all press-fit anterior cruciate ligament (ACL): programs A and B. (**A**) Program A allows complete extension on the first day after surgery. Patient and physiotherapist start rapidly with active and passive exercises. (**B**) Program B limits extension for 2–4 weeks in a brace (24 h/day). A standard program typically after healing response of femoral ACL reinsertion or, for example, osteopenic bone. Co-exercises of quadriceps muscle simultaneously in knee flexion with ischiocrural muscles (hamstrings) (Fig. 11.1) are suggested

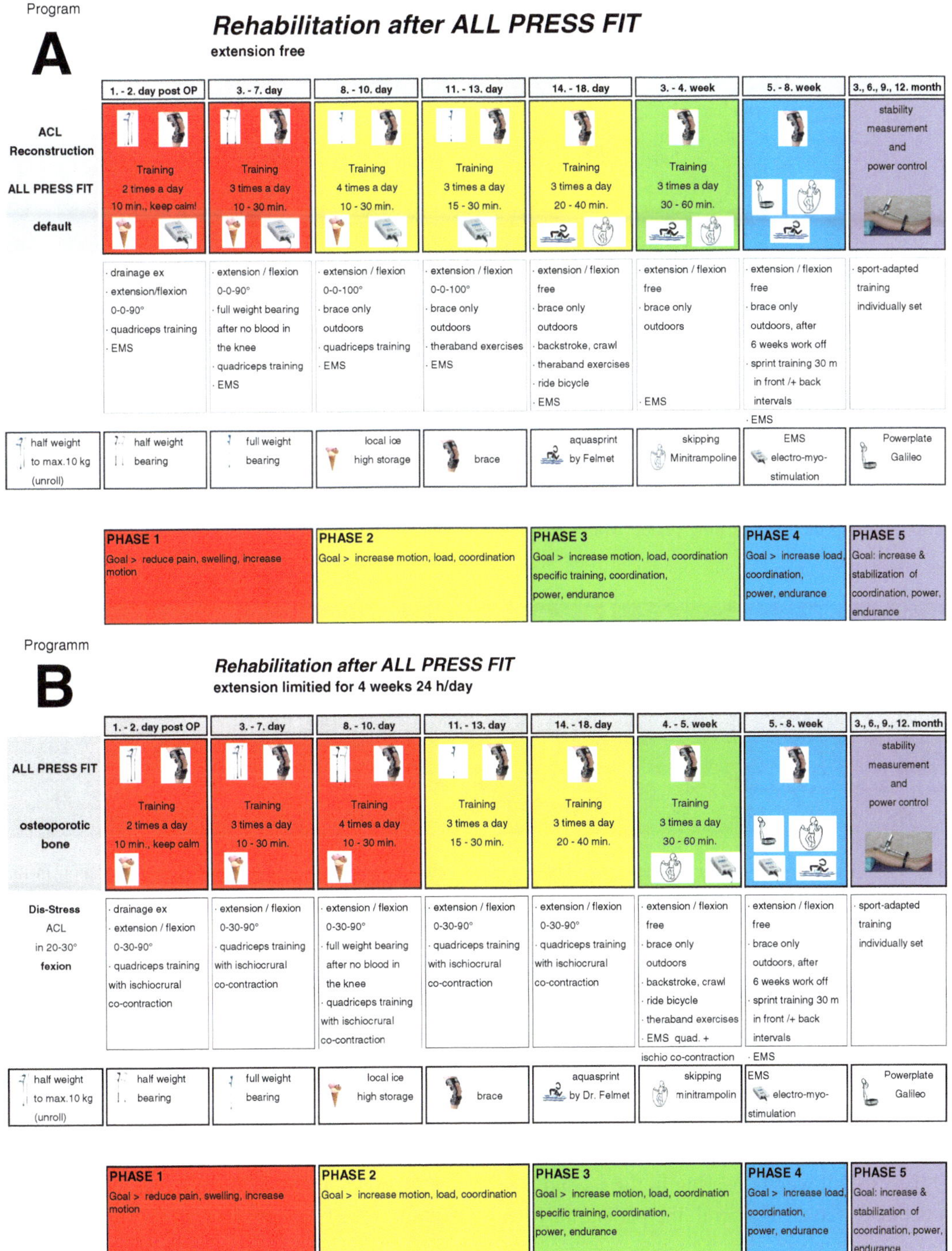

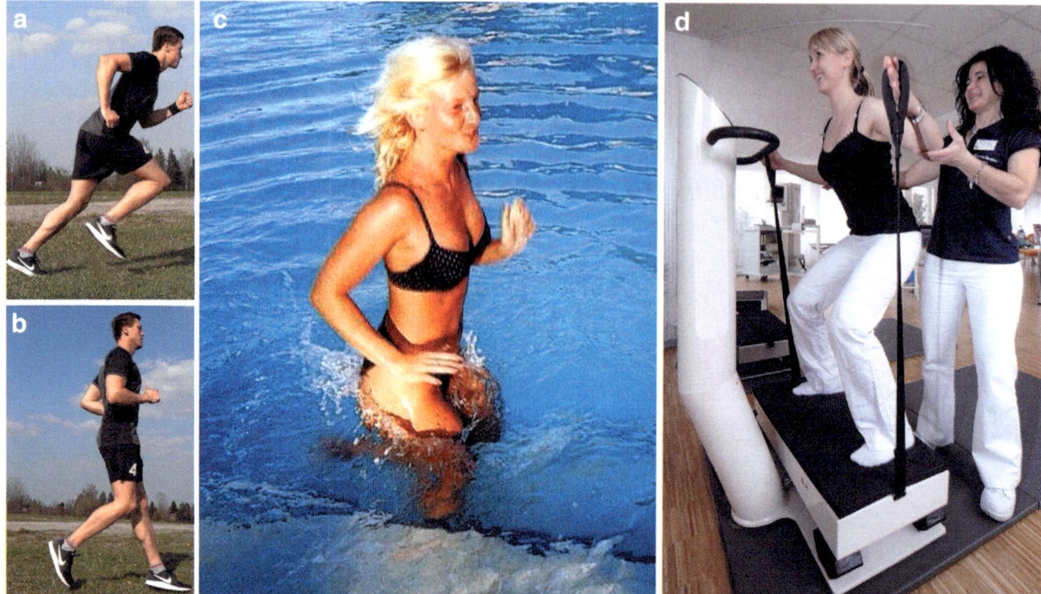

Fig. 11.3 Slightly skipping; later short sprints forward (quadriceps muscle) (**a**), backward running (more for the ischiocrural muscles) (**b**), and aqua-sprint (in knee- to hip-deep water) against water resistance can be started after finishing the early healing period. Water resistance stabilizes like a brace (**c**) [43]. Proprioceptive vibration training can be included to support reinforcement of the quadriceps muscle and vastus medialis and may prevent further bone loss (**d**) [42]

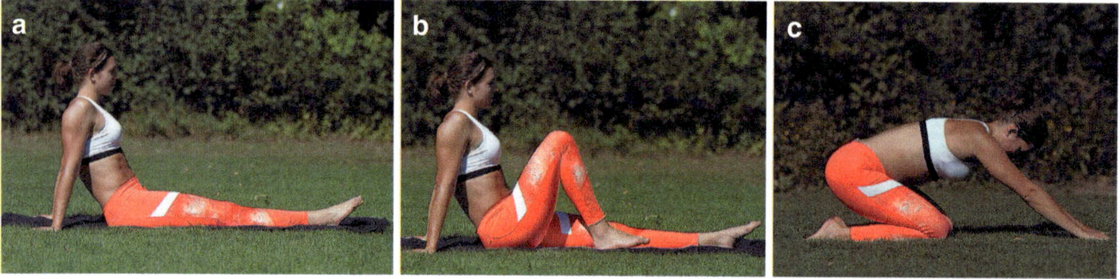

Fig. 11.4 Knee mobility. 1. Heal slides: extend the leg as far as possible and push the knee to the ground in order to regain full extension (**a**). Use a brace if range of motion (ROM) is limited. Bend the knee as far as possible without feeling pain (**b**). Please note that ROM limitation in the first week is 90° and in the second and third weeks it is 140°. 2. Regaining the final degrees of knee flexion in a kneeling position (**c**)

11.3.2.2 Weight Shifting

In order to start functional and strength training as soon as possible an increase in weight bearing should be trained every 2–3 h per day, starting from low weight bearing of 15–20 kg in the first 2 days to 50% of body weight between 3 and 7 days to full weight bearing in the second post-operative week. In general, the patient may load the leg until pain occurs. The exercise should be done 6–8 times per day, for 45–60 s, and three sets (Fig. 11.6).

11.3.2.3 Quadriceps Contraction

Many patients have problems with quadriceps contraction after the ACL injury and surgery with negative feed-back-mechanics [46, 47]. Voluntary

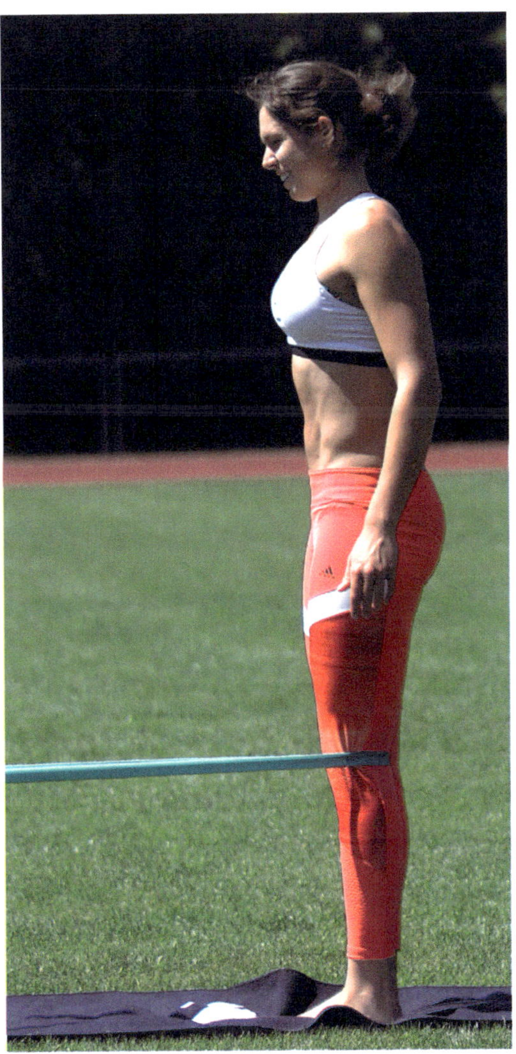

Fig. 11.5 Knee extension in standing against resistance band to enhance knee extension. Knee must be pushed into full extension

contraction of the quadriceps should be trained once per hour. Isometric contraction of the healthy side first may help, as well as the Jendrassik maneuver for reinforcement [37, 38] (Fig. 11.1a). In the case of limited extension (program B) isometric exercises as co-contraction simultaneously with the ischiocrural muscles are helpful, raising hips and supporting the heels with the knees bent (Figs. 11.1b and 11.6). Neuromuscular electrical stimulation is helpful against loss of quadriceps. Anode (+) and cathode (−) can be used side to side, stimulating the injured side by the healthy side in the later period (a). Quadriceps and Ischiocrural muscle stimulation can work in parallel [40] (Fig. 11.2).

11.3.3 Postoperative Days 3–7

11.3.3.1 Mini Squats

Mini squats should be introduced early. Squats are important as the basis for progressive exercises such as double-legged jumps, single-leg squats, and functional movements [48, 49]. As stated in the biomechanical (Sect. 1.2), squatting exercises causes a low level of stress to the ACL [7]. ROM is dependent on tissue limitation and pain.

It is suggested that speed should be low to reduce stress: starting with 3–5 s for eccentric contraction/1 s hold/1 s concentric contraction [44]. In particular, the eccentric phase should be addressed, as it leads to faster growth of quadriceps strength and better functional results [50, 51]. The following aspects should be considered:

1. Athletic position—feet are shoulder width apart and point forward. They may have a slight outward rotation. Pressure should be equally distributed between the legs and under the foot. The knees are positioned over the middle of the foot and under the hip joint. Knees should never collapse inward! Back should be parallel to the lower legs (Fig. 11.7).
2. Half squats should be reached after 3–4 weeks. Deep squats may be trained later on if there are no patellar or meniscal problems. Training a proper deep squat to enhance mobility and muscle control over full ROM is recommended but not obligatory [52, 53].
3. Reaching a 90° increase in load may start as much as tolerated [7].

Further exercises to strengthen the gluteus maximus muscle, abductor muscles, and external rotators of the hip should be carried out to improve the leg axis [54, 55]. In addition, squats training should include double-legged exercises such as good mornings, the bridge, the clam

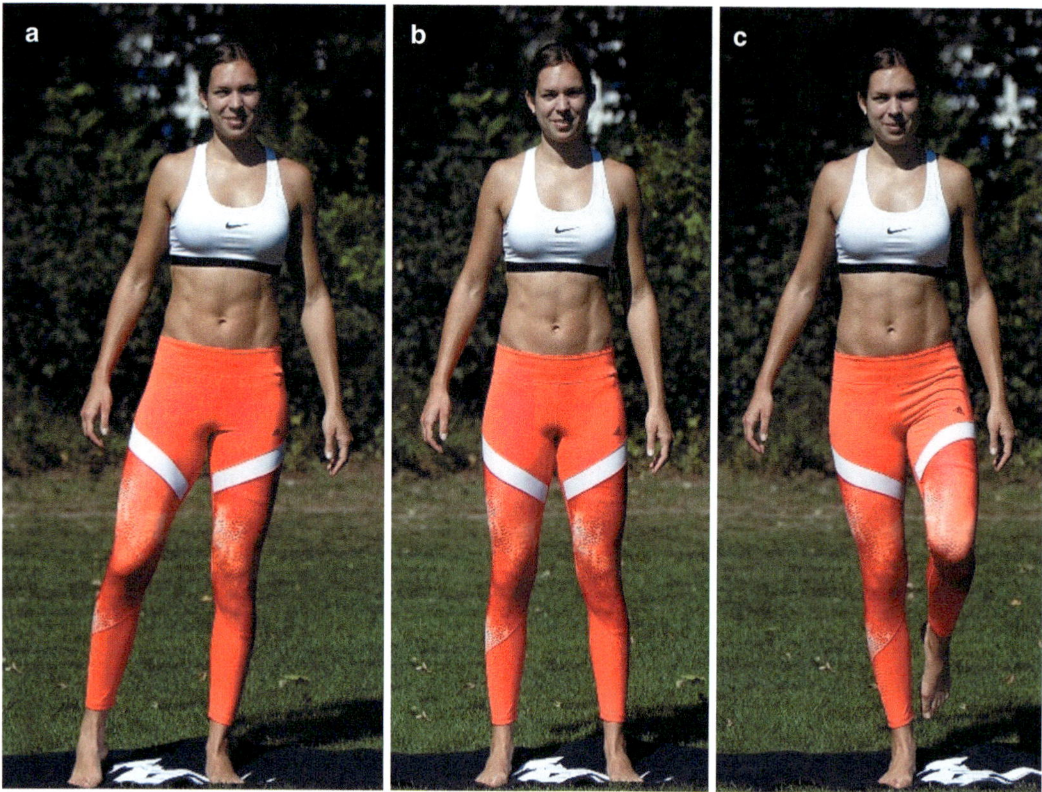

Fig. 11.6 Weight shifts. Start with most of the weight on the involved leg (**a**), reach the same weight distribution (**b**), and finally stand on the operated leg alone (**c**)

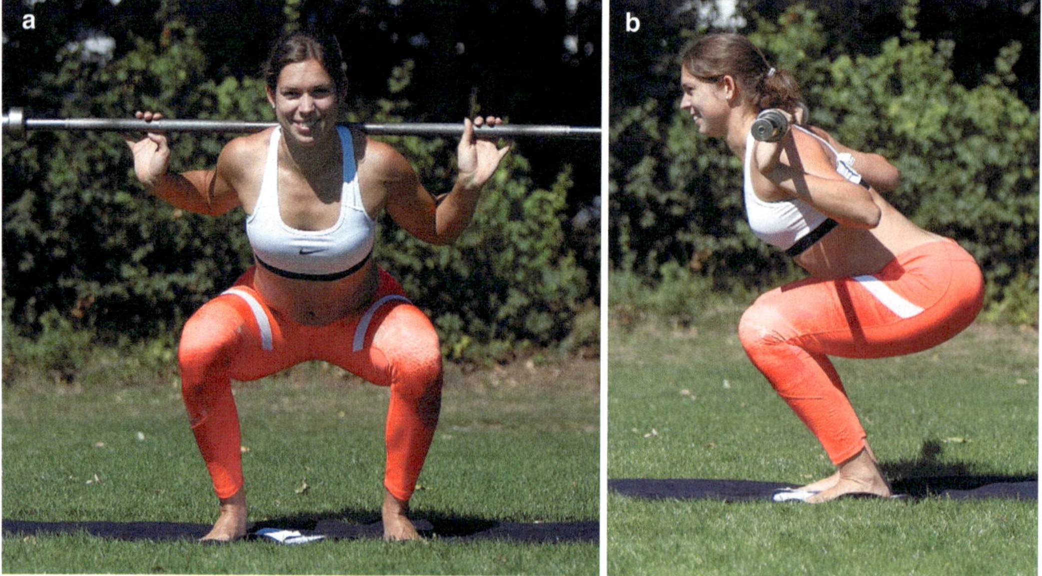

Fig. 11.7 Athletic position and squats. Foot, knee, and hip should be in one line under each other (**a**). In the squatting exercise hip-dominant variations should be preferred (**b**)

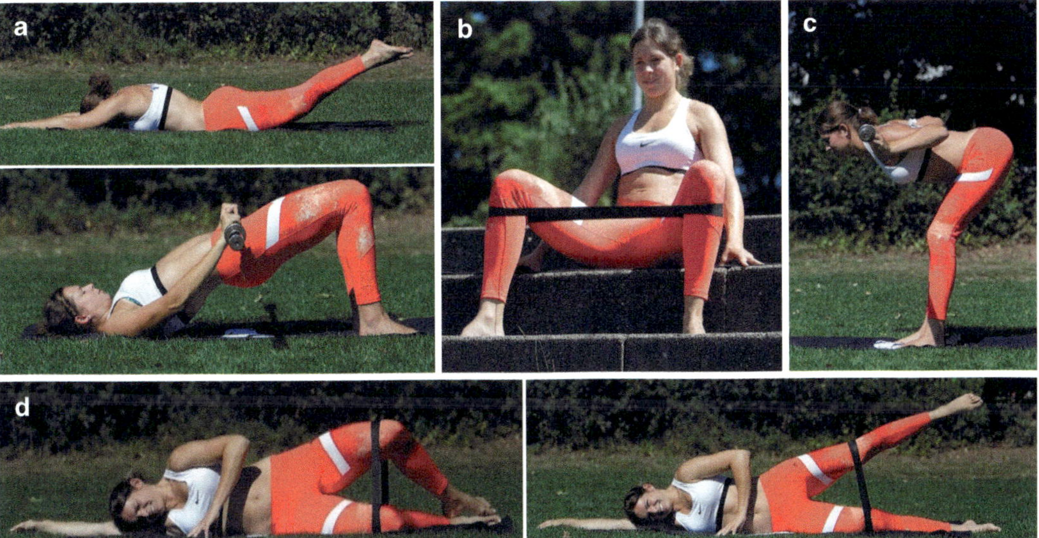

Fig. 11.8 Hip-dominant, nonweight-bearing and double-legged exercises in early anterior cruciate ligament rehabilitation: hip extension in lying and in bridging (**a**), hip abduction in sitting in 45° hip flexion and lying (**b**, **e**), and good morning (**c**)

shell, side-lying hip abduction, and calf raises [56]. Knee extension exercises should be avoided in the first 6 weeks as they place a high level of stress on the ACL [7] (Fig. 11.8).

11.3.4 Second Postoperative Week

Loading in everyday activities might be increased to full weight bearing. Therefore, the weight shifts should be done several times per day. The patient should be able to stand comfortably on his/her operated leg before taking the crutches away. Functional training may start with one-legged exercises such as step ups and downs, single leg dead lifts, and lunges. As all close-chain exercises involve high activation of the hamstrings the ACL is not under much of a load [57, 58]. TheraBands and mini bands may be included in training to enhance resistance or facilitate movement through guiding. The main focus of all exercises should be on the mechanical axis. The single-leg squat (SLS) is one of the most important exercises in rehabilitation and should be used carefully [59, 60].

11.3.4.1 Single-Legged Squats

Dynamic valgus is the most common reason for ACL injury [18]. SLQs are an important screening tool regarding return to sport and injury prevention. The SLQ correlates with biomechanical landing, cutting, and running patterns [60–62]. Nearly half of ACL patients show a poor performance on SLQs 6 months postoperatively [31]. Those functional deficits are also obvious in the hop test and correlate with problems in returning to sports [63–65].

Progression to SLQs include step ups and step downs, split squats, and Bulgarian split squats. SLQs are important to control the knee into the frontal axis (Fig. 11.9).

11.3.4.2 Core Training

Core stability plays an important role in injury prevention, because a weak core cannot withhold the forces produced by the limbs. As a result quality of limp coordination is inhibited and injury risk increases [66, 67].

Exercises for the lower abdominal muscles such as pelvic rises and the Russian twist to stabilize the lower core for enhancing gluteal activa-

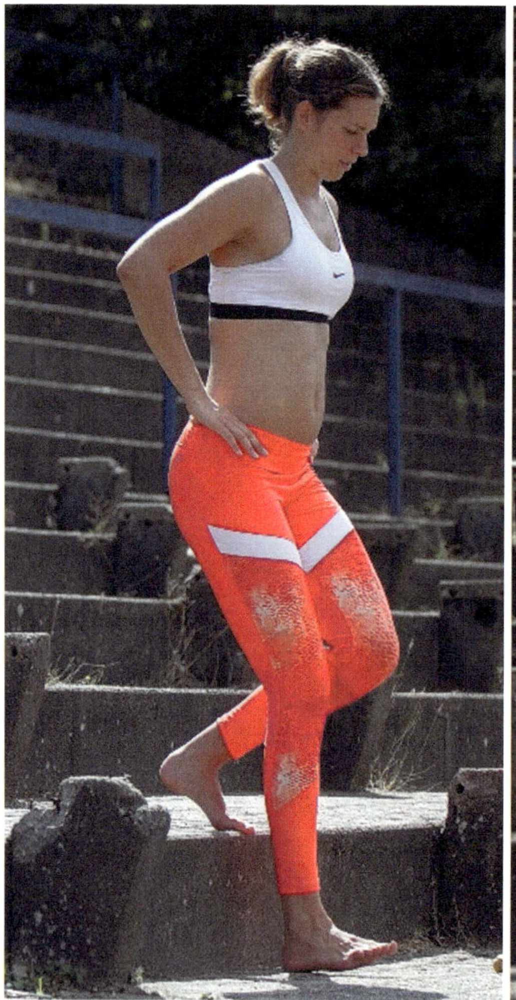
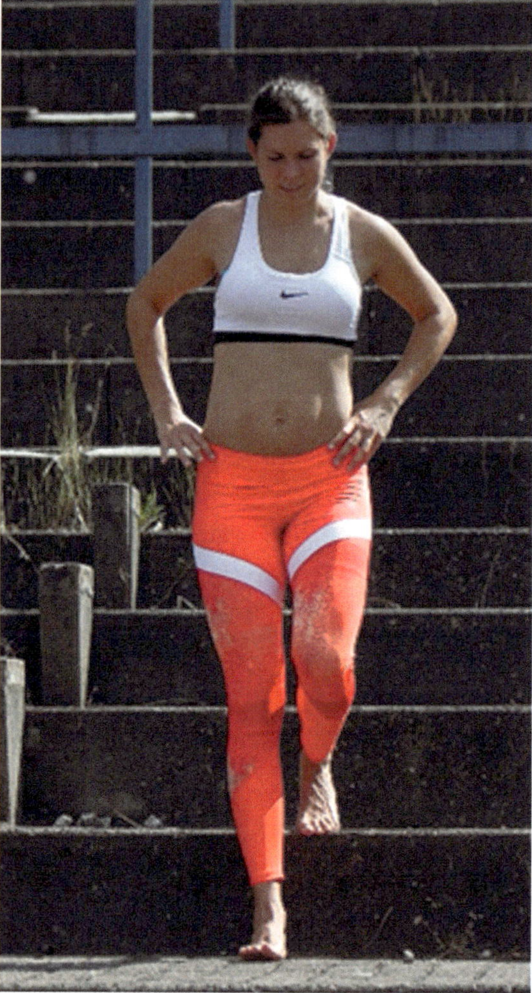

Fig. 11.9 Single-leg step down: foot, knee, and hip form a line. Upper body is vertical to the ground; no side-tilt is allowed. Hip is parallel to the floor. Knee may go forward to enhance eccentric quadriceps contraction (knee dominant); later on, hip dominant exercises should be included to train hip control

tion are recommended to decrease lower limb pathological conditions [68, 69]. Core stability is mainly assessed through tilting of the trunk, pelvic drop, and pelvic rotation in hopping and cutting maneuvers [66, 70, 71] (Fig. 11.10).

11.3.4.3 Stability Training

Several studies indicate that stability training on uneven surfaces contributes to ACL injury prevention and enhances performance [72, 73]. Stability training enhances neuromuscular control, which is defined by Griffin as "the unconscious activation of the dynamic restraints surrounding a joint in response to sensory stimuli" [74]. Sensorimotor training may help to improve proper muscle activation strategies in incidence and leads to favorable adaptations in movement strategies of landing tasks [75, 76]. Traumatic incidence and the operative reconstruction of the ACL reduces sensorimotor abilities of the joint and the surrounding muscles; neuromuscular training is important [77].

Stability training is included in one-legged exercises and can be aggravated by unstable platforms such as wobble boards, wobble cushions, BOSU balls, slack lines, bars, sofa cushions, old towels, yoga mats, etc. A mixture of different training tools is recommended to set different stimuli (Fig. 11.9).

11.3.4.4 Cycling

Cycling can be started about 2–3 weeks after the all press-fit reconstruction and 4 weeks after healing response. Variations occur because of other ROM limitations. Staring with slow velocity at 30 turns/min with middle then high resistance. Turns per minute should increase steadily from 30 to 40 to 50, etc. [78].

11.3.5 Three to Four Weeks: Dynamic Lunges

Dynamic exercises should be integrated into training to prepare for jumping and running drills. Owing to forefoot activity and low impact drills from the runner's ABC can prepare for fast drills such as sprinting, cutting, and jumping [79]. It enhances muscle physiology and coordination, reducing hamstring strains. TheraBands and mini bands can be integrated into training to increase difficulty.

At this point forefoot drills may involve (Fig. 11.9):

1. Standard ABC running drills
2. Step variations at the stairs or at a stepper (not jumps yet)
3. Coordination letter

Proprioceptive vibration training such as PowerPlate, Galileo, or similar devices, support reinforcement and muscle power [42]. "Aquasprint" is a dynamic training in 40- to 90-cm-deep water. Water resistance stabilizes the knee like a brace (Fig. 11.3). Pain is reduced and dynamic training with drainage of the periphery occurs. A positive influence on the vastus medialis of the quadriceps muscle is described [43] (Fig. 11.9). Freestyle crawl swimming in the belly position or backstroke are also useful as exercises in an open chain.

Static lunges may be started as soon as one-legged stands are possible. Dynamic lunges may be started 3–4 weeks after the operation. Further progressions are lunge walks (also with added weights). To train eccentric contraction of the hamstrings lunges are performed, pushing the foot to the floor. This variation is important for jumping exercises and prepares the hamstring for eccentric contraction while landing. Dynamic lateral lunges prepare for cutting maneuvers. Training intensity should be 2–3 times/week and 3–5 repetitions to develop maximal strength or 6–8 repetitions for increasing tissue quality per set. Sets are dependent on performance. As soon as three or six repetitions cannot be performed properly any longer the exercise should be stopped. Muscular endurance is exhausted (Figs. 11.10 and 11.11).

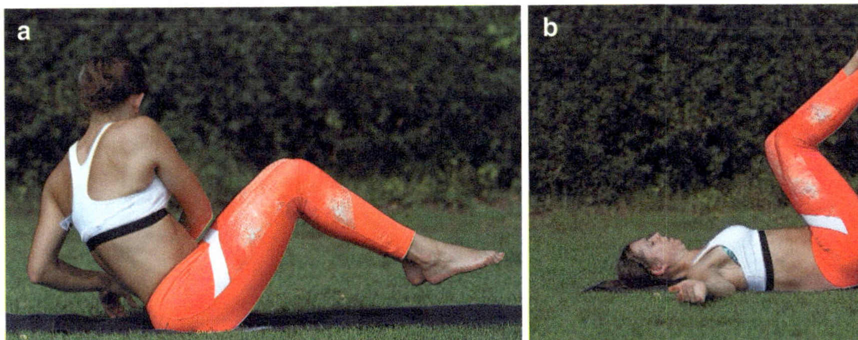

Fig. 11.10 Training of trunk muscles. Rotating from side to side to enhance muscle activation of the oblique abdominals (**a**). Lifting hip from the floor to train lower abdominals (**b**)

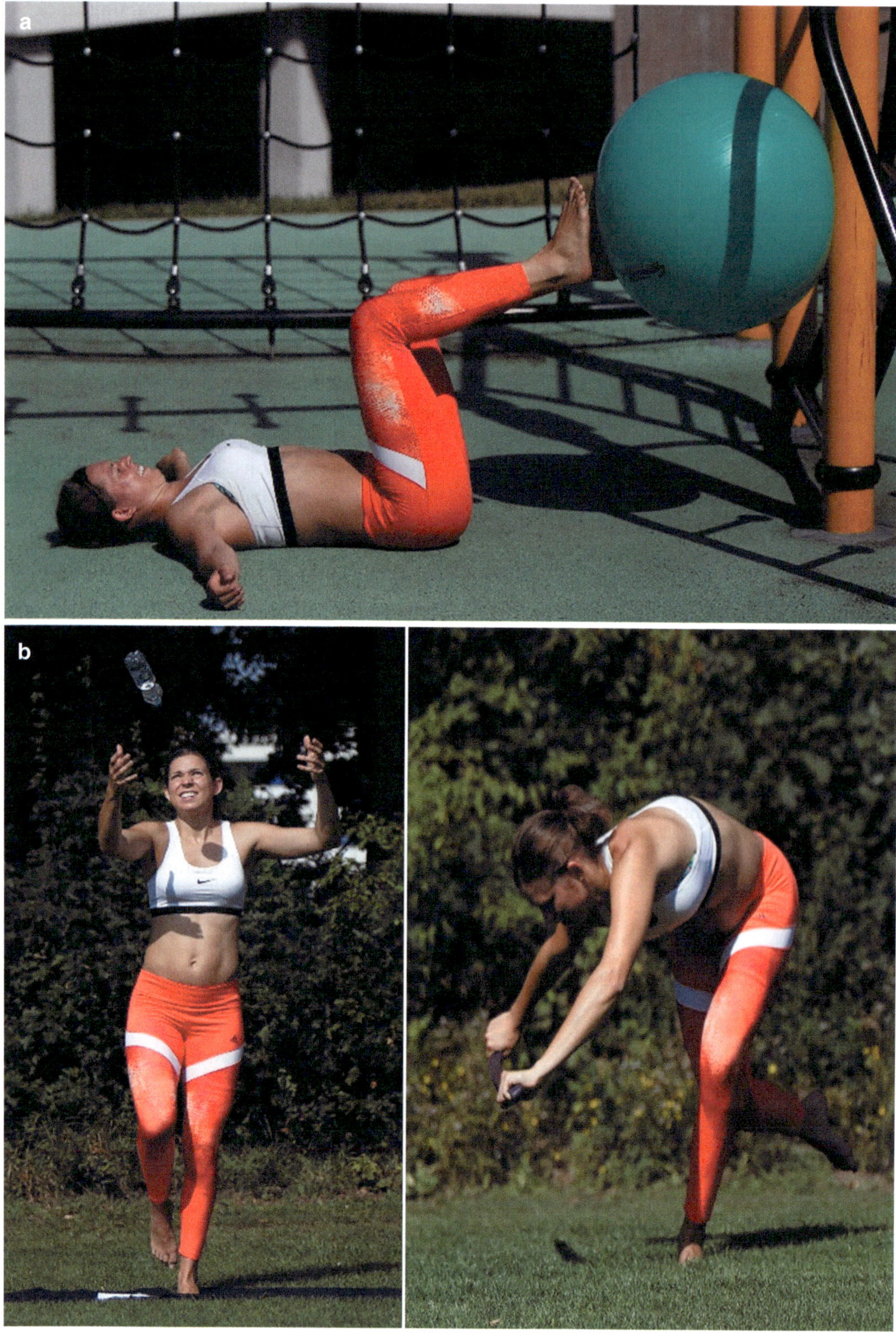

Fig. 11.11 Stability training lying with a Pezzi ball (**a**) and single-leg standing (**b**) as well as in single-leg standing with rotation

11.3.6 Five to Eight Weeks: Jump Trainings

Jump performance and quality is directly linked to risk of ACL injury [20]. There is also a lack of performance in comparison with the uninvolved side [64]. Functional scores from operated patients are even worse than those of patients with ACL-deficient knees [63, 64]. Furthermore, patients with abnormal scores tend to develop pain, swelling, and giving way, especially in recreational activities, as well as re-ruptures [65, 80].

Most return-to-play criteria involve different hop tests for those skills [32]. The main goal of jumping exercises should be to regain symmetrical power and re-educate jumping and landing kinematics, so that a valgus no longer occurs/PREVENT-X [63].

Double-legged jumps can be introduced much earlier than one-legged jumps. Squats with the focus on maximal speed (1 rep/s) prepare the muscles for faster movements and should be initiated 3 weeks before jump training. Weight decreases with increasing speed. After 2–3 weeks of double-legged jump training, one-legged jumps may be preferred [62].

Within 2–3 months twice per week landing kinematics can be altered [81]. Recovery time is recommended every 72 h after explosive work outs [82]. Athletes who start with jump training 2–3 months after the operation may need 2 months or more to get back to ~70% of their non-injured side.

Many athletes have trouble with jumping, because of a lack in the sensorimotor system [83]. The knee does not react as fast as desired and landing feels strange, especially in one-leg jumps. Table 11.3 provides a sequence of jump training and progress. The knee should prevent a dynamic valgus; the hip tilt and the upper body tilt are over the standing leg side (Table 11.3) (Figs. 11.11, 11.12, 11.13, and 11.14).

Table 11.3 Jump training

Exercise	Execution	Intensity
Double-legged jumps Entry criteria: Squat on maximal speed (1 rep/s)		
Squats with maximal speed	Pay attention to athletic position Small break between each rep to get air is allowed	6–8 repetitions 3–4 sets
Box jumps double	Starting from a squatting position the athlete jumps onto a box (30 cm high, for example)	
Drop jump double	Starting from a box the athlete jumps down and lands in a squatting position. This exercise serves to lose fear of landing and control the leg axis while decelerating	
Squat jumps	Starting from a squatting position the athlete jumps and lands in a squatting position	6–8 reps 3–4 sets
Single-legged jumps Often 2–3 weeks after start of double-legged jumps		
Box jump single	Starting from a single-leg stance the athlete jumps onto a stepper (10 cm in height is usually sufficient; most athletes have the biggest problems with this step)	3–4 reps 2–3 sets
Drop jump single	Starting from a height of 10 cm the athlete jumps and lands in light knee flexion and a stable leg axis. Progress to the height of the box jump in order to start vertical jumps	3–4 reps 2–3 sets
Single-leg vertical jump	Vertical jumps on one leg	3–4 reps 3 sets
Jumping forward/backward	Hops for a distance are added into the program. Within 2 months after the initial start of jump training, the athlete should reach 70% of the contralateral side. Within 3–4 months they should reach 90–100%	3–4 reps 3 sets
Jumping sideways	Goals are decreasing contact time and increasing jumps per minute	
Jumps with rotation	Starting with rotation of 90° and increasing to 180°	

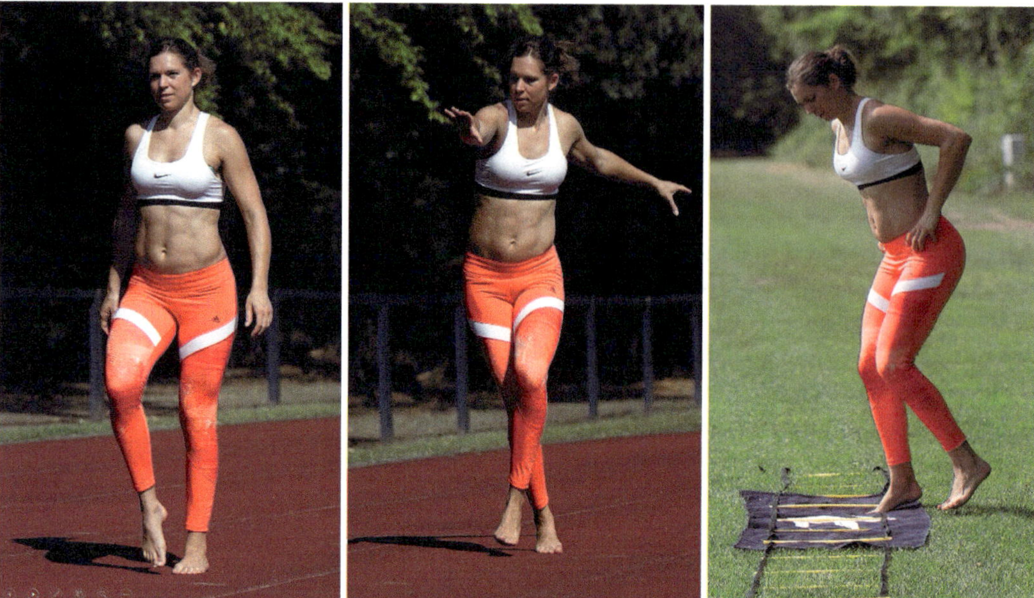

Fig. 11.12 Agility drills on the forefoot

11.3.7 Six to Eight Weeks: Running Technique

Before starting endurance and sprint training, running technique should be addressed by running drills. Furthermore, the athlete should be able to perform a hop for distance with 70% of the uninvolved leg and he/she should have the full extension back [84]. Running speed and distance should comply with subjective estimation. Running should not cause pain for a maximum length of 100 m.

11.3.8 Three Months: Sprint-Training

Skipping and short distance sprints may be tested slowly after 3–4 weeks. Sprint training can be started roughly 2–3 months postoperatively. The pre-stretch test and wall drills can be used to determine the eccentric power and speed performance. If eccentric power is too weak (<+15%) in comparison with concentric power, the athlete is at a higher risk of muscle pulling [85]. Furthermore, he/she should feel comfortable running on the forefoot.

Three to five short sprints in the beginning should be increased individually.

11.3.9 Four Months: Cutting Movements

Many ACL injuries occur by falling into a sudden dynamic valgus with cutting [18]. In the beginning many athletes tend to push out the leg in order to unload it in cutting.

SLQ: studies show a moderate to strong correlation between the biomechanics of the SLQ and cutting [60].

Dynamic lateral lunges: the dynamic lateral lunge is the basic movement for cutting. If the athlete hesitates to load the leg in this exercise or falls into a valgus position, he/she is not ready for cutting maneuvers.

Side hops: side hops should be performed without any hesitation and the patient should feel safe on his/her leg. He/she should have an LSI of >70% (Table 11.4) (Fig. 11.14). Shuffles are integrated (Fig. 11.15).

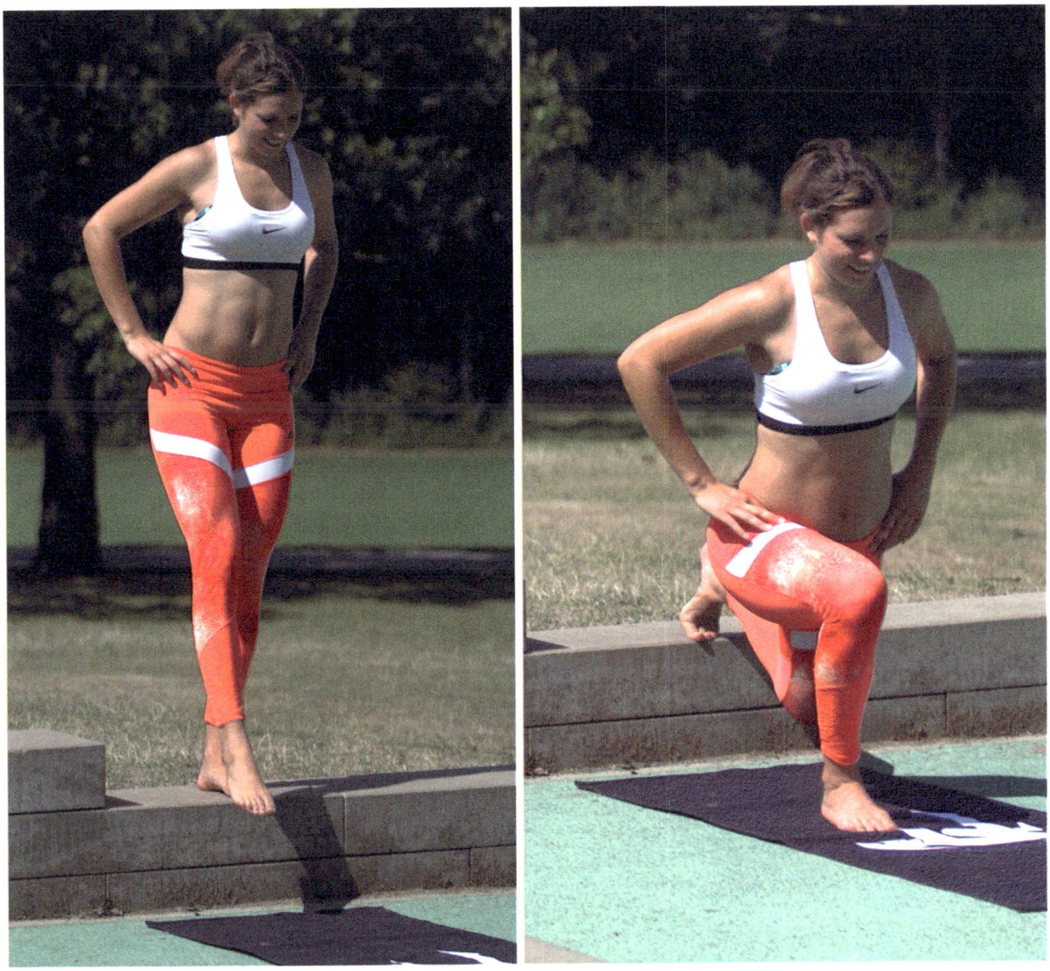

Fig. 11.13 Dynamic lunges. Dynamic progression of lunges in order to train eccentric strength and withstand higher impulses on the knee

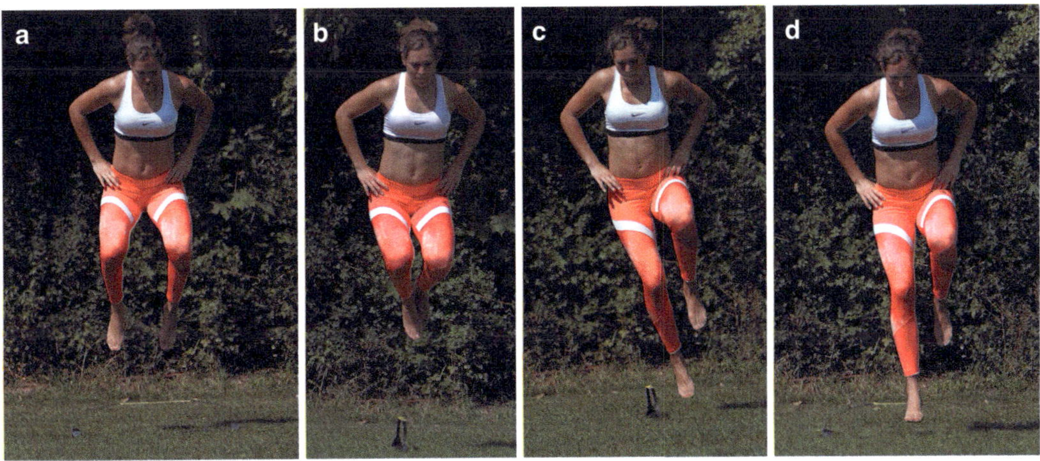

Fig. 11.14 Jumps. Double-legged jump from athletic position (**a**, **b**), jump over hurdle (**c**), and single-leg jump (**d**)

Table 11.4 Shuffle training

Shuffles	
Side step and stop Double/ triple steps	Starting from a base position the athlete moves one/two/three step(s) to the side and lands in the base position again
Cut from base position	Starting from a base position the athlete performs one cut
Side step with cut	Starting from a base position the athlete does one or two side steps and cuts
Run and shuffle	Run 3–5 m in one direction and land in the base position
Run and cut	Run 3–5 m in one direction and cut

11.3.10 Five Months: Jogging

Starting with jogging.

These tests help to determine the athlete's readiness:

- *One-legged jump* with approximately 70% quality of his/her contralateral side [60, 84].
- *Drop hop test* from a 15-inch-high box and land stable on one leg in the proper leg axis (Fig. 11.16a).
- *Double-legged spreads* train to prevent X-legged landing and activate the gluteal dynamic function (Fig. 11.16b).

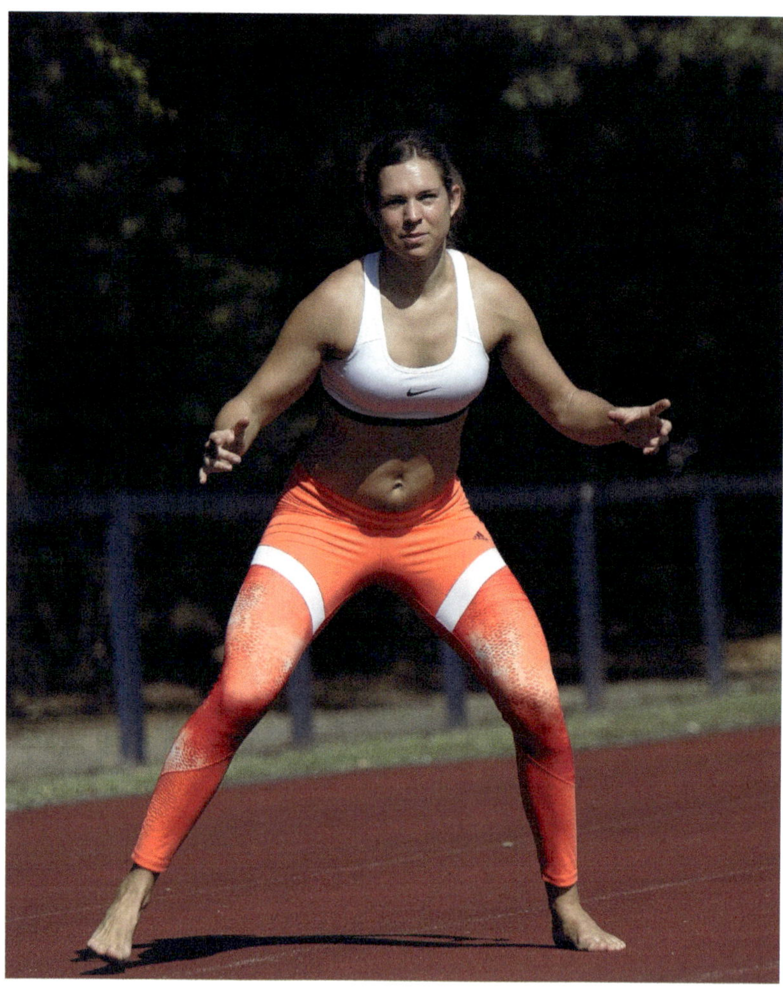

Fig. 11.15 Shuffles

- Ischiocrural test should be type B (Chap. 3).
- Vastus medialis test should be type B (Chap. 3).

Backfoot running is stressful for the ACL whereas the external knee flexion moments push the tibia forward. Forefoot running is recommended to reduce ACL stress in the long distance and secure performance [86].

Training intensity differs:

1. 100-m runs at a low speed of 1 km in 6 min. Speed is chosen by running performance and lactate production. The leg axis should be stable; a harmonic running pattern and no limping should be visible. The athlete should not get out of breath and should be able to breathe pleasantly. Breaks should take about 30–60 s in between. 5–6 reps are mostly sufficient in the beginning. Training volume can be increased daily if the knee does not cause problems and muscles are not overtraining.
2. Jogging can be integrated.
3. In the middle phase short interval training sessions of 1–3 min to enhance basic endurance is more effective than longer runs. Training volume should be around 2–3 sets, which can be increased at each training session [44, 87, 88].

11.3.11 Five to Six Months: Sport-Specific Drills

Sport-specific skills are assembled gradually by exposing the athlete to the specific demands of his/her sport. Training should evolve from close skill exercise to open skill exercises [89]. In the first phase this can imply dribbling a ball, skating, or handling a racket at low intensities. The second phase increases and anticipated changes of directions are included. In the third phase anaerobic endurance and unanticipated changes of directions are trained. In the last phase the athlete is exposed to opponent contact [90]. In all phases correct landing and cutting movements should be focused upon. Complex movements such as overhead throwing, unanticipated change of direction, fatigue, and contact with an opponent lead to more risky injury patterns [91–97].

In this phase sport-specific drills are essential to stabilize neuromuscular competence and psychological readiness. Loss of mechanoreceptors of the ligament cause changes in the primary sensory cortex and gamma-motor neuron feedback loops of long latency reflexes. The need for increased input to the motor cortex may lead to

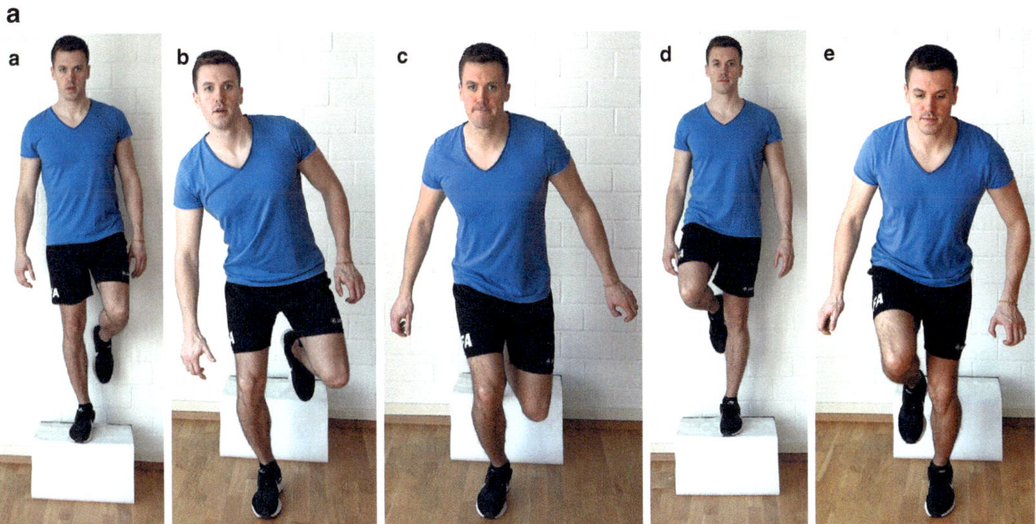

Fig. 11.16 (**A**) One-leg drop-hop test from a step (a, d) with unstable landing in varus (b), in valgus (c), and straight stable landing (e). The aim is to prevent valgus (c) and land in a stable varus (b) or stable straight position (e). (**B**) Jump up (a) and spread out (b) and land in bow legs on both sides (c); later, land single leg as prevention cross training. Helpful after a failed single-leg jump test

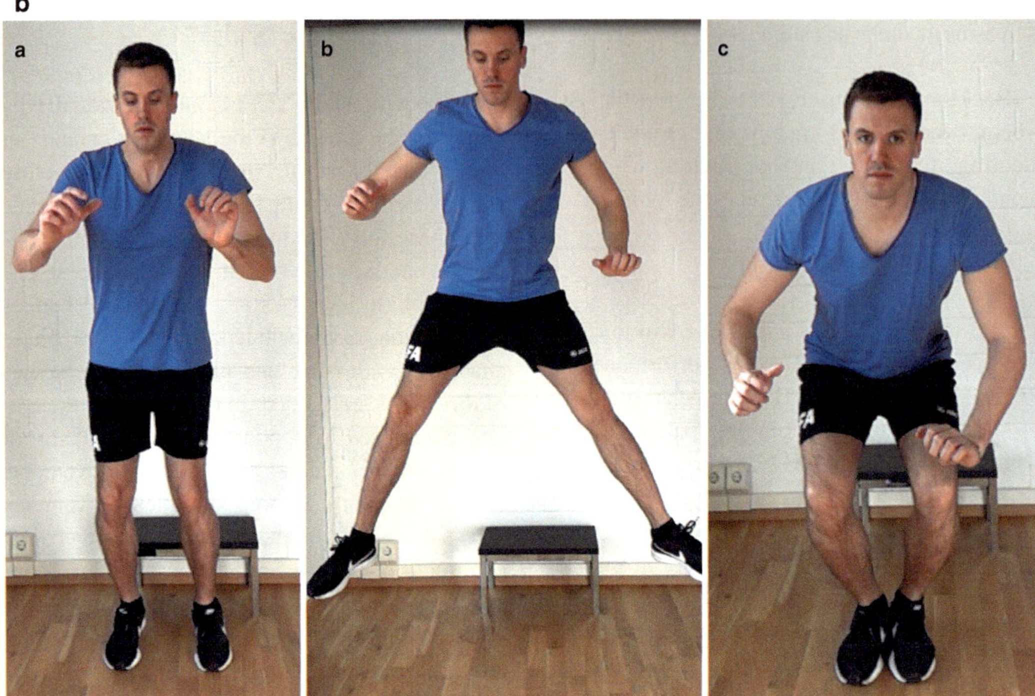

Fig. 11.16 (continued)

sensory-motor nervous system compensations such as additional visual feedback and spatial awareness in motor planning. Highly competitive skill need intensive individual sport-specific training to regain the original competence [98].

11.3.12 Return to Play

Determining the point of return to sports is a difficult issue and widely discussed in the literature. In recent years the interest in return to sport has grown owing to high re-rupture rates. The shift from graft-related time-based criteria to functional testing has resulted in a wide range of testing procedures [99].

Current tests can be divided up into three categories:

1. Basic tests for strength, proprioception and movement quality
2. Basic tests for dynamic drills, reaction, speed and movement quality
3. Sport-specific tests

Decision making should be based on tests from all three categories. Tests start from basic to complex movements adapted to sport-specific needs. Squatting and lunging are common movements in almost any sport, e.g., double-legged landing at a net or cutting maneuvers, also possible under laboratory control to be compared with reference values [91, 100, 101] (Table 11.5).

Dynamic tests differ in performance and sport. Basketball players jump in general much higher than soccer players. Soccer players may run the agility tests much faster than a volleyball player to escape their opponent (Fig. 11.17). Different sports have different limitations for determining the point of return for an individual. Tests help to decrease reinjury rates up to 84% and are an important screening tool. Even though they are not able to prevent every ACL injury, they prevent most of them [102–104]. Therefore, many researchers suggest comparing performance with the contralateral side, such as the limb-symmetry index (LSI) [103]. The non-injured side often loses performance because of the injury too. Hence, comparing the injured side with the

Table 11.5 Examples of mobility drills

Exercise	Intensity		
Mobility drills			
Foot circle	10 reps		
90/90	10 reps	Heel sit	10 reps
Pretzel	10 reps	Scorpion	10 reps
Movement preparation			
Warm up stretching exercises	4 reps	Hand walks	4 reps
Backward lunge with lateral rotation	4 reps	Partner plank	30 s
Drop lunge	6 each leg	Single leg stance	30 s
Lateral walk with mini band hip AR	10 reps	Mini band lateral walk	10 to each side
Rabbit runs	2 × 5 s		
Plyometric			
In line-hurdle double-legged jumps (18 cm in height)	5 each leg	12 in line single-legged hops (12 cm in height)	5 each leg
12 lateral hops (12 cm in height)	5 each leg	Hops with 45° rotation	5 each leg
Movement skills			
Wall drills	5 sets	Linear skip in place	8 s
Fall to sprint	2 sets at 10 reps	Ankle skips	5 m
Straight leg shuffles	5 m	Straight leg skips	5 m
Power block			
Nordic hamstring curl	5 reps	Partner squats	8 reps
Single-legged dead lifts	8 reps each	Push-ups	8 reps

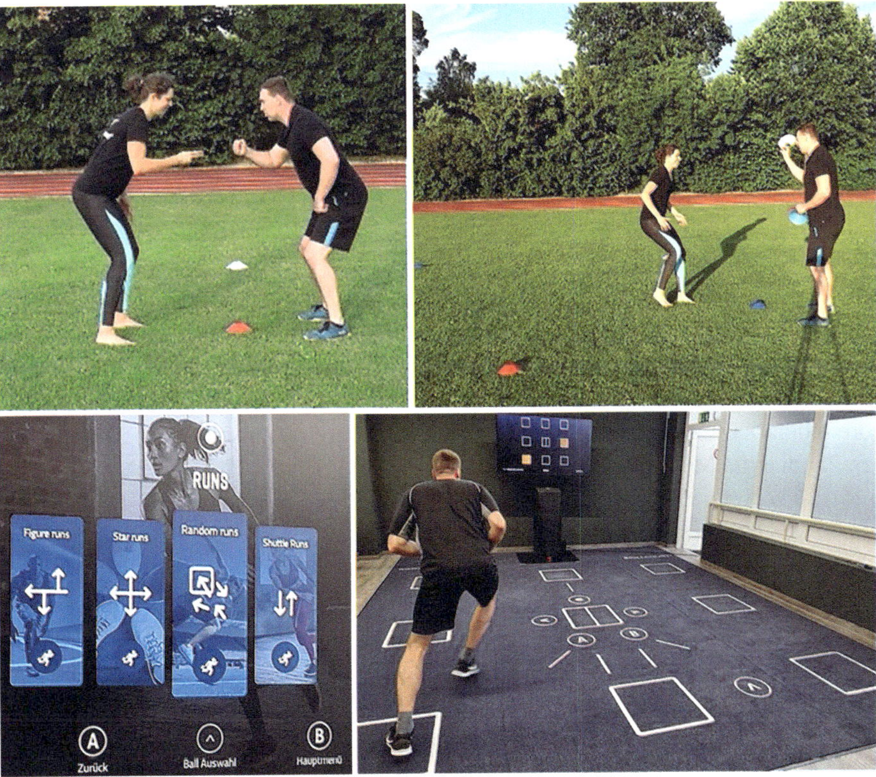

Fig. 11.17 Agility, reaction, and individual skills training and tests include different sports. Here with few technical equipment and a skill court with computer program and evaluation

non-injured side before an injury increases the prediction of second ACL injuries [105].

Common tests involve Drop Jumps, Side Hops, Hops for Distance, running or hopping a certain figure like a cross or an figure of eight (Table 11.5). A sum of seven established tests is the Knee Santy Athletic Return to Sport (K-STARTS) test for functional improvement for return to sports after ACL reconstruction [106].

Biomechanical parameters such as strength, coordination, functional movement and basic neuromuscular control should be combined [107]. Decision making, reactions under time pressure, performance under fatigue, and movement screening with opponent contact show evidence for a high impact on the central nervous system, thus inducing an injury [83]. This can be imitated by simple games such as rock-paper-scissors: the athlete needs to react to visual cues like a cone with a certain color and runs to a cone with the same color lying on the floor. The speed court is a conventional biomechanical tool to test reaction times and ground reaction forces in cutting. (Fig. 11.17). Other tests and courses are established with technical equipment with optical and acoustic sensors to push or touch and change the direction of movement.

Determining a confidence interval of a favorable or less favorable movement, has a coverage of 95% and only 5% of being wrong. Even though an athlete exhibits predisposing factors that may place them at a high risk for ACL injury, there is no guarantee of an ACL tear or not [108]. There are only a few studies examining reference values for different exercises. Even though there is a strong correlation between most screening tools (camera in 2D, Inertial Measurement Unit in 3D, or Vicon 3D), they produce different values of the same motion, which makes it even harder to compare the results [109–111].

Although there are no clear references for examining sport-specific movements, those testing show up technically reproducible biomechanical parameters in movement [95]. Similarly, volleyball-specific tasks such as a spike jump and block jump were carried out with highly technological devices (Fig. 11.18). Motion capturing (knee flexion angle, trunk lean, hip rotation, etc.) with external sensors helps to detect current deficits [112–115]. Developments such as functional near-infrared spectroscopy, transcranial magnetic stimulation (TMS), and electro-encephalography (EEG) may provide a deeper insight into neurological changes and adaptions under injuries [116]. A few studies have investigated somatosensory and motor cortex neuroplasticity using EEG and TMS in athletes with ACL injuries [117]. Experiments with TMS conclude that the excitability of descending cortical pathways is reduced, especially in cortical areas. Larger stimuli are needed to excite descending cortical neurons, leading to reduced performance in motor control. These findings indicate that in the long term cortical measurements could be useful to determine readiness to return to sport [118, 119].

Psychological readiness and tests are to be integrated [120–122]. Research indicates that fear can increase the ACL-injury rate by over 13 times [103, 123]. Higher motivation during rehabilitation was associated with returning to the pre-injury sport activity [122]. The social area of tension such as family, friends, colleagues, sponsors, training and work, setting goals, and dealing with the club and/or coach and/or team. Social entrapment between coach, athlete, motivation, and mentality must be considered in its complexity [124] (Fig. 11.19). The cascade of the algorithm shows the complexity of steps to return to sports and competition (Fig. 11.20).

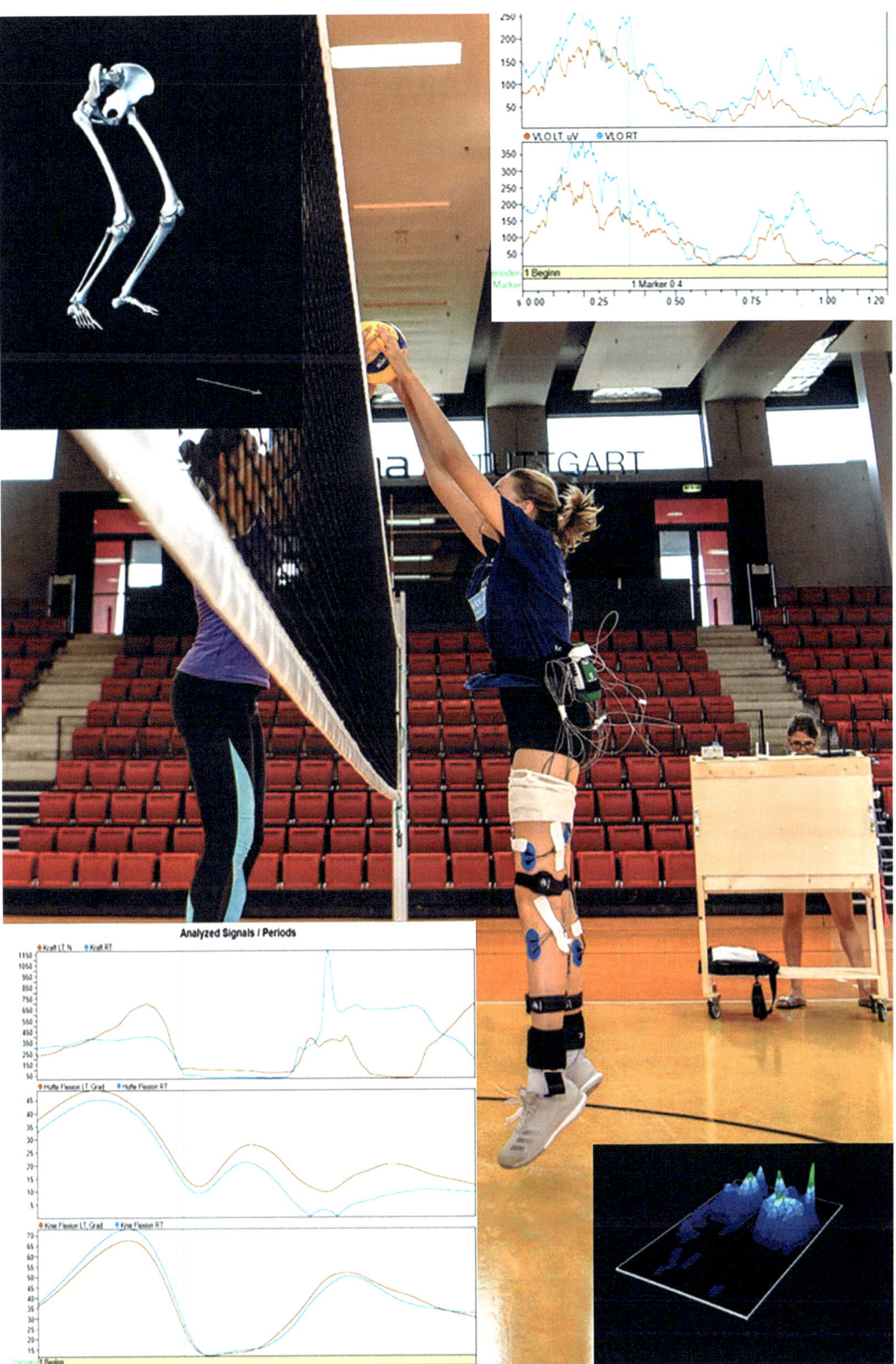

Fig. 11.18 Volleyball-specific tasks such as a spike jump and block jump were carried out with highly technological equipment and recording

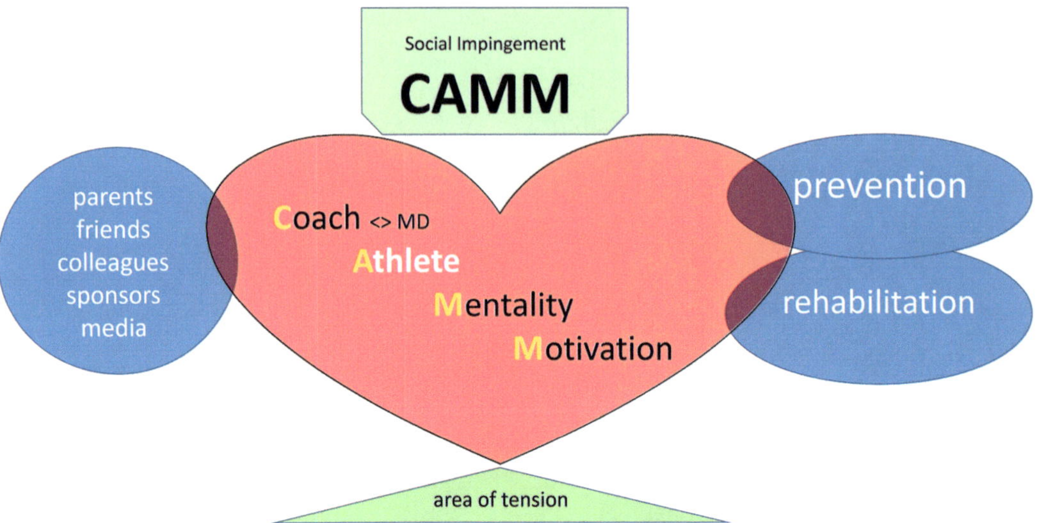

Fig. 11.19 A social area of tension such as family, friends, colleagues, sponsors, media, training and work, setting goals, and dealing with the club and/or coach and/or team and/or medical doctor. Social entrapment between coach, athlete, motivation, and mentality must be considered in its complexity (CAMM) [133]

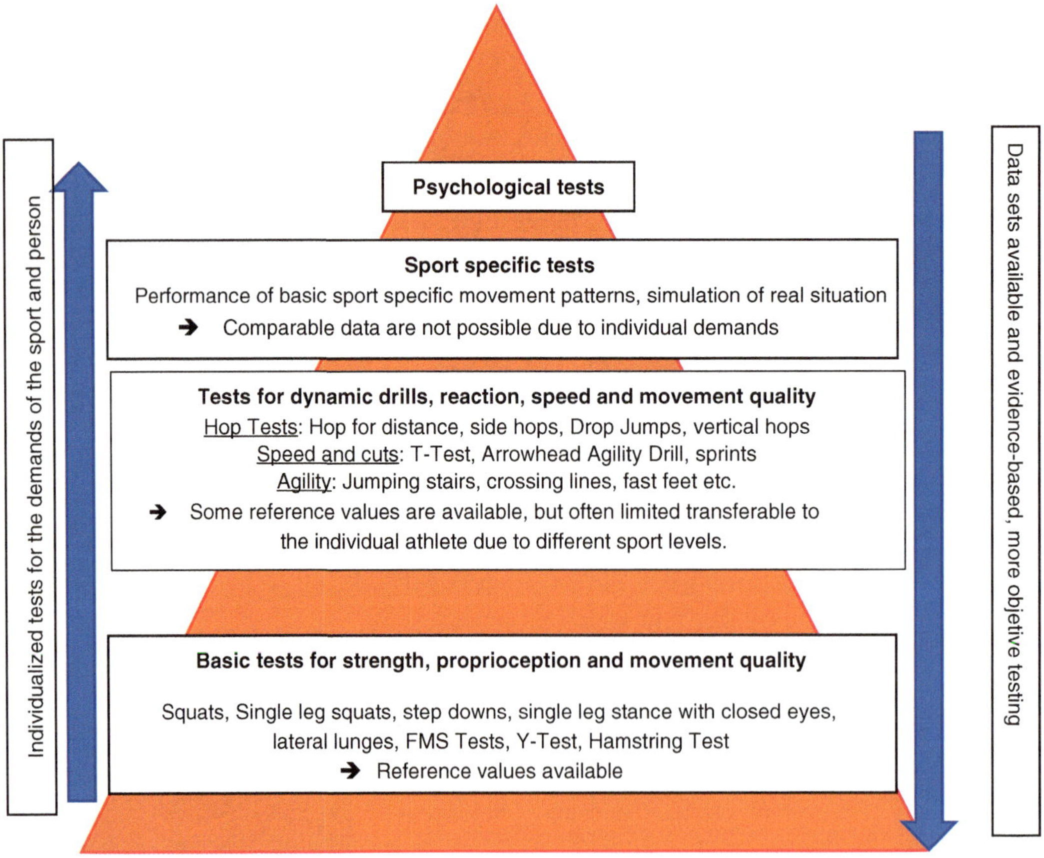

Individualized tests for the demands of the sport and person

Psychological tests

Sport specific tests

Performance of basic sport specific movement patterns, simulation of real situation

➔ Comparable data are not possible due to individual demands

Tests for dynamic drills, reaction, speed and movement quality

Hop Tests: Hop for distance, side hops, Drop Jumps, vertical hops

Speed and cuts: T-Test, Arrowhead Agility Drill, sprints

Agility: Jumping stairs, crossing lines, fast feet etc.

➔ Some reference values are available, but often limited transferable to the individual athlete due to different sport levels.

Basic tests for strength, proprioception and movement quality

Squats, Single leg squats, step downs, single leg stance with closed eyes, lateral lunges, FMS Tests, Y-Test, Hamstring Test

➔ Reference values available

Data sets available and evidence-based, more objetive testing

Fig. 11.20 Algorithm for tests and readiness for making the decision to return to sport

11.4 Prevention

11.4.1 Effects of Prevention Programs

There is evidence that prevention programs have a positive effect on decreasing injury rates. This effect was induced by the FIFA 11+ prevention program, which has a substantial injury-preventing effect by reducing football injuries by 39% [125]. An injury reduction of 87% through training on unstable surfaces for 20 min per day could be shown [126]. In a Norwegian intervention group, in which jump and proprioceptive training were combined, injury rates decreased by 50% and athletic performance increased [127]. Programs are advocated for improving balance, lower extremity biomechanics, muscle activation, functional performance, strength, and power, as well as decreasing landing impact forces. A multicomponent injury-prevention training program should, as a minimum, provide feedback on movement technique: strength, plyometrics, agility, balance, and flexibility [128].

11.4.2 Example: Basic Structure of a Prevention Warm-Up Program

Warm-up programs differ. Here is an example following strength, plyometrics, agility, balance, and flexibility [128]. In addition to running exercises, which activate neuromuscular pathways, prepare the muscles for high endurance or explosive workouts, stimulate the important muscle groups, and optimize movement strategies. The warm-up program can be split into different categories:

1. *Mobility drills:* mobility drills enhance movement quality and are aimed at improving ROM by moving from the neutral zone into the end zone.
2. *Movement preparation:* these drills are a combination of stretching and muscle activation. They involve fast and slow dynamic movements combined with rotations or flexion to maximal ROM. Mini bands and TheraBands are useful to increase resistance and enhance activation.
3. *Plyometric block:* these drills are aimed at increasing power, explosive force and speed by improving the stretch-shortening cycle. In warm-up programs the focus is on movement quality. Different jumping drills should be included to cover a broad range of movements.
4. *Movement skills:* these exercises enhance quality of movement by dissolving coarser movement patterns into fine specific differentiated ones.
5. *Power block:* the last block serves to enhance the strength and power of certain muscle groups: thigh (quadriceps and ischiocrural) muscles, hip abductor, extensors, and outward rotators, as well as exercises for trunk stability, are important with regard to ACL injury prevention.

Rehabilitation starts with prevention and a clever training program. Coaches are role models and idols, as are the top athletes that young people emulate. "*Prevention first*": a sympathetic program, which, like other books, can make this book superfluous.

Many activity programs of knee injury prevention have been established on the internet, such as those against obesity. They should be started early in young athletes [129–132] at school and be repeated every day in the media, such as on radio and television. For children, specialization in top-class sports should take place as late as possible. Children should play and find their own individual way out of a wide range of physical activities. "*Only what you do can make you successful*"!

Acknowledgment Acknowledgment goes to Christina Frese, Scientific Assistant and PhD student at the University of Stuttgart, Germany, who supported with exercises, pictures and discussion.

References

1. Jagodzinski M, Friederich NF, Müller W. Das Knie [the knee]. 2nd ed. Berlin, Heidelberg: Springer; 2016.
2. Klein P, Sommerfeld P. Biomechanics of the human joints. Special Edition: Joints and Spine. 2012.
3. DeMorat G, et al. Aggressive quadriceps loading can induce noncontact anterior cruciate ligament injury. Am J Sports Med. 2004;32:477–83.
4. Nicholettos A, Barcellona MG, Morrissey MC. The immediate effects of open kinetic chain knee extensor exercise at different loads on knee anterior laxity in the uninjured. Knee. 2013;20(6):500–4.
5. Perriman A, Leahy E, Semciw AI. The effect of open- versus closed-kinetic-chain exercises on anterior tibial laxity, strength, and function following anterior cruciate ligament reconstruction: a systematic review and meta-analysis. J Orthop Sports Phys Ther. 2018;48(7):552–66.
6. Ucar M, et al. Evaluation of open and closed kinetic chain exercises in rehabilitation following anterior cruciate ligament reconstruction. J Phys Ther Sci. 2014;26(12):1875–8.
7. Escamilla RF, et al. Anterior cruciate ligament strain and tensile forces for weight-bearing and non-weight-bearing exercises: a guide to exercise selection. J Orthop Sports Phys Ther. 2012;42(3):208–20.
8. Li G, et al. The importance of quadriceps and hamstring muscle loading on knee kinematics and in-situ forces in the ACL. J Biomech. 1999;32(4):395–400.
9. Beynnon BD, et al. Anterior cruciate ligament strain behavior during rehabilitation exercises in vivo. Am J Sports Med. 1995;23:24–34.
10. Toutoungi DE, et al. Cruciate ligament forces in the human knee during rehabilitation exercises. Clin Biomech. 2000;15:176–87.
11. Markolf KL, et al. Combined knee loading states that generate high anterior cruciate ligament forces. J Orthop Res. 1995;13:930–5.
12. Hame SL, Oakes DA, Markolf KL. Injury to the anterior cruciate ligament during alpine skiing: a biomechanical analysis of tibial torque and knee flexion angle. Am J Sports Med. 2002;30:537–40.
13. Meyer EG, Haut RC. Anterior cruciate ligament injury induced by internal tibial torsion or tibiofemoral compression. J Biomech. 2008;41:3377–83.
14. Ballal MS, et al. Rotational and peak torque stiffness of rugby shoes. Foot (Edinb). 2014;24(3):107–10.
15. Bittencourt NFN, et al. Foot and hip contributions to high frontal plane knee projection angle in athletes: a classification and regression tree approach. J Orthop Sports Phys Ther. 2012;42:996–1004.
16. Beckett ME, et al. Incidence of hyperpronation in the ACL injured knee: a clinical perspective. J Athl Train. 1992;27:58–62.
17. Loudon JK, Jenkins W, Loudon KL. The relationship between static posture and ACL injury in female athletes. J Orthop Sports Phys Ther. 1996;24:91–7.
18. Alentorn-Geli E, et al. Prevention of non-contact anterior cruciate ligament injuries in soccer players. Part 1: mechanisms of injury and underlying risk factors. Knee Surg Sports Traumatol Arthrosc. 2009;17(7):705–29.
19. Cochrane JL, et al. Characteristics of anterior cruciate ligament injuries in Australian football. J Sci Med Sport. 2007;10:96–104.
20. Hewett TE, et al. Biomechanical measures of neuromuscular control and valgus loading of the knee predict anterior cruciate ligament injury risk in female athletes: a prospective study. Am J Sports Med. 2005;33:492–501.
21. Myer GD, Ford KR, Hewett TE. High knee abduction moments are common risk factors for patellofemoral pain (PFP) and anterior cruciate ligament (ACL) injury in girls: is PFP itself a predictor for subsequent ACL injury? Br J Sports Med. 2015;49:118–22.
22. Shin CS, Chaudhari AM, Andriacchi TP. The effect of isolated valgus moments on ACL strain during single-leg landing: a simulation study. J Biomech. 2009;42:280–5.
23. Charvet B, Ruggiero F, Le Guellec D. The development of the myotendinous junction. A review. Muscles Ligaments Tendons J. 2012;2(2):53–63.
24. Novak ML, Koh TJ. Macrophage phenotypes during tissue repair. J Leukoc Biol. 2013;93(6):875–81.
25. Docheva D, et al. Biologics for tendon repair. Adv Drug Deliv Rev. 2015;84:222–39.
26. Biau DJ, et al. ACL reconstruction: a meta-analysis of functional scores. Clin Orthop Relat Res. 2007;458:180–7.
27. Anderson MJ, et al. A systematic summary of systematic reviews on the topic of the anterior cruciate ligament. Orthop J Sports Med. 2016;4(3):2325967116634074.
28. Ardern CL, et al. Return to sport following anterior cruciate ligament reconstruction surgery: a systematic review and meta-analysis of the state of play. Br J Sports Med. 2011;45:596–606.
29. Gerber JP, et al. Safety, feasibility, and efficacy of negative work exercise via eccentric muscle activity following anterior cruciate ligament reconstruction. J Orthop Sports Phys Ther. 2007;37:10–8.
30. Petersen W, et al. Return to play following ACL reconstruction: a systematic review about strength deficits. Arch Orthop Trauma Surg. 2014;134:1417–28.
31. Hall MP, et al. Neuromuscular evaluation with single-leg squat test at 6 months after anterior cruciate ligament reconstruction. Orthop J Sports Med. 2015;3:2325967115575900.
32. Abrams GD, et al. Functional performance testing after anterior cruciate ligament reconstruction: a systematic review. Orthop J Sports Med. 2014;2:2325967113518305.
33. Kjaer M, et al. From mechanical loading to collagen synthesis, structural changes and function in human tendon. Scand J Med Sci Sports. 2009;19(4):500–10.

34. Cook JL, et al. Revisiting the continuum model of tendon pathology: what is its merit in clinical practice and research? Br J Sports Med. 2016;50(19):1187–91.
35. Rio E, et al. Tendon neuroplastic training: changing the way we think about tendon rehabilitation: a narrative review. Br J Sports Med. 2016;50(4):209–15.
36. Thomopoulos S, et al. Mechanisms of tendon injury and repair. J Orthop Res. 2015;33(6):832–9.
37. Ertuglu LA, et al. Jendrassik maneuver effect on spinal and brainstem reflexes. Exp Brain Res. 2019;237(12):3265–71.
38. Gregory JE, Wood SA, Proske U. An investigation into mechanisms of reflex reinforcement by the Jendrassik manoeuvre. Exp Brain Res. 2001;138(3):366–74.
39. Simonsen EB. Contributions to the understanding of gait control. Dan Med J. 2014;61(4):B4823.
40. Nozoe M, et al. Efficacy of neuromuscular electrical stimulation for preventing quadriceps muscle wasting in patients with moderate or severe acute stroke: a pilot study. NeuroRehabilitation. 2017;41(1):143–9.
41. Mundermann A, et al. Comparison of volumetric bone mineral density in the operated and contralateral knee after anterior cruciate ligament and reconstruction: a 1-year follow-up study using peripheral quantitative computed tomography. J Orthop Res. 2015;33(12):1804–10.
42. Felmet, G. The significance of proprioceptive vibration training in postoperative treatment after ACL reconstruction. In: DGOOC. Berlin; 2004.
43. Felmet G. "Aquasprint" in the early functional rehabilitation program after ACL reconstruction. In: Frenzel G, Wuschech H, editors. Arthroskopische Gelenkchirurgie, Gestern-Heute-Morgen Standortbestimmung. Berlin: Kongress compact Verlag; 2002. p. 188–96.
44. Van Wingerden BAM, van Erp AJ. Bindegewebe in der Rehabilitation. 1998.
45. Petsche TS, Hutchinson MR. Loss of extension after reconstruction of the anterior cruciate ligament. J Am Acad Orthop Surg. 1999;7:119–27.
46. Hueter-Becker A, Dölken M. Biomechanik, Bewegungslehre, Leistungsphysiologie, Trainingslehre. 2011.
47. Haus J, Halata Z. Innervation of the anterior cruciate ligament. Int Orthop. 1990;14:293–6.
48. Wisløff U, et al. Strong correlation of maximal squat strength with sprint performance and vertical jump height in elite soccer players. Br J Sports Med. 2004;38:285–8.
49. Donohue MR, et al. Differences and correlations in knee and hip mechanics during single-leg landing, single-leg squat, double-leg landing, and double-leg squat tasks. Res Sports Med. 2015;23(4):394–411.
50. Gerber JP, et al. Effects of early progressive eccentric exercise on muscle size and function after anterior cruciate ligament reconstruction: a 1-year follow-up study of a randomized clinical trial. Phys Ther. 2009;89:51–9.
51. Risberg MA, Holm I. The long-term effect of 2 postoperative rehabilitation programs after anterior cruciate ligament reconstruction: a randomized controlled clinical trial with 2 years of follow-up. Am J Sports Med. 2009;37:1958–66.
52. Bloomquist K, et al. Effect of range of motion in heavy load squatting on muscle and tendon adaptations. Eur J Appl Physiol. 2013;113(8):2133–42.
53. Morton SK, et al. Resistance training vs. static stretching: effects on flexibility and strength. J Strength Cond Res. 2011;25(12):3391–8.
54. Khayambashi K, et al. Hip muscle strength predicts noncontact anterior cruciate ligament injury in male and female athletes: a prospective study. Am J Sports Med. 2015;44(2):355–61.
55. Palmer K, Hebron C, Williams JM. A randomised trial into the effect of an isolated hip abductor strengthening programme and a functional motor control programme on knee kinematics and hip muscle strength. BMC Musculoskelet Disord. 2015;16:105.
56. Reiman MP, Bolgla LA, Loudon JK. A literature review of studies evaluating gluteus maximus and gluteus medius activation during rehabilitation exercises. Physiother Theory Pract. 2012;28:257–68.
57. Escamilla RF, et al. Cruciate ligament tensile forces during the forward and side lunge. Clin Biomech. 2010;25:213–21.
58. Kulas AS, Hortobágyi T, Devita P. Trunk position modulates anterior cruciate ligament forces and strains during a single-leg squat. Clin Biomech. 2012;27:16–21.
59. Ugalde V, et al. Single leg squat test and its relationship to dynamic knee valgus and injury risk screening. PM R. 2015;7:229–35.
60. Alenezi F, et al. Relationships between lower limb biomechanics during single leg squat with running and cutting tasks: a preliminary investigation. Br J Sports Med. 2014;48:560–1.
61. Atkin K, et al. The relationship between 2D knee valgus angle during single leg squat (SLS), single leg landing (SLL), and forward running. Br J Sports Med. 2014;48:563.
62. Fox AS, Bonacci J, Mc Lean S. The relationship between performance on a single-leg squat and leap landing task: moving towards a netball-specific acl injury risk screening method. In: 25th congress of the international society of biomechanics. Aaron Fox; 2015.
63. Gustavsson A, et al. A test battery for evaluating hop performance in patients with an ACL injury and patients who have undergone ACL reconstruction. Knee Surg Sports Traumatol Arthrosc. 2006;14:778–88.
64. Itoh H, et al. Evaluation of functional deficits determined by four different hop tests in patients with anterior cruciate ligament deficiency. Knee Surg Sports Traumatol Arthrosc. 1998;6:241–5.
65. Barber SD, et al. Quantitative assessment of functional limitations in normal and anterior cruciate

ligament-deficient knees. Clin Orthop Relat Res. 1990:204–14.
66. Zazulak BT, et al. Deficits in neuromuscular control of the trunk predict knee injury risk: a prospective biomechanical-epidemiologic study. Am J Sports Med. 2007;35:1123–30.
67. Myer GD, et al. Trunk and hip control neuromuscular training for the prevention of knee joint injury. Clin Sports Med. 2008;27:425–48.
68. Elphinston, J., Stability, sport, and performance movement: great technique without injury. 2008. p. 33–4.
69. Panayi S. The need for lumbar-pelvic assessment in the resolution of chronic hamstring strain. J Bodyw Mov Ther. 2010;14:294–8.
70. Hewett TE, Boden B. Video analysis of trunk and knee motion during non-contact anterior cruciate ligament injury in female athletes: lateral trunk and knee abduction are combined components of the injury mechanism. Br J Sports Med. 2009;43:417–22.
71. Houck JR, Duncan A, Haven KED. Comparison of frontal plane trunk kinematics and hip and knee moments during anticipated and unanticipated walking and side step cutting tasks. Gait Posture. 2006;24:314–22.
72. Cerulli G, et al. Proprioceptive training and prevention of anterior cruciate ligament injuries in soccer. J Orthop Sports Phys Ther. 2001;31:655–60; discussion 661.
73. Hewett TE, et al. The effect of neuromuscular training on the incidence of knee injury in female athletes: a prospective study. Am J Sports Med. 1999;27:699–706.
74. Griffin LY, et al. Noncontact anterior cruciate ligament injuries: risk factors and prevention strategies. J Am Acad Orthop Surg. 2008;8:141–50.
75. Sheth P, et al. Ankle disk training influences reaction times of selected muscles in a simulated ankle sprain. Am J Sports Med. 1997;25:538–43.
76. Hewett TE, Ford KR, Myer GD. Anterior cruciate ligament injuries in female athletes: part 2, a meta-analysis of neuromuscular interventions aimed at injury prevention. Am J Sports Med. 2006;34:490–8.
77. Gokeler A, et al. Proprioceptive deficits after ACL injury: are they clinically relevant? Br J Sports Med. 2012;46:180–92.
78. Van Wingerden BAM. Physiologie und Pathophysiologie des Knorpel. Bad Pyrmont; 2013.
79. Pratama NE, Mintarto E, Kusnanik NW. The influence of ladder drills and jump rope exercise towards speed, agility, and power of limb muscle. J Sports Phys Educ. 2018;5(1):22–9.
80. Paterno MV, et al. Biomechanical measures during landing and postural stability predict second anterior cruciate ligament injury after anterior cruciate ligament reconstruction and return to sport. Am J Sports Med. 2010;38:1968–78.
81. Irmischer BS, et al. Effects of a knee ligament injury prevention exercise program on impact forces in women. J Strength Cond Res. 2004;18:703–7.
82. Davies G, Riemann BL, Manske R. Current concepts of plyometric exercise. Int J Sports Phys Ther. 2015;10(6):760–86.
83. Needle AR, Lepley AS, Grooms DR. Central nervous system adaptation after ligamentous injury: a summary of theories, evidence, and clinical interpretation. Sports Med. 2017;47(7):1271–88.
84. Rambaud AJM, et al. Criteria for return to running after anterior cruciate ligament reconstruction: a scoping review. Br J Sports Med. 2018;52(22):1437–44.
85. Whitehead NP, et al. Damage to human muscle from eccentric exercise after training with concentric exercise. J Physiol. 1998;512:615–20.
86. Marquardt M, Ansah P. Laufen und Laufanalyse. 2012.
87. Billat V, et al. Interval training at VO2max: effects on aerobic performance and overtraining markers. Med Sci Sports Exerc. 1999;31:156–63.
88. Gibala MJ, McGee SL. Metabolic adaptations to short-term high-intensity interval training: a little pain for a lot of gain? Exerc Sport Sci Rev. 2008;36(2):58–63.
89. McCormick B. Task complexity and jump landings in injury prevention for basketball players. Strength Condition. 2012;34:89–92.
90. Capin JJ, et al. On-ice return-to-hockey progression after anterior cruciate ligament reconstruction. J Orthop Sports Phys Ther. 2017;47(5):324–33.
91. Trulsson A, et al. Altered movement patterns and muscular activity during single and double leg squats in individuals with anterior cruciate ligament injury. BMC Musculoskelet Disord. 2015;16:28.
92. Di Stasi S, Myer GD, Hewett TE. Neuromuscular training to target deficits associated with second anterior cruciate ligament injury. J Orthop Sports Phys Ther. 2013;43:777–92, A1–11.
93. Paterno MV, et al. Incidence of second ACL injuries 2 years after primary ACL reconstruction and return to sport. Am J Sports Med. 2014;42:1567–73.
94. Brown TN, Palmieri-Smith RM, McLean SG. Sex and limb differences in hip and knee kinematics and kinetics during anticipated and unanticipated jump landings: implications for anterior cruciate ligament injury. Br J Sports Med. 2009;43(13): 1049–56.
95. Ford KR, et al. Use of an overhead goal alters vertical jump performance and biomechanics. J Strength Conditioning Res (Allen Press Publishing Services Inc). 2005;19:394–9.
96. Borotikar BS, et al. Combined effects of fatigue and decision making on female lower limb landing postures: central and peripheral contributions to ACL injury risk. Clin Biomech. 2008;23:81–92.
97. McLean SG, Lipfert SW, van den Bogert AJ. Effect of gender and defensive opponent on the biomechanics of sidestep cutting. Med Sci Sports Exerc. 2004;36(6):1008–16.
98. Grooms DR, et al. Neuroplasticity associated with anterior cruciate ligament reconstruction. J Orthop Sports Phys Ther. 2017;47(3):180–9.

99. Webster KE, Feller JA. A research update on the state of play for return to sport after anterior cruciate ligament reconstruction. J Orthop Traumatol. 2019;20(1):10.
100. Chmielewski TL. Asymmetrical lower extremity loading after ACL reconstruction: more than meets the eye. J Orthop Sports Phys Ther. 2011;41:374–6.
101. Yamazaki J, et al. Differences in kinematics of single leg squatting between anterior cruciate ligament-injured patients and healthy controls. Knee Surg Sports Traumatol Arthrosc. 2010;18(1):56–63.
102. Grindem H, et al. Simple decision rules can reduce reinjury risk by 84% after ACL reconstruction: the Delaware-Oslo ACL cohort study. Br J Sports Med. 2016;50(13):804–8.
103. Paterno MV, et al. Clinical factors that predict a second ACL injury after ACL reconstruction and return to sport: preliminary development of a clinical decision algorithm. Orthop J Sports Med. 2017;5(12):2325967117745279.
104. Wiggins AJ, et al. Risk of secondary injury in younger athletes after anterior cruciate ligament reconstruction: a systematic review and meta-analysis. Am J Sports Med. 2016;44(7):1861–76.
105. Wellsandt E, Failla MJ, Snyder-Mackler L. Limb symmetry indexes can overestimate knee function after anterior cruciate ligament injury. J Orthop Sports Phys Ther. 2017;47(5):334–8.
106. Blakeney WG, et al. Validation of a composite test for assessment of readiness for return to sports after anterior cruciate ligament reconstruction: the K-STARTS test. Sports Health. 2018;10(6):515–22.
107. Rambaud AJM, et al. Criteria for return to sport after anterior cruciate ligament reconstruction with lower reinjury risk (CR'STAL study): protocol for a prospective observational study in France. BMJ Open. 2017;7(6):e015087.
108. Hewett TE, et al. Mechanisms, prediction, and prevention of ACL injuries: cut risk with three sharpened and validated tools. J Orthop Res. 2016;34(11):1843–55.
109. McLean SG, et al. Evaluation of a two dimensional analysis method as a screening and evaluation tool for anterior cruciate ligament injury. Br J Sports Med. 2005;39(6):355–62.
110. Cesar G, Pfeifer C, Burnfield J. 3-dimensional versus 2-dimensional comparison of knee valgus collapse during vertical jump: clinical implications for ACL risk of injury assessment. J Sports Med Ther. 2017;2:32–8.
111. Al-Amri M, et al. Inertial measurement units for clinical movement analysis: reliability and concurrent validity. Sensors (Basel). 2018;18(3):719.
112. Filippeschi A, et al. Survey of motion tracking methods based on inertial sensors: a focus on upper limb human motion. Sensors (Basel). 2017;17(6):1257.
113. Rabuffetti M, Scalera GM, Ferrarin M. Effects of gait strategy and speed on regularity of locomotion assessed in healthy subjects using a multi-sensor method. Sensors (Basel). 2019;19(3):513.
114. Ueberschaer O, et al. Measuring biomechanical loads and asymmetries in junior elite long distance runners through triaxial inertial sensors. Sports Orthop Traumatol. 2019;35:296–308.
115. Wang Q, et al. Interactive wearable systems for upper body rehabilitation: a systematic review. J Neuroeng Rehabil. 2017;14(1):20.
116. Curtin A, et al. A systematic review of integrated functional near-infrared spectroscopy (fNIRS) and transcranial magnetic stimulation (TMS) studies. Front Neurosci. 2019;13:84.
117. Schilaty ND, Nagelli C, Hewett TE. Use of objective neurocognitive measures to assess the psychological states that influence return to sport following injury. Sports Med (Auckland, NZ). 2016;46(3):299–303.
118. Koenraadt KL, et al. Cortical control of normal gait and precision stepping: an fNIRS study. NeuroImage. 2014;85(Pt 1):415–22.
119. Gramigna V, et al. Near-infrared spectroscopy in gait disorders: is it time to begin? Neurorehabil Neural Repair. 2017;31(5):402–12.
120. Forsdyke D, Gledhill A, Ardern C. Psychological readiness to return to sport: three key elements to help the practitioner decide whether the athlete is REALLY ready? Br J Sports Med. 2017;51(7):555–6.
121. de Mille P, Osmak J. Performance: bridging the gap after ACL surgery. Curr Rev Musculoskelet Med. 2017;10(3):297–306.
122. Sonesson S, et al. Psychological factors are important to return to pre-injury sport activity after anterior cruciate ligament reconstruction: expect and motivate to satisfy. Knee Surg Sports Traumatol Arthrosc. 2017;25(5):1375–84.
123. Paterno MV, et al. Self-reported fear predicts functional performance and second ACL injury after ACL reconstruction and return to sport: a pilot study. Sports Health. 2018;10(3):228–33.
124. Felmet G. Rehabilitation and return to sports but, mostly, prevention! What could we do to avoid tendon injury? In: ESSKA speciality days, sports injuries. New concepts! Madrid: European Sports Medicine Associates (ESMA); 2019.
125. Thorborg K, et al. Effect of specific exercise-based football injury prevention programmes on the overall injury rate in football: a systematic review and meta-analysis of the FIFA 11 and 11+ programmes. Br J Sports Med. 2017;51(7):562–71.
126. Caraffa A, et al. Prevention of anterior cruciate ligament injuries in soccer. A prospective controlled study of proprioceptive training. Knee Surg Sports Traumatol Arthrosc. 1996;4:19–21.
127. Myklebust G, et al. Prevention of anterior cruciate ligament injuries in female team handball players: a prospective intervention study over three seasons. Clin J Sport Med. 2003;13:71–8.
128. Padua DA, et al. National Athletic Trainers' association position statement: prevention of anterior cruciate ligament injury. J Athl Train. 2018;53(1):5–19.
129. Ardern CL, et al. 2018 International Olympic Committee consensus statement on prevention,

diagnosis and management of paediatric anterior cruciate ligament (ACL) injuries. Br J Sports Med. 2018;52(7):422–38.
130. Myer GD, et al. Sports specialization, part II: alternative solutions to early sport specialization in youth athletes. Sports Health. 2016;8(1):65–73.
131. Myer GD, et al. Sport specialization, part I: does early sports specialization increase negative outcomes and reduce the opportunity for success in young athletes? Sports Health. 2015;7(5):437–42.
132. Jayanthi NA, et al. Health consequences of youth sport specialization. J Athl Train. 2019;54(10):1040–9.
133. Zantop T, et al. Anterolateral rotational knee instability: role of posterolateral structures. Winner of the AGA-DonJoy Award 2006. Arch Orthop Trauma Surg. 2007;127(9):743–52.

GPSR Compliance

The European Union's (EU) General Product Safety Regulation (GPSR) is a set of rules that requires consumer products to be safe and our obligations to ensure this.

If you have any concerns about our products, you can contact us on ProductSafety@springernature.com

In case Publisher is established outside the EU, the EU authorized representative is:

Springer Nature Customer Service Center GmbH
Europaplatz 3
69115 Heidelberg, Germany

Batch number: 10371063

Printed by Printforce, the Netherlands